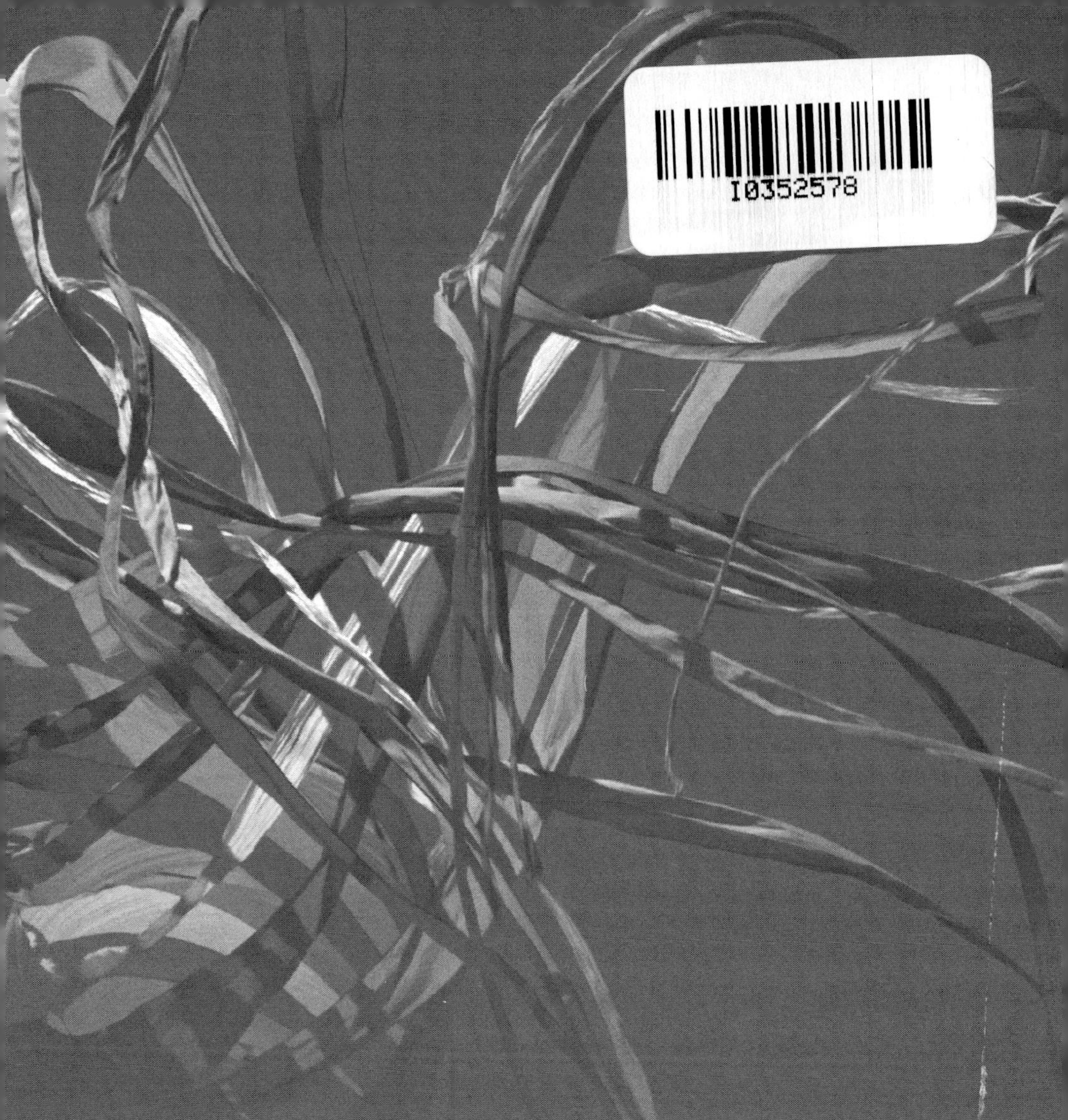

Creativity and Mental Health

A Cognitive Analytic Approach to Integrating Play and Imagination in Psychotherapy, Supervision and Training

INNOVATIONS in CAT

Edited by Yvonne J. Stevens

Creativity and Mental Health:
A Cognitive Analytic approach to integrating play and imagination in psychotherapy, supervision and training.

© Pavilion Publishing & Media

The authors have asserted their rights in accordance with the Copyright, Designs and Patents Act (1988) to be identified as the authors of this work.

Published by:

Pavilion Publishing and Media Ltd
Blue Sky Offices, 25 Cecil Pashley Way, Shoreham by Sea,
West Sussex, BN43 5FF

Tel: +44 (0)1273 434 943
Email: info@pavpub.com
Web: www.pavpub.com

Published 2024

All rights reserved. No part of this publication may be reproduced, stored in a retrieval system, or transmitted in any form or by any means, electronic, mechanical, photocopying, recording or otherwise, without prior permission in writing of the publisher and the copyright owners.

A catalogue record for this book is available from the British Library.

ISBN: 978-1-803882-46-8

Pavilion Publishing and Media is a leading publisher of books, training materials and digital content in mental health, social care and allied fields. Pavilion and its imprints offer must-have knowledge and innovative learning solutions underpinned by sound research and professional values.

Editor: Yvonne J. Stevens
Cover design: Phil Morash, Pavilion Publishing and Media Ltd
Page layout and typesetting: Emma Dawe, Pavilion Publishing and Media Ltd
Printing: Independent Publishers Group (IPG)

INNOVATIONS in
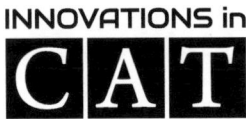

Available now in the *Innovations in CAT* series:

Conversations in Later Life
(edited by Michelle Hamill, Ellen Khan and Paul Catlin)

Innovative Practice in Forensic Settings
(edited by Jenny Marshall and Jamie Kirkland)

Working Relationally with Young People
(edited by Nick Barnes and Lee Crothers)

Reflective Practice in Forensic Settings
(edited by Jenny Marshall and Jamie Kirkland)

For ***BEJ***

Still singing Galway Bay …

Contents

Series preface
Foreword
About the editor
Preface
Contributors

Introduction
    Yvonne J. Stevens 15

PART 1: Mental health and the capacity to play 21
    Chapter 1: CAT, creativity and mental health
        Yvonne J. Stevens 25

    Chapter 2: The neurobiological benefits of novelty and play
        Suzanne Lyons and Yvonne J. Stevens 45

    Chapter 3: The zone of playful proximal development
        Paul Sullivan 51

PART 2: Creative psychotherapy in practice 67
    Chapter 4: Working with objects as a key to unlocking complex trauma
        Suzanne Lyons 71

    Chapter 5: Dramatherapy and playful relationality
        Vicky Petratou 93

    Chapter 6: Beyond your wildest dreams
        Sophie Rushbrook and Nicola Coulter 111

    Chapter 7: Enabling change through metaphor and imagery
        James Turner 127

    Chapter 8: Relational dialogues with the inner child
        Louise Yorke 143

    Chapter 9: Innovative approaches within a learning disability service
        Sarah Nicholas and 'Col' 167

    Chapter 10: Neurodivergence and the Multiple Self States Model
        James Randall 193

PART 3: Bringing our creative selves to therapy 217
    Jak Smith 219

    Chapter 11: Reflection as a creative process within supervision
        Vicky Petratou 221

    Chapter 12: Human development and Shakespeare's 'Seven Ages of Man'
        Jason Hepple 245

    Chapter 13: The roots and heart of Cognitive Analytic Music Therapy (CAMT)
        Stella Compton Dickinson 259

    Chapter 14: Training films for psychotherapeutic education
        Kathryn Pemberton 283

    Chapter 15: Bringing our stories to life through animation
        Rhona Brown 293

    Chapter 16: Well-being workshops for CAT therapists
        Steve Potter, in conversation with Annalee Curran and Elizabeth Wilde McCormick 313

    'The Jigsaw aka The Battle of Humpty'
        Louise Yorke 321

    Afterword
        Yvonne J. Stevens 323

    Glossary of CAT terms 325

Appendices 331
    Appendix 1: The Psychotherapy File 333

    Appendix 2: Describing self-states 343

    Appendix 3: Restrictions on capacity for reflexivity 344

    Appendix 4: The House of Self States template 345

    Appendix 5: Six-Part Story Method template 346

    Appendix 6: Reciprocal Roles – ways of relating to self and others 347

    Appendix 7: Creative tasks for trainee therapists and clients 348

References 351

Series preface

The *Innovations in Cognitive Analytic Therapy* book series aims to offer helpful but also challenging accounts by practitioners in various fields of theoretical development and clinical work based on Cognitive Analytic Therapy (CAT). The editors and contributors are experts in their fields who have undertaken innovative and exploratory work using the CAT approach – the presentation of which, in our view, is long overdue. We hope that these books will make important and compassionate contributions to our understanding of and approaches to a range of clinical and other problems and presentations – contributions that will be helpful and thought-provoking not only for colleagues already familiar with CAT, but also for many others. The series builds on and complements previous overviews by the late Anthony Ryle, creator of the CAT model, and other wide-scope multi-author volumes.

A distinctive feature is a predominantly relational and socio-cultural conceptualisation of mental health problems, or of distress and 'disorder', and correspondingly of therapeutic approaches to them. A fundamental emphasis throughout, based on understandings derived from years of psychotherapy outcome research, Vygotskian activity theory and more recent research in infant psychology, is the importance of a (genuinely) collaborative and co-creative approach to treatment. This long-standing emphasis in CAT will be evident in, for example, descriptions of the co-creative process of reformulation, both written and diagrammatic ('mapping'). These in turn will emphasise recognising and working on enactments of internalised early relational patterns ('reciprocal roles') in life generally, but also between both clinicians and clients. They will also emphasise the gradual internalisation of new, more benign relational experience. This is regrettably far from being the case for many individuals currently in therapy or, especially, undergoing treatment within public health services, despite its recognised importance as a key 'common factor' in outcomes.

As well as offering practically helpful accounts of developing and innovative work in often challenging clinical fields, we aspire for these books also to contribute to the ongoing development of the CAT model, including as a general framework for understanding and treating mental health problems. This will be important for its own validity and vitality as well as more generally to advance the field of mental health. Anthony Ryle, who created the CAT model during a long and avowedly integrative evolutionary process, certainly always welcomed such developments. We look forward to the *Innovations in Cognitive Analytic Therapy* series promoting productive debate, and being part of an open, creative dialogue between practitioners of CAT and colleagues from other approaches and disciplines in support of a versatile, integrative and relational approach to mental health in general.

Ian. B. Kerr and Steve Potter
Series Editors

Foreword

This is a scholarly and compassionate read. It celebrates the uniqueness and originality available when our imaginative selves are invited to be expressed within a safe structure; and that, through harnessing the power of this creative world, we are all more available for healing. The book is a really great addition to the existing literature on the work of Cognitive Analytic Therapy in different settings. It offers therapists from many different backgrounds examples of how the CAT structure may be used within their speciality. Each of the many contributors offers detailed and thorough examples from their therapeutic work with patients. This includes dramatherapy; music therapy; artwork and painting; working with dreams, objects, metaphor, and the inner child.

In Part 1 Yvonne Stevens writes about CAT, creativity and mental health, and she and Suzanne Lyons write about the neurobiological benefits that arise from the invitation to be playful and creative in therapy. Creative approaches to therapeutic work with people who have experienced trauma in childhood are illustrated, and also creative therapeutic work within CAT for people with learning difficulties and autism. Yvonne Stevens illustrates how different creative approaches may also be used in supervision so that therapists may strengthen their own understanding of their own learned patterns. She writes: *'creativity can be woven in from the beginning to the end through the CAT process.'*

The power of personal narrative through reformulation is central to the structure of CAT, read aloud to the patient at session four with an invitation to reflect and join in the written narrative over the next couple of sessions. The book illustrates how this basic CAT sharing may be enhanced by different creative specialities – especially helpful for patients with few verbal skills, or who struggle with a borderline structure, when naming the 'parts' through painting, music, drama or objects helps to illustrate a whole picture.

Throughout all the chapters of this really interesting and often moving text we meet the creative versatility of the CAT structure in many different forms, all supported by examples and references.

Elizabeth Wilde McCormick MA psych; Dip. Psych. Soc. Psych.
Psychotherapist and author; Founder member and life member of ACAT

In Memoriam

Dr Louise Yorke (1965-2024)

DClinPsych. CPsychol. AFBPsS

It was with great sadness that we learned of the passing of Louise Yorke shortly before this book went to press. Louise was such a positive supporter of this project, including contributing her own chapter on the relational technique she developed on working imaginatively with the inner child in Cognitive Analytic Therapy. Her contribution to developments in CAT are widely known.

In her career of over more than twenty years in both the NHS and the private sector, Louise achieved leadership roles in her clinical, teaching, and supervisory work. In both operational and strategic management, she contributed published papers and book chapters and was an invited conference speaker.

From 2015, Louise specialised in CAT and taught on the doctorate course at the University of Exeter. She was an active member of the Association for Cognitive Analytic Therapy (ACAT) and served as co-editor of their journal, *Reformulation*.

Her focus and influence on innovative psychology and psychological therapy services, the training of psychologists and on service development was well recognised. Louise's dedication to psychology and psychotherapy and her creative inspirational work in training and supervision will be her lasting legacy.

About the editor

Yvonne J. Stevens

Yvonne is a CAT psychotherapist, supervisor and psychotherapy lecturer, having trained with Dr Anthony Ryle in London. She has supervised and taught CAT trainees throughout the southwest of the UK. Yvonne works in the NHS and is Course Director for the embedded CAT Foundation Training at the University of Exeter psychology doctorate, and an associate psychotherapy lecturer with the Peninsula Medical School. Yvonne is currently Chair of the ACAT Examination Board and ACAT Vice-Chair for Supervisor Training. Yvonne contributed to *Cognitive Analytic Supervision: A relational approach* (2017) and the *Oxford Handbook of Cognitive Analytic Therapy* (2024). Yvonne's passion is bringing creativity to psychotherapy and training. Yvonne co-convenes the annual ACAT Trainers and Supervisors Event with Jason Hepple and supports the ACAT Relational Skills Training run by Steve Potter. Yvonne shares her West Country family home with four cats.

Preface

"Forget your perfect offering, there is a crack, a crack in everything, that's how the light gets in." – Leonard Cohen, *'Anthem'*[1]

The first ideas for this book began to emerge and take shape during the COVID pandemic lockdowns. The loss of normal routine and the upside-downness of how we were living, seemed to create spaces for new thoughts. The book was then made possible by Steve Potter and Ian Kerr, through their proposal to launch a series of books exploring developments in Cognitive Analytic Therapy (CAT). I thank and applaud them for their visionary 'build it and they will come' approach, which is gathering steam and now has several books in process, and some already in bookshops and online. This book arose initially from a collaboration between a number of CAT therapists – Stella Compton Dickinson, Rosanna Cooper and Julia Coombes – with whom Vicky Petratou and I wrote a chapter on Creativity and CAT for the *Oxford Handbook of Cognitive Analytic Therapy* (Brummer et al, 2024).

Our feeling during that process was that there was so much more we wanted to say and so many more ways to use creativity and imagination to enrich the practice of CAT to share with the wider CAT and therapeutic community. I am indebted to Vicky who has again so skilfully brought her voice to this book and to Stella for her wealth of practice and experience, and all the other authors for the particular gifts that they have brought to this 'creative festival' of CAT and for their commitment to this project. I know there is much more about the creativity of CAT practice to capture – but as in any creative endeavour, you need to start somewhere and know the limits of what you can achieve.

I have been particularly fortunate over the course of my career in mental health and psychotherapy to have worked alongside and been inspired by many therapists, trainers, supervisors, mental health professionals and trainees who have enriched my own personal and professional development and psychotherapy practice as we have struggled and felt challenged together in our work. I continue to feel grateful for the extraordinary courage and creativity of people who have sat across from

---

1   From 'The Future' (Columbia Records, 1992)

me in the therapy room or, more recently, on phones and computer screens, and who have trusted me to steer the therapeutic processing of their narrative towards acceptance, healing and recovery. And the creative process is often such a surprise! Paul Sullivan, in Chapter 3, talks about how out of two or more minds coming together, the most unexpected and creative of things can happen. Stories of precious *polyphonic* therapeutic moments of spontaneity are threaded through this book. I talk about the liberating and healing nature of creativity in the therapeutic process with individuals with whom I have worked.

My interest in the politics of mental health has led me to consider how psychotherapists commit to liberating the minds of their clients, by also freeing their own minds. There are no limits on the imagination, so as such creativity has no limits. Analyst Carl Jung and poet Diane di Prima consider this:

> *'Without this playing with fantasy no creative work has ever yet come to birth. The debt we owe to the play of the imagination is incalculable.'* – Carl Jung (1916) *'Psychological Types'*, p.88, Routledge.

> *'... the imagination is not only holy, it is precise*
> *it is not only fierce, it is practical*
> *men die everyday for the lack of it,*
> *it is vast & elegant.'*
> – Diane di Prima *Revolutionary Letters* No 75 p.104 (City Lights)

At the point of collating this book, the world feels an even less safe, less welcoming and less hopeful place than when we all set out on this creative journey, and we may have all emerged from the COVID pandemic more connected with our human vulnerability and with our own share of the collective trauma. The work we do in psychotherapy, the processing of the unbearable memories that we seek to meet with our creative techniques and imaginative ideas, are needed more than ever to help us make sense of and survive the distress not only of individual past and present trauma, but also for our emotional survival of global experiences of international conflict, racial and cultural oppression, civil war and climatic disaster.

Judith Herman (1992) linked the intrapersonal, interpersonal, family and cultural/state/political experiences of powerlessness and trauma in her book *Trauma and Recovery*, which resulted in the new diagnosis she coined 'complex post-traumatic stress disorder (CPTSD)'. It took another 25 years for this to be accepted as a diagnostic description in psychiatry and in mental health services, but it is a theme that runs through the pages of this book, and one which links the embodied experience of trauma, psychotherapeutic ways of understanding distress and creative interventions and healing, and the possibility of hope – and even joy – in the darkest of times.

Regarding that mention of hope and joy – I must share my delight at a report on BBC Radio 4 of a description of lonely pet parrots who had learned to video call each other and how they used these social moments to dance and sing with and to each other – becoming more and more animated – although also at times needing to switch off and have some quiet time. For that creative dialogic relationship within myself, I value dearly that childhood immersion in a kaleidoscope of colour and the nurturing quality of dance and music and song and fairy tales and poetry. For that, I need to thank my mother, the artist, who even into her 90s, sought out the creative, the colourful and the playful, and engendered this playfulness in me, both for myself as a mother and as a therapist. My father, the engineer, lived life as a pathway of possibilities; he introduced me to the stars in the night sky and he modelled how to plan projects and execute ideas with precision, and the importance of artefacts and tools – an outing to the beach was an expedition! So, I thank him for gifting me the skills needed to plan and project manage this book.

This book does not attempt to be inclusive of the creative within CAT, or indeed anywhere near, but rather has shown how one might pick up and follow a thread or a glint of something that catches our eye and may be woven into our practice. I hope the reader is inspired and encouraged by the authors' personal stories of their creative journeys and their own creative paths, and so recognize opportunities as they present themselves. Maybe there is a dance therapist out there who might explore and choreograph the relational and dialogic of the CAT process?

There are people and chapters missing from this book that could have been – again, the creative process compels us to let go of some things, allowing space for other things take shape. The size and shape of this book has ebbed and flowed like the tide at Newlyn and has settled in its present form as my own creative self met with other creative selves. Perhaps if there are future editions, any one of you readers might become an author…

"Keeping CAT alive" (Ryle, 2007)

This book, and the contributors to it, are as varied as CAT itself, which has always been such a broad church, with thanks to Anthony Ryle's open and welcoming stance to anyone who showed genuine interest and curiosity. At his memorial gathering in 2017, the word that was most referred to of Tony was his *generosity*. He was encouraging of creativity, and in our work with trainees and with clients and colleagues, this requires generosity and giving of space and time to the other. Some of the voices of clients and trainees are here because of their reciprocated generosity and enthusiasm about being able to contribute to this project:

> *'Freely given to gratefully received.'*

I first met Anthony Ryle in 1989 at St Thomas's Hospital. I was seeking training in psychotherapy and was handed a leaflet on CAT by a colleague Frances, to whom I owe so much, as CAT has been the beacon of my career ever since. I felt an affinity with Tony's humanity and compassion in his work, his capacity to be alongside the people he sought to help, his recognition of the impact of trauma, poverty and economic and social deprivation on mental health and well-being. These values underpin the CAT model.

Yvonne J. Stevens
Somerset
June 2024

Contributors

Rhona Brown is a CAT Practitioner and Clinical Psychologist working in Manchester NHS services with adults from a rich diversity of communities. She has longstanding interests in social context and inequalities, working across cultures, and how therapeutic approaches can be adapted to enhance relevance and accessibility to people with differing needs. She currently works in an occupational health service for NHS staff, alongside training activities with Catalyse and supporting ACAT in its public engagement initiative. In this role she has helped to develop accessible online content about CAT.

Stella Compton Dickinson is an independent consultant supervisor, Fellow of The Institute of Mental Health, Nottingham, and Alumna of King's College London and Anglia Ruskin University Cambridge. She followed a successful career as a classical musician and recording artist (Royal Academy of Music), then as a music therapist (Guildhall School of Music), later gaining accreditation as a CAT therapist. She was awarded the Ruskin Medal 2016 for her doctoral research at Anglia Ruskin University. Stella has authored numerous chapters, papers and two books, she speaks regularly at international conferences and provides workshops and training for healthcare charities and the NHS.

Nicola Coulter is an Occupational Therapist in the Intensive Psychological Therapies Service, Branksome Clinic, Dorset NHS. Her work in occupational therapy and as a CAT Therapist, Supervisor and Trainer is in a tertiary NHS service with people who have complex trauma and also in independent practice

Annalee Curran is a Founder Member of ACAT, was its first Chair and is a Life Member. She has been working using CAT ideas since 1985. She worked for many years in primary care in the NHS as well as supervising and teaching in the UK and abroad. She is now retired from the NHS and has a private practice. Annalee has always felt that creativity in CAT can greatly enhance the understandings and the experience of therapy.

Jason Hepple is Honorary Psychotherapist with Somerset NHS Foundation Trust and an ACAT life member, psychotherapist, supervisor and trainer. He has published and taught internationally on CAT in later life, CAT in groups, CAT in obsessionality and the dialogic heart of CAT. He has a background in directing amateur drama, and he has used Shakespeare's insights as a stimulus for reflection and creative engagement in therapy.

Suzanne Lyons is a Chartered Clinical Psychologist, CAT psychotherapist and supervisor in private practice and in NHS adult mental health services. She was director of the Dorset CAT course. Her experiences of training in EMDR and attending ACAT conference workshops have informed her of the importance of embodiment and bringing creative to her work with clients for the processing of trauma and developing a greater sense of self. She has enjoyed supporting supervisees in developing their own skills and confidence in this area and she suspects that this approach may also help to prevent burnout amongst therapists.

Sarah Nicholas is Clinical specialist Occupational Therapist for Dorset Healthcare University NHS Foundation Trust and has over twenty years' experience of working in NHS services for people with learning disabilities and more recently in Intensive Psychological Therapy services and inpatient mental health. Sarah's clinical expertise is in specialist therapeutic interventions for people learning disabilities and complex mental health needs. She is trained in Cognitive Analytic Therapy, EMDR and DBT, and has a MSc in Sensory Integration Therapy

Kathryn Pemberton is a Clinical Psychologist, CAT practitioner and supervisor who has worked in the NHS and private practice and has extensive experience as a CAT trainer. Before training as Clinical Psychologist, Kathryn worked as an actor and director.

Vicky Petratou is a CAT Psychotherapist, Dramatherapist, Clinical Supervisor and Trainer working in private practice, the NHS including South London & Maudsley, Oxleas & Hertfordshire NHS Trusts, various London schools and charities, and with individual therapists. Her passion for creative CAT psychotherapy has been influenced by her love of and commitment to Physical Theatre, Playback Theatre and Dramatherapy and the inspiration she gained from the inherent creativity of the people she has had the privilege to work with. These experiences have enriched her understanding and clinical CAT practice since her first forays into CAT in 1993.

Steve Potter is an independent CAT psychotherapist, supervisor and trainer and ACAT life member. He is a past chair of ACAT and the International Association of Cognitive Analytic Therapy and co-editor of the *International Journal of Cognitive Analytic Therapy and Relational Mental Health* (www.internationalcat.org/journals), and is the author of two books on CAT and its relational and integrative approaches and various chapters and articles (www.mapandtalk.com). He is chair of his local residents' association in East London. He is keen to see CAT's relational tools and concepts applied in and beyond the therapy room with teams, organizations and in wider society and has spent the last twenty years developing an approach to reflective practice called Map and Talk.

James Randall is a vegan, tattooed Clinical Psychologist, and a newly qualified CAT practitioner working in CAMHS & Social Care. He works with children and young people within the NHS and social services (looked-after context). His specialist interests professionally include complex and developmental trauma, neurodiversity and social context. James is editor of the book *Surviving Clinical Psychology: Navigating personal, professional and political selves on the journey to qualification* (2020).

Sophie Rushbrook is a Consultant Clinical Psychologist and Head of Service in the Intensive Psychological Therapies Service, Branksome Clinic, Dorset NHS. Sophie leads a tertiary, specialist service in the NHS for people with complex trauma and longstanding difficulties. She has been practicing CAT for the past twenty years and is also an accredited CAT supervisor.

Jak Smith is an ACAT accredited CAT practitioner, supervisor and trainer working as part of Cumbria, Northumberland, Tyne and Wear NHS Foundation Trust CAT Service within The Centre for Specialist Psychological Therapies. Alongside this, he is an accredited psychotherapist with the British Association for Counselling and Psychotherapy (BACP) and holds a special interest in creatively adapting and developing CAT, to work with people across neurological and physical health settings.

Paul Sullivan is a Reader in Psychology and has worked at the University of Bradford since 2004. Originally from Cork, Ireland, he specializes in the creative responses that imbue dialogical processes. He has written extensively on qualitative methods to help understand this and applied a dialogical approach to a variety of contexts including organization studies, mental health and education. He is significantly inspired by the work of Vygotsky and Bakhtin.

James (Jim) Turner is Associate Professor of Mental Health and Wellbeing at Sheffield Hallam University. He is a CAT Practitioner and clinical supervisor with thirty-eight years' experience of ward, community, psychological therapies, senior nurse leadership, and senior academic roles. He has local, regional, national and international networks and consultations. As a researcher, nurse and therapist, Jim has strong foundations, investigating a range of topics such as end of life care, the therapeutic encounter, clinical supervision, young people's mental health, and well-being through sport; teaching and researching therapeutic interventions as applied to mental health and well-being in general.

Elizabeth Wilde McCormick joined the CAT project with Tony Ryle at Guy's Hospital in 1984 and later became a Trustee of ACAT and a Life member in 2014. After forty years in clinical practice, she has now retired as a psychotherapist and supervisor. She is the author of a number of psychological self-help books including the CAT self-help book *Change for The Better*, now in its fifth edition, and a trilogy of novels about the work of psychotherapist Dr Max Maxwell.

Introduction

Yvonne J. Stevens

For those of you who are confidently creative in the therapy room and have a well-stocked therapy tool kit, I hope you will find something new of interest in these pages. For those of you who perhaps don't know where to start and may feel anxious, perhaps even awkward or uncomfortable using creative techniques with your clients, perhaps not knowing how to broach this, I hope you will find encouragement in some of the detailed guides to integrating creative techniques in your therapeutic work with your clients. These chapters will help you take the courage to dip your toes in the water. You may find it helpful to bring some of the ideas in this book to discuss in your supervision group or with your supervisor and incorporate some of the suggestions in your therapies. There are useful resources in the appendices at the back of the book to support creativity in CAT practice, supervision and training.

The intention of this edition is by no means to be a comprehensive source book of creative techniques in CAT. Readers may feel that there are some missing names, although the threads of their voices may be woven like warp and weft through the fabric of these pages as they have influenced many of us through their pioneering work in the early days of CAT, and others are now forging innovation and renewing of the model. The final shape and content of this book has had its own lived experience of a creative process of false starts, the misshapen clay thrown back on the wheel, the dropped stitch unpicked, and the dissonant note scratched out, which has left some holes and under-explored themes, like a melody unheard, and the 'decisive moment' of a photograph missed.

The ripples of all the contributors' lives, therapeutic and learning experiences inform this book, which draws on their invention and innovation. Some with greater experience and others newer to CAT, each one shares how they have approached the CAT model with openness, creativity and imagination to develop their own practice and expertise and made meaningful connections with their clients, trainees and supervisees. I hope that their creative process will speak to the imaginative in all of us, as we interact with and respond to the relational dialogue with both our inner selves and our social and cultural environment. Each chapter stands on its own as a creative endeavour, in some cases the product of decades of passionate work by the author, while in others representing an emerging integration of different aspects of the author and their clinical practice through the medium of the CAT model.

Two previous publications on CAT deserve a particular mention. Elizabeth Wilde McCormick's *Change for the Better* (2017), now in its fifth edition, has been mindfully guiding people through relational self-discovery for over three decades, and her insights, workshops and writing have inspired many of the authors in this book. The other is Julie Lloyd's and Philip Clayton's *Cognitive Analytic Therapy for People who have an Intellectual Disability and Their Carers* (2014). The CAT literature on the use of creativity was much enriched and enhanced by both of these books. The latter is full of innovative practice describing creative and imaginative adaptation and adoption of CAT tools developed by therapists working with people with intellectual disabilities. Lloyd and Clayton reference Dr Ros King (2005), where she describes her development of the therapeutic relationship with her clients using colour to represent emotion, early versions of emojis to reflect mood and feelings, and objects to represent relationships, and she adapted CAT tools to collaboratively share the framework and structure of CAT, counting down the sessions and working towards ending. These ideas are described in practice (see Sarah Nicholas Chapter 9, this volume) and further developed with the CAT Multiple Self States Model (MSSM) by James Randall (Chapter 10, this volume).

Artists and writers speak to us across hundreds of years; oral traditions hand down fables and myths, from the Ramayana and the Akan tales of Anansi, from the Arabian Nights to Rumi and Shakespeare; playwrights, poets and painters engage our minds, hold our gaze – what I hear, what I see, what I feel, what I have made of it. We see the best and worst of our humanity reflected back to us in art and literature, representations of ourselves laid bare for examination. These pages reach back in time to the ways in which humans across cultures have always sought to find expression of their lived experience in the visual, narrative and dramatic, and through the development of language and music. And it moves forward through the ages to our most recent scientific understandings of our emotional, psychological and embodied experiences through discoveries in neuroscience, neurobiology and neuropsychology. Some of the authors explore these links for example between what is cathected onto our aural experience of music, our tactile experience of objects and the corresponding neural development and limbic activity.

About this book

The book is in three parts. The first sets the scene and context of creativity and play as an aspect of mental health. Then part two thinks about the creative as a therapeutic model such as drama therapy, or as an active method for accessing, expressing and healing trauma, with detailed techniques to integrate into the CAT framework. The third part follows some very individual and personal ways in which CAT trainers and supervisors have merged their interests and creative gifts with the CAT model. The focus is on communicating their understandings and meaning-making in CAT supervision and training, making space within CAT supervision and CAT training for the creativity of polyphonic minds in the dialogue of supervision process – sharing moments, events, experiences and memories through literature, dramatic techniques, metaphor and film and literature. The book concludes with reflections on the well-being and nurturing of the creative therapist, and how we restore, nurture and heal ourselves in our capacity for play.

Part 1:

- **Chapters 1 and 2:** Yvonne Stevens and Suzanne Lyons introduce CAT and creativity, mental health and play, drawing on the literature on CAT and creativity and the use of creative techniques, and exploring the evidence for the utility of creativity in mental health services. Suzanne and Yvonne further discuss the relationship between play, creativity and developments in neuroscience and how CAT has sought to maximize opportunities for interpersonal neurobiology to be engaged in the cause of increased well-being both developmentally for children and for adults in therapy.

- **Chapter 3:** Paul Sullivan introduces the 'zone of playful proximal development' as a new perspective on the 'zone of proximal development' (ZPD) and considers how spontaneity and play are mediated through dialogical polyphonic minds, and how this then relates to the therapeutic understanding of multiple voices in CAT.

Part 2:

- **Chapter 4:** Suzanne Lyons describes the benefits of working creatively in therapy with objects to promote an embodied connection and to enhance the use of CAT tools, with a focus on the effects of trauma and the integration of self-states. Suzanne brings her many years of experience developing this integrated approach to treating trauma and complex PTSD, incorporating CAT with creative techniques. Suzanne offers a useful and detailed guide on these techniques.

- **Chapter 5:** Vicky Petratou explores how Dramatherapy can enrich and enhance the therapeutic presence and playful relationality in CAT, and how the imaginative and performative can reach beyond the limitations of words. She vividly illustrates how dramatherapy techniques such as role play can promote a sense of experimentation to access a meaningful integration of different self-states.

- **Chapter 6:** Nicola Coulter and Sophie Rushbrook offer an elegant introduction to understanding how dreams can be understood from an embodied relational CAT perspective and linked to the 3Rs of reformulation, recognition and revision, with clear guidance on how to integrate dreamwork into your CAT tool kit. They reveal the depth and breadth of the different parts of the self that may be embodied through dreamwork with fascinating and at times dramatic and moving verbatim transcripts as examples of the process.

- **Chapter 7:** James Turner introduces us to how the use of metaphor, image and embodied improvisation work can provide useful vehicles for unspoken or unspeakable feelings, numbed senses, and traumatic memories and experiences that perpetuate the fear that shuts down curiosity and playfulness. James describes how shared metaphors created in the therapy room, can then be reflected on in the reformulation letter and diagram and later may offer signposts to exits offering ways of integrating different parts of the self.

- **Chapter 8:** Louise Yorke (1965-2024) has left us her legacy in this chapter. Louise brings her passion for working creatively in a relational and trauma-focused way to this thoughtful work on relational dialogues with the 'inner child', offering detailed guidance on a technique for accessing and working with traumatized clients within a CAT framework, and includes the experiences of therapists, trainees and clients who have followed this technique.

- **Chapter 9:** Sarah Nicholas presents a case study from when she was a trainee CAT therapist using creative approaches in CAT, within an intellectual disability service. Sarah reflects on the process of finding a voice through moments of therapeutic engagement. The therapeutic narrative that unfolds is a beautiful and moving account of vulnerability and change through therapy using many of the techniques in practice described in Chapters 4 and 7. For those new to CAT, this case study offers a good introduction to the CAT tools and structure of a sixteen-session CAT therapy.

- **Chapter 10:** James Randall explores the Multiple Self States Model in CAT for neurodivergent individuals with dissociated and pluralized identities. He describes how imaginative representations of 'special interests' can offer new insights. Descriptions of heroic characters in fairy tales, film characters, literary themes and gaming culture offers opportunities for dialogical perspectives on multi-voiced selves, family relationships and life experiences. James introduces us to three people who have brought their individual creativity to the therapeutic space, and in doing so he gently challenges us to review our therapeutic skills and our assumptions about the therapeutic process and ultimately the goals of therapy.

Part 3

- **Chapter 11:** Vicky Petratou reflects on the creative process and asks how creativity and imaginative action can enrich the practice of CAT and psychotherapy supervision. I think that perhaps those who have been supervisors for a while will find inspiration through Vicky's chapter and consider the ways in which we can enhance the supervision experience for our supervisees, and maybe enrich the training of new supervisors. I suspect that my supervisees may expect more from me once they have read this chapter.

- **Chapter 12:** Jason Hepple brings two of his passions together in his chapter – Shakespeare and CAT – reflecting deeply on human development through the voice of one of Shakespeare's more acerbic characters, Jason seeks out a more reparative and dialogical interpretation of our journey from birth to death through a CAT lens. Anyone who has had the good fortune to be taught by Jason or to have attended one of his workshops will be familiar with Jason's fluidity in weaving a dialogical perspective on Shakespeare's perceptiveness about human passions, failings and frailties into his teaching days – you will know what to expect. For those who have not – enjoy!

- **Chapter 13:** Over the past twenty years, classical musician Stella Compton Dickinson has been the sole pioneer in developing the Cognitive Analytic Music Therapy (CAMT) model. Stella's unrelenting hard work, therapeutic integrity and at times dogged persistence were rewarded with acceptance of her RCT of CAMT within a forensic setting in 2017. More recently, Stella's dedication to innovation in her clinical practice was rewarded by her acceptance by the World Federation of Music Therapy of CAMT as a recognized model of music therapy. Stella is now able to supervise music therapists in the CAMT model, working with both children and adults.

- **Chapter 14:** Kathryn Pemberton's chapter about CAT training films. I am most grateful to Kathryn for her generosity in writing this chapter, which offers an insightful and engaging window into the process of producing psychotherapy training videos and films. Trainees coming to courses these days are much more attuned to visual media and often voice their expectations for training days to include videos and films as well as standard teaching materials, and these films from Catalyse have proved popular.

- **Chapter 15:** Rhona Brown has written a moving personal account of how a creative process and the ensuing journey can emerge from times of crisis and displacement. For Rhona, from a happenstance alongside a traumatic time in her personal life, emerged an interest in how storytelling through animation might be engaged with and applied to the therapy process. Rhona imagines and captures future possibilities for developments in CAT. And at the end of the chapter, you get to meet the Pilemonster!

- **Chapter 16:** Bringing their decades of wisdom and experience as international CAT trainers and psychotherapists, ACAT life members Elizabeth Wilde McCormick and Annalee Curran engage in inspiring conversation with Steve Potter to discuss well-being workshops they have facilitated for decades for CAT therapists using creative and mindfulness techniques.

PART 1: Mental health and the capacity to play

Daisy's[1] reflections on the experience of therapy

"The parting of the ways" (abridged)

So now we stand together looking at the fork in the road
For now, it is the time for us to take a different way
We have journeyed along the same road for a moment in time
And the shared experience has shaped and formed us both as we meet today

It has been a journey of ups and downs; pauses and movement
But I thank you for journeying with me and giving me a chance
Thank you for your knowledge and experience
which has helped me in my thinking
Has challenged my perceptions and given me new steps to dance

I know I am different having journeyed the road with you
I can see changes in me by the meeting of our minds
I understand more of myself and what makes me tick
The identities I created and the voices which define

I see what I became by the need to survive in my childhood
I see the wounds that I received from those who should have shown care
I see behaviours and attitudes which covered over my deep pain
And now it is time to move on and it is now time to dare!

The journey together means that now I am not the same
You have equipped me with the tools I need to help along the way
To listen to self, to soothe, to parent and to care,
To have self-compassion and make time for me to play!

Printed with permission

---

1 Pseudonym

Chapter 1:
CAT, creativity and mental health

Yvonne J. Stevens

> *'You can learn more about a person in an hour of play than a year of conversation.'* – Plato

Introduction

Reflections in this chapter are borne of decades of working therapeutically in the NHS and mental health services. As Suzanne Lyons notes in Chapter 4, rather like magpies we have collected skills and techniques from workshops, conferences and colleagues over the decades of our mental health and psychotherapeutic practice. We are aware of the risks of a disjointed eclecticism in psychotherapy. However, the CAT framework and the strength of the reformulation process offer hooks and hangers for the integration of a variety of means of accessing and working with unmanageable feelings, trauma and fragmented states. In addition, the shared and collaborative therapeutic frame of working within the CAT model offers scaffolding for exploration – to try things out – in ways that might be informed by a person's map and indicated exits, so that each therapy is in effect custom-created for each client according to the therapist's skills. CAT offers opportunities for creativity with the process of change through the 3Rs of recognition, reformulation and revision, holding in mind the importance of the metaphorical and the imaginative of the creative mind's expansive altered states and potential for peak experiences.

An overview of the creative in CAT practice

In *The Value of Written Communications in Dynamic Psychotherapy* (1983), Anthony Ryle says:

> 'The main arguments in favour of the greater use of written communication are to do with complexity and economy. Learning to recognize and change oneself in respect of modes hitherto unrecognized or unquestioned is difficult. Writing provides a means of articulating issues and of achieving distance and objectivity, and written material is available for repeated consideration. As a patient in once-weekly therapy is with the therapist for less than one per cent of his waking life, these considerations are of some importance.'

Ryle tried to pull together what mattered, wanting to help by creating an integrated framework for therapy. His creative focus was on the power of the written word; however, Ryle welcomed the integration of creative skills and techniques into his new model of psychotherapy. Ryle himself synthesized his exploration of the human condition through poetry, literature, philosophy, politics and anthropology and integrated this with his therapeutic approach, teaching and understanding (Stevens & Petratou, 2024). With the CAT model, Ryle created a heuristic device to work in the room, and he saw the need to continually develop, expand and explore with creativity.

In his brief address to the CAT community on 'Keeping CAT Alive', Ryle (2007, pp 4-5) said:

> 'CAT theory is not a doctrine. There is no inner circle of disciples charged with preserving its purity to whom, imitating Freud, I have given rings. Every practitioner has the right and duty to observe and report how the theory makes sense of what they see and how well it guides what they do. If it turns out that they have misunderstood the theory, it is likely that so have many others and that the theory needs clarification. If it turns out that the theory is wrong or does not work in some circumstances, then describing this will contribute to its further growth. Having said all that it should be noticed that 2006 brought two very welcome developments of CAT theory and practice:

> Stella Compton Dickinson. 2006. Beyond body, Beyond words: Cognitive Analytic Music Therapy in forensic psychiatry–new approaches in the treatment of personality disordered offenders. [See Chapter 13 in this volume.]
>
> Rose Hughes. 2007. An enquiry into an Integration of Cognitive Analytic Therapy with Art Therapy.'

I would add to this Petratou, V. (2007) *Bringing Drama to Dialogue: The use of Dramatherapy methods in Cognitive Analytic Therapy.'* (See Chapter 5 in this volume.)

It could be suggested that only therapists accredited in creative arts psychotherapies should use creative techniques in therapies, but through our exploration of working in this way beyond the usual therapeutic conversation, we are learning from each other and our clients, and it has led to therapeutic gains for clients and rewarding therapy experiences for therapists. Therefore, it behoves therapists to equip themselves with a better toolbox. CAT creates a supportive and gentle framework to hold and contain the abstract and unspoken which can be accessed creatively. I know that many CAT therapists are and have been using creative techniques with their clients integrated with the 3Rs of CAT, and I hope that they will find recognition, affirmation and some inspiration from the authors in the following chapters.

I have included here some of the contributors to the Association for Cognitive Analytic Therapy's (ACAT) *Reformulation* journal, who have shared their creative explorations and journeys, but also there have been many novel dissertations and essays submitted by CAT trainees describing their creative practice within the CAT model. Sarah Huish's dissertation for her CAT psychotherapy training, *Ways of Seeing – when words are a second language*, (2022, unpublished) explores how images can be helpfully integrated into CAT diagrams and bring a client's inner world into dialogue in the therapy room when words may fall short; it can be hard for some people to find words that describe what they see, maybe poetry comes close in its use of metaphor. Huish wonders whether 'CAT is too abrupt with its use of words, and whether more space should be given to states of mind and embodied images'. Huish reported that 'CAT therapists are more likely to use the observing eye, "healthy island" or colour coordinate their maps than use other forms of images.' Barriers to using images she identified as being a 'lack of training, images not being used in their own personal therapy.'

Furthermore, Sarah Supple (2022) from her own position of being registered blind, describes the challenges of finding the creativity within what she encountered as a text-dominated CAT model, to feel included rather than excluded, as might be experienced by clients and therapists due to any issues of difference or disability. Supple continues with an exploration of the ways in which the use of metaphor, popular imagery, current media memes, objects and the body might offer more creative vehicles for inclusive reformulation that are accessible and within both therapists' and clients' zone of proximal development (ZPD). (See Lyons Chapter 4, Turner Chapter 7, Randall Chapter 10, Compton Dickinson Chapter 13 this volume.) One musical client composed and performed her goodbye letter on a flute, others have written poems, painted pictures and created collages. The CAT tools and diagrams lend themselves to creative representation dramatically, pictorially, musically and related to through the body, as is described throughout this volume.

Gregory and Wilde McCormick (pp. 33-35, 2019) explore the poetic narrative in the dialogue of CAT as enabling the expression of core emotions and experiences:

> *'This matching of words to feelings is the task of poetry. Helping patients explore feelings by joining them in a dialogue about feelings and by using the body to deepen contact with feelings can change understanding – such as when what is thought of as anger, can in fact be sadness. And so, a completely different dialogue begins… CAT theory names the myriad ways in which human beings learn to survive an often-difficult early life that masks the "healthy self". Working with intention to reveal and nourish this healthy self is the business of psychotherapy. Some poems do speak to the potential for a healthy self within each of us. In R S Thomas' poem "The Bright Field" (Thomas, 1990) he writes about seeing the sun break out over a field one day, but he "goes on his way" and forgets it. Later he knows that he must give his all to remember and connect with that precious moment. "For that is the Pearl of Great Price." My reading of his poem is that the poet is inviting us to notice and nourish those moments of real connection, inner and outer, that help begin the process of healing.'*

The keystone of the reformulation letter in CAT provides a coherent, integrating experience of a person's previously fragmented or vague or unreflected-upon narrative – like a jigsaw with pieces missing. Often, lost childhood traumas are remembered following the reading of the letter – one client remembered a childhood experience of abuse while bedbound during an illness, another being the young confidante to a parent's marital betrayal, another running away from their fearful life at boarding school. Sometimes, these felt like the lives lived by another person, so distant does that traumatized child seem from the adult-self. Dickens (1861) wrote of Pip in *Great Expectations* when in the criminal Magwitch's clutches that 'few people know what secrecy there is in the young under terror… I was in mortal terror of my interlocutor with the iron leg; I was in mortal terror of myself from whom an awful promise had been extracted … I am afraid to think of what I might have done in requirement, in the secrecy of my terror.' Louise Yorke (Chapter 8, this volume) offers ways to connect with that child within therapy and to understand and witness what fears, hurts and terrors may lie there. That Pip, perceived by others as a 'difficult child', was in truth a 'child in difficulty'. People who have been silenced as a child have also related to Tove Janson's story of *The Invisible Child* (1962), in which a young a girl has slowly disappeared, her presence reduced to just the tinkle of a bell, through cruel and neglectful treatment. Through the compassion and acceptance by the Moomin Family, feeling loved and accepted, she gradually finds her voice and then her anger, and becomes a complete child again.

Ryle (1994) considered that which has not been kept as available for conscious reflective thought as a key focus for attention in CAT (see Appendix 3). Rather than explain this through the concept of the structural unconscious, Ryle considered ideas about consciousness, the 'reflected-upon' and 'unreflected-upon' mind, along with our emerging understandings from neuroscience which reflect philosophical understandings from Zen and Buddhism of meditation and mindfulness practice that focus on the expansion of reflexivity and self-awareness. Ryle suggested that these forms of restrictions on the capacity for reflexivity are derived from both trauma and deprivation, and frequently co-exist (see Appendix 3). The therapeutic task is to describe and name these restrictions on the capacity to reflect on the self in the reformulation letter and map, and address through the therapeutic relationship and through the creation of alternative narratives and 'targeted interpersonal activity'. Below, and in the rest of the book, are some ways in which CAT therapists have sought to enhance the capacity for self-reflection through the activity of imaginative creativity.

The power of narrative

In our work with clients and as trainers and supervisors, we often draw on shared cultural narratives to illustrate human dilemmas, whether that is the latest cliffhanger from 'Eastenders', a well-worn childhood text, or tales and myths from world folklore. Great stories in literature and oral traditions of the Global South explore our capacity for naivety, recklessness, narcissistic pre-occupation, murderous rage, and revenge, as well as courage, generosity and love, for example Shakespeare's *Troilus and Cressida* (Nehmad, 1997) and *King Lear* (Hepple, 2012). In teaching the narrative construction of the reformulation letter, Alison Jenaway (2019) chooses Cinderella, a popular choice from among fairy tales. Here is an extract of her letter:

> *Dear Cinderella,*
>
> *Your childhood was very difficult. Your mother died when you were very young, and you have no real memories of her. People told you that she loved you very much and that she was a wonderful person, always loving and giving. You grew up with your father, who can be quite difficult and demanding at times. It felt important to you to be kind like your mother, and you vowed to be like her – always caring and helping out, never thinking about yourself or your own needs… When your father remarried and your stepmother came to live with you, bringing her two daughters, you continued this same pattern. You spent every moment trying to please them and do what they wanted, hoping that they would love you like your mother did… Feeling not worthy and not good enough, meant that you did not look after yourself well. Instead, you still tried desperately to please your family. They took advantage of this and made you feel even less worthy, pushing back down to the bottom of the diagram we drew together. We called this the 'what more can I do for you' cycle…*

We have some idea about how the story might unfold for Cinderella, but Jenaway creates a new 'happy ever after' ending/beginning for her protagonist where 'perhaps this therapy can be the start of you getting to know yourself and what you want. It might help you learn how to be as kind and compassionate towards yourself as you try to be towards others.'

Jason Hepple[2] devised a therapeutic and training narrative to illustrate the experience of dread some may feel and enact in compulsive repetitive thoughts and rituals. The story of 'The Burden' invites people to write the ending of the story of the young boy visited by an angel in the dead of night and given 'the burden' of protecting his family from harm. He acquiesces and becomes a dedicated servant, and then a prisoner, to his pledge, with the sense of dread should he fail growing with every year until it consumes him completely. Hepple describes our responses to this story in terms of 'insideness', our empathy for the boy, which is concerned with our authentic 'experience of the commonality of human suffering', and 'outsideness' with seeing from a distance the role 'the individual usually unwittingly plays in the perpetuation of their own suffering'. In the therapeutic relationship, Hepple (2006) explains 'this encourages a dialogical position of seeing the self as the other sees us, as in Bakhtin: "The way in which I create myself is by means of a quest. I go out into the world in order to come back with a self," (Clark & Holquist, 1984). Through the creation of these images, it is possible to communicate how the layers, parts, and voices of the person can become visible and heard in the eyes of another, witnessed perhaps for the first time.'

The mythologies, folklore and fairy tales we share in from our very early years with our families and communities communicate powerful and profound truths about relationships, our past, present and future, about love and death, through the use of powerful archetypes, often with a simplicity and brevity that are accessible to all. Archetypal alters can now be accessed digitally through AI-generated avatars in gaming such as 'Dungeons and Dragons'; an avatar may be an electronically generated image, as in a 3-D video game or virtual reality (VR) experience, that represents and may be manipulated by gamers, enabling them to role play new narratives in the alternative reality of the metaverse. See Randall (Chapter 10, this volume) for how AI created alters might be used within the CAT Multiple Self States Model (MSSM).

Jefferis (2011) describes reasons for drawing attention to the relevance of stories to CAT:

---

2   For a copy of The Burden exercise contact Jason Hepple via: admin@acat.me.uk
Further information on the exercise can be found in: Hepple J (2019) Cognitive Analytic Therapy (CAT), obsessions and overvalued ideas: Developing a model and a method. International Journal of Cognitive Analytic Therapy and Relational Mental Health 3, 51-68. Journal CAT 3 PAGES 9 (internationalcat.org)

> '*First, CAT employs narrative as a key tool of understanding and therapeutic change. The power of the Reformulation Letter largely comes from its narrative form, its status as a (particular type of) story. Mindful that it is a reformulation – there is already a story, a narrative by which the person understands their predicament – in CAT we develop that story and consider different ways of telling it. This fits with the notion that life is a narrative form – "we enter a stage which we did not design and we are already part of the action; each of us is a main character in his own drama, plays subordinate parts in the drama of others, and each drama constrains the others" (or in CAT terms we might say "is in dialogue with the others") (MacIntyre, 2007: 213). Second, creativity is encouraged in CAT, as seen in the frequent use of creative techniques such as imagination and visualisation work (Wilde McCormick, 2008), and in the potential for experiment and flexibility in what takes place in the session, rather than adherence to manualised or standardised techniques. Third, these ideas would appear to fit with CAT theory, especially the Vygotskian and Bakhtinian elements.*' (p.29-33)

Rachel Pollard (2012) reflects through her dialogical analysis of the film 'Blade Runner' how 'stories can carry the social and cultural meanings of a particular time and place and thus can be *formative of the self*; dialogue about stories can be a form of *joint activity*; stories potentially act as a *shared tool* for understanding. Narrative itself can be a catalyst for memory and learning.'

Jefferis (2011), captures the potential for powerful identification with narratives:

> '*Stories are abundant with imagery and rich language which may offer powerful "signs" which can mediate learning. They carry meaning of previous dialogues – for example, myths carry a long history of human experience within themselves, and Leiman (1994a) thinks it is this richness which gives them their power in psychotherapy to transform peoples' experience and understanding of their own situation. Stories may "transform" the therapeutic dialogue by opening new possibilities for making meaning of the personal experiences brought by the client. Stories sometimes communicate something about the nature of personal experience which may be*

hard to attain by other means; the therapeutic moment when a word or a nickname (such as one from a story) is found to describe a particular state – when both client and therapist know that it's the "right" description – can be a powerful one.' (Jefferis, pp.29-33)

Make space for the creative in the therapy room

"This writer is of the firm belief that our tears become holy in the form of ink on a page. Once we have spoken our saddest story, we can be free of it. And then all that's left behind is the tortured poetry."

Taylor Swift, The Tortured Poets Department, (2024).

For a client's creativity to truly emerge within the busy-ness of the CAT reformulation process, it needs the therapist to make space within the therapeutic frame. Encouraging a person's imaginative and creative acts – a word, an image, lyrics of a song, a fairy tale or a story - may be remembered together with an emotion.

Elia and Jenaway (2007), in considering creating a space to think and imagine, suggest that 'we listen carefully if patients talk about their favourite film, song, or play. Ask them about their identification with created roles or suggest something for them to view, read, or listen to. It may sometimes be easier and less threatening to first identify Reciprocal Roles in creative contexts and to use created roles as shared signs in therapy to promote meaningful dialogue.'

Some clients come to therapy as journal keepers, with volumes of thoughts never revealed before – this can be brought into the service of the therapeutic process, and perhaps changed – the journalling voice may change, the focus of the notes may change. Some people find this an invaluable way to describe memories, express their thoughts and convey feelings as a transition to sharing these in dialogue. I have always tended to promote the value of self-reflection or between-session tasks for myself and for my clients and recommended this for trainees and supervisees to use with their clients.

Dynamic genograms and timelines that tell stories become shared collaborative tools with opportunities for noticing generational relational roles and repetitions of trauma or neglect and difficulties. In Ryle's early days as an

East London general practitioner, he looked for patterns in familial patterns of mental health distress and trauma which sowed the seeds of the CAT understanding of relational transfer and the repetition of Reciprocal Roles.

Clients bring their own dialogical and creative selves to the creative process in therapy. One client in her 70's brought a roll of lining paper which she rolled out across the floor of the consulting room – with her decades of gains and losses, times of joy and despair drawn out in felt pen. Complex life stories can be traced across the page on a winding road to fill in as the sessions go by – filling in the forgotten and the disavowed and the unspeakable – maybe leaving a mark on the timeline to go back to when the therapeutic space feels safe enough and ready to contain and witness what has felt unbearable to speak of before. The sanctity of the therapy room is where words come into being that have never been said before – except perhaps repeated again and again in the ruminations of the internal critical voice.

Creativity can be woven in from the beginning to the end through the CAT process. For some clients, the invitation to bring their creative selves to therapy provokes a shyness, while for others it is pushing on an open door – lengthy goodbye letters, filling volumes of journals and artwork, stick figures, self-portraits, cartoons, paintings, origami self-states, collage triptychs, poetic explorations of despair and the fantasies of secret alter-egos emerge, that have never been spoken of before. Each has created artefacts of meaning and importance and relevance to them within the CAT reformulation, recognition and revision process.

For the uniqueness and originality in our imaginative selves, as Pollard (2012) refers to, there are also archetypal and cultural shared themes and language (perhaps tapping into something akin to Jung's idea of the collective unconscious) as images and metaphors represent commonly held human experiences (see Turner Chapter 7, this volume). Islands, fortresses, caves and bunkers are places to hide away; feeling lost in a fog or at the bottom of a pit or well, cut off from the self and loved ones; hidden feelings are locked away in a box, or behind a firmly bolted door, which might be opened slightly to peep inside and then firmly shut again. Overwhelming feelings erupt from volcanoes, pans of boiling potatoes overflow, atomic bombs and grenades threaten anyone close. These metaphors often have bodily correlations – the closed box of unmanageable memories and feelings seems to reside in the anterior of the brain, terror and dread in the pit of the guts, and loss and sadness bring an aching to the heart and fear and anxiety tighten the throat, with panic constricting the voice. For one client, a gruesome toad sat just behind her shoulder whispering cruel words in her ear, often the voices of monstrous bullies are just out of sight, in the corner of one's eye, manifestations of the inner critical voice. Drawings of tentacled beasts, demonic faces and menacing shadowy presences while a small child huddles in their bed in terror may give the first inklings of the historical trauma the person sitting across from you has endured.

From these narratives there may be a familiar pathway of heroic endeavour and challenge and triumph which has been etched into our psyche through novels, plays and stories, which may be retold through the Six-Part Story Method (Dent-Brown, 2011) (see Appendix 5) revealing the potential aims and exits of self-actualization. A creative and flexible CAT is accessible, inclusive and responsive to meet the client in their world and to integrate these experiences.

Elsa wrote her journal after every therapy session: 'My mind is like a scribble which converges into a straight line through the medium of a pen.' Through the course of a lengthy CAT therapy in recovery from anorexia she described the emergence of the 'New Elsa' in constant stand-offs with 'Old Elsa'. We had both watched and talked about the film 'Inside Out' (2015) from Pixar Animation Studios, and in her journal, Elsa introduced her anorexia as a new character:

> 'So, I'm panicking and if I refer back to my or our "Inside Out" analogy – every emotion that there ever has been is running around in a blind panic pressing all the buttons, screaming with their hands in the air, jumping out of windows, setting off alarms, trying to do something, anything, to help. Usually at this point Anorexia sweeps in nonchalantly ignoring the chaos around her, takes her seat, puts her feet up on the desk, legs crossed at the ankles, leans back, lights a cigarette, inhales deeply and, as she blows it slowly and deliberately in the faces of Joy, Fear, Anger, Disgust and most of all Sadness, she smiles slightly and says "Showtime".'

> '…I have Old Elsa trying her damnedest to sabotage New Elsa … Old Elsa is intent on killing herself one way or the other because she is worthless and invisible and alone … trying to remind me of the fun we had when all we had to worry about was how many pieces we could cut a lettuce leaf into and eat piece by piece with a cocktail stick.'

'...I don't want to attempt suicide because I now have so much to live for. Yes, at the moment I'm panicking and scared and sad and all those things, but I've survived the worse. Psychotherapy has been hideous on many occasions, but we've got through it and look where those hideous sessions have got me, look at who I've become ... well maybe not look at the shambles that I am at the moment, but this is a minor blip – it is a blip if I deal with it effectively, in the New Elsa mode. I'm so wise on paper and so calamitous in practice...'

Elsa was able to use her emerging reflective and independent self and her 'observing eye' to notice when Old Elsa tried to sabotage her new life. Elsa created a CAT 'playlist' as we went through the therapy. The song by The Waterboys, 'The Whole of the Moon, became an important anthem for Elsa's exits.

Daisy and I worked together using the CAT Multiple Self States Model and the states description questions first devised by Hilary Beard with Anthony Ryle at St Thomas' Hospital which then became incorporated into the CAT States Description Procedure (SDP) (see Appendix 2). Daisy wanted to understand how it was that she often felt hurt and out of control, or angry and rejected (and rejecting) in her relationships with herself and others. She wanted to better understand these different states as they seemed to sometimes change quite suddenly and affect how she felt about herself and others. At times, how Daisy felt about me as her therapist might also change quite suddenly and unexpectedly and threaten to derail our relationship and end our sessions. Daisy felt that 'state changes' had caused problems in her relationships and had significantly affected her life chances. For a few weeks, Daisy worked on these creative descriptions of states between our sessions (see Figure 1.1) which she had constructed from online cartoons and filled them out in response to the states' questions (Appendix 2). We were able to refer to these descriptions and create an integrated Multiple Self States Map for Daisy to connect up these states and feel more understanding and compassion towards herself, and to explain herself better to others and to negotiate how to better express her needs in her relationships. Daisy's poem at the beginning of this section reflects her recognition of these changes in herself.

Chapter 1: CAT, creativity and mental health

Figure 1.1: Daisy's (pseudonym) self-states descriptions

How did I get into this State?
My need is not seen or heard; anticipated or understoon
I feel I have been belittled, undermined or dismissed
I have not been listened to or heard
I have been treated unfairly or unjustly
I have not been given an opportunity to explain myself
When boundaries are changed without consultation, negotiation or explanation
When I try to accomplish a task and it doesn't work
When I fail to be who I want to be
When people demand things of me when I am tired

What do I do when I am in this State?
Shout
Scream
Rage
Hit G
Ruminate
Have conversations in my head with the person
Throw things
Smash things
Run away

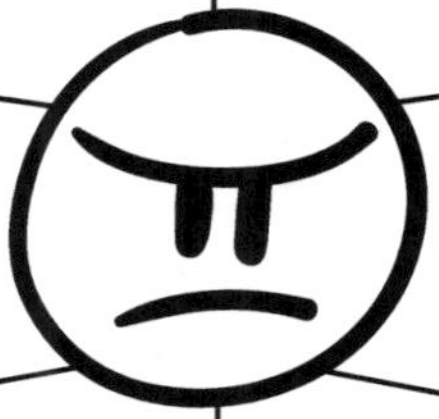

Bodily feelings
Red face
Blood boils
Muscles tense especially in my head
Stomach constricts

What do others feel about me
Scared
Walking on egg shells
Disgusted
Dislike
Disapproving
Critical

How do I get out of this State?
Thump pillow
Express the anger
Process in my journal – try and work out why I am angry and find an assertive course of action
Talk to a trusted friend
Self parent – listen to hurt and pain, empathise, love, care

Conclusions/questions
Anger can be spontaneous so still spills out
No + exit strategy
Can't stop or control triggers

Chapter 1: CAT, creativity and mental health

How did I get into this State?
I am scared of this
I can't do this
This is too much for me
I am going to mess up/fail
This is out of my control
People will discover I am a fraud, incapable
If I don't do x people may be angry, displeased, disapprove, criticise
I have to get this right/succeed
I will be punished if I get this wrong or don't do it
I will lose affirmation, acceptance and approval I need

What do I do when I am in this State?
Drive self and strive to succeed
Work too hard and too long
Forget self care and time for play
Frenetic activity
Hypervigilance
Aim high
Perfectionist expectations
Beat self up
Criticise self
Judge self

What do others feel about me
Annoyed at my neediness
Concerned for me
Confused

Bodily feelings
Agitation
Sleeplessness
Brain works overtime
Stomach tense
Tense
Butterflies in stomach

How do I get out of this State?
Work until I feel on top of things but detrimental to self – can end up crying as exhausted
Occasionally I find a voice that says enough is enough; do not worry; take time and space for self/ value self

Conclusions/questions
??? Struggle with + exit strategy

How did I get into this State?

- My needs were not met or anticipated
- I got angry first and then slipped into this state
- When I feel overlooked
- When I feel invalidated
- When I compare myself to others and am left wanting
- When I have tried really hard and do not get approval, affirmation, praise
- When people do not recognise my efforts
- When I cannot get the outcome that I desire

What do I do when I am in this State?

- Negative internal dialogue
- Beat self up
- Crush self
- Self-castigation
- Negative inner beliefs whirl around e.g. you are not making progress; you are a nothing and a nobody
- Run away, hide, lock myself in a room, cry

What do others feel about me

- I think others will dislike me, reject me, be angry at me
- M – compassionate, caring, gentle, able to hold me emotionally
- G – kind, gentle, caring, compassionate
- Others feel sad I am feeling so low and want to help

Bodily feelings

- Excruciating pain in stomach
- Sensation in vagina???
- Shaking
- Tensed muscles

How do I get out of this State?

- Talk to people I know love and support me for who I am and as I am
- Hug Teddy or Panda
- Use journal to process feelings and thoughts
- Replace CIV with + inner dialogue
- Sit, relax, breathe
- Engage in adult conversation
- Pray/remind self of Scriptures

Conclusions/questions

- Can I avoid getting into this state?
- Can I change reactions once triggered?

Chapter 1: CAT, creativity and mental health

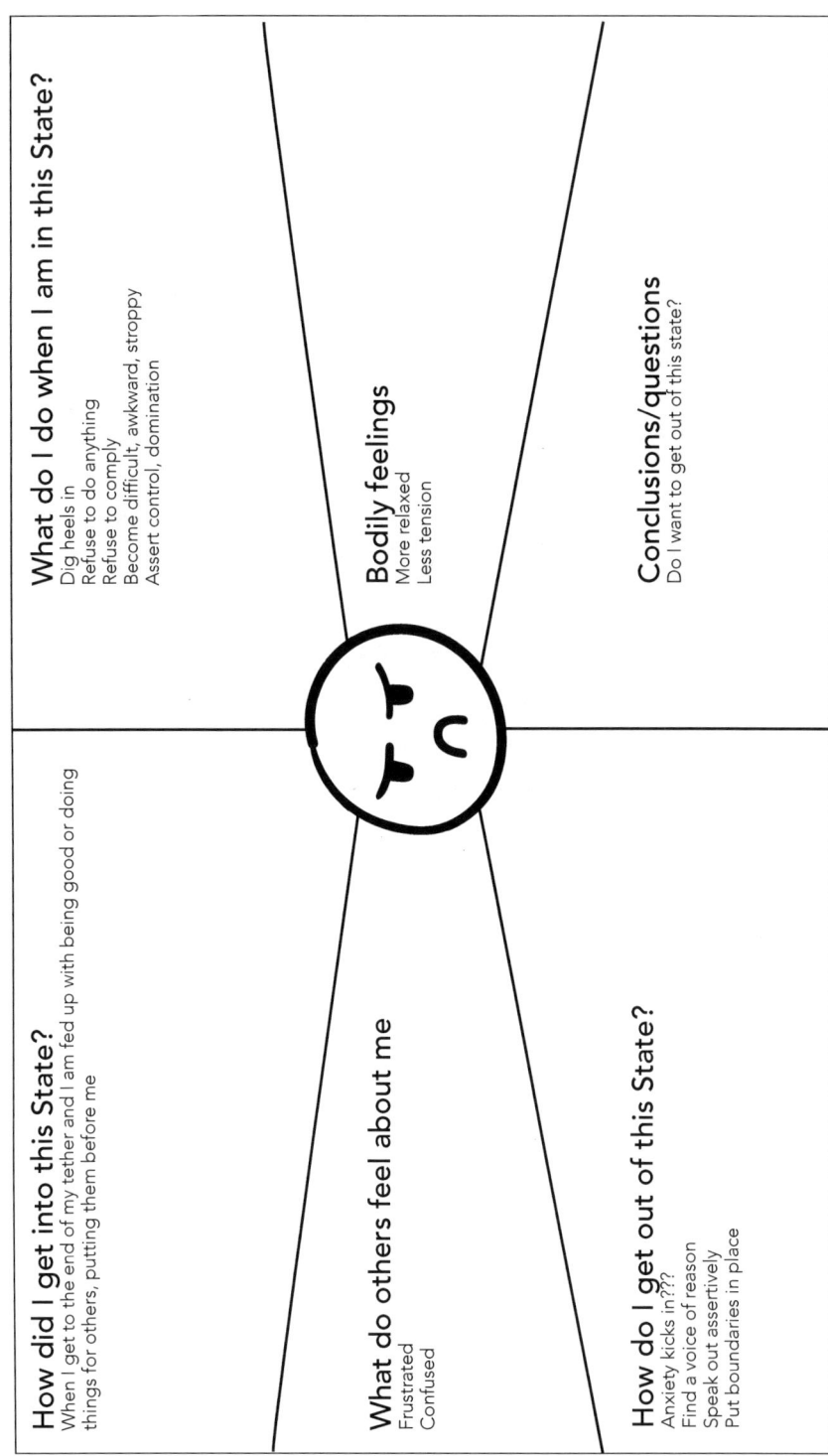

Chapter 1: CAT, creativity and mental health

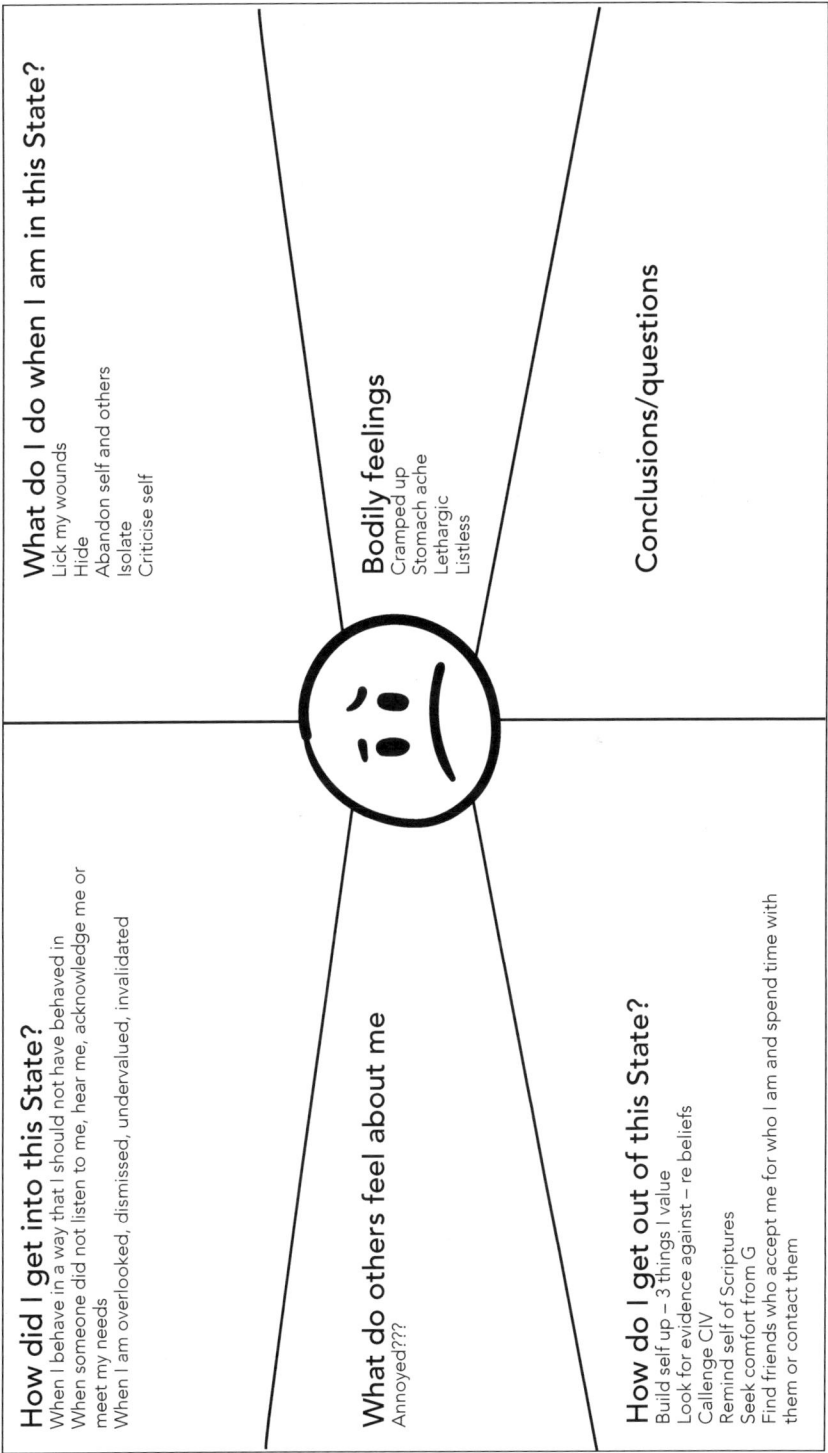

What do I do when I am in this State?
Lick my wounds
Hide
Abandon self and others
Isolate
Criticise self

Bodily feelings
Cramped up
Stomach ache
Lethargic
Listless

Conclusions/questions

How did I get into this State?
When I behave in a way that I should not have behaved in
When someone did not listen to me, hear me, acknowledge me or meet my needs
When I am overlooked, dismissed, undervalued, invalidated

What do others feel about me
Annoyed???

How do I get out of this State?
Build self up – 3 things I value
Look for evidence against – re beliefs
Callenge CIV
Remind self of Scriptures
Seek comfort from G
Find friends who accept me for who I am and spend time with them or contact them

Chapter 1: CAT, creativity and mental health

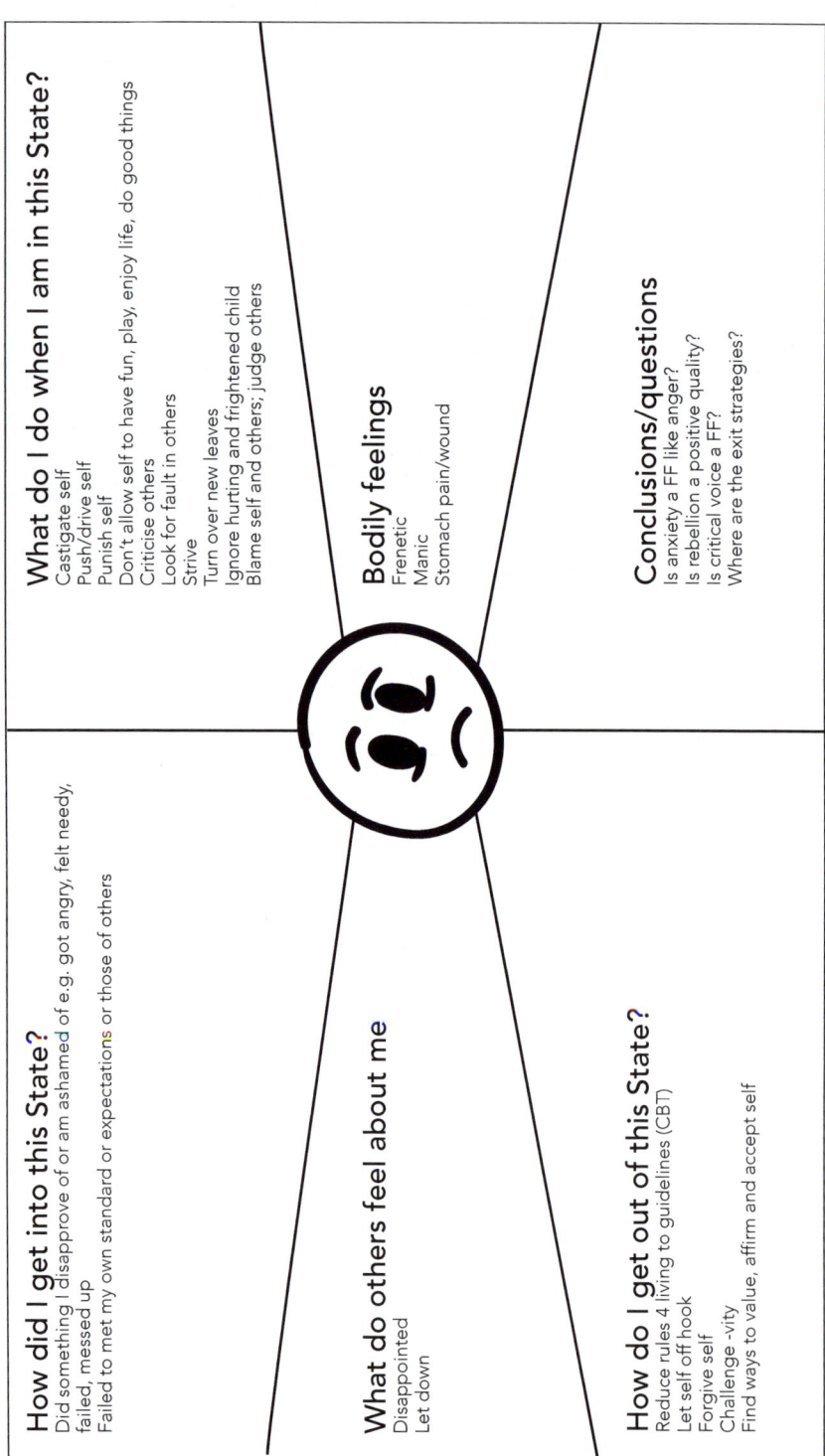

How did I get into this State?
Did something I disapprove of or am ashamed of e.g. got angry, felt needy, failed, messed up
Failed to met my own standard or expectations or those of others

What do I do when I am in this State?
Castigate self
Push/drive self
Punish self
Don't allow self to have fun, play, enjoy life, do good things
Criticise others
Look for fault in others
Strive
Turn over new leaves
Ignore hurting and frightened child
Blame self and others; judge others

Bodily feelings
Frenetic
Manic
Stomach pain/wound

What do others feel about me
Disappointed
Let down

How do I get out of this State?
Reduce rules 4 living to guidelines (CBT)
Let self off hook
Forgive self
Challenge -vity
Find ways to value, affirm and accept self

Conclusions/questions
Is anxiety a FF like anger?
Is rebellion a positive quality?
Is critical voice a FF?
Where are the exit strategies?

Finding space for creativity in mental health services

- Creativity as the journey.
- Creativity as the treatment.
- Creativity as the exit.

In a care home I worked in for people with dementia, when we sang the old Vera Lynn and music hall songs, the residents who no longer knew their names and had long since forgotten their children, would sing along, their eyes bright with recognition and tears. Engaging with arts as a therapeutic experience has been shown to lessen depression and dementia in older adults; ('Just One Long Thing', Michael Mosely on Radio 4; 4.1.24).

Across cultures we invest in and value art, artefacts and anthropological collections, and performance of stories and music – these vital human activities bring our sense of ourselves and our ancestors alive. When integrated into our understanding of mental health practice – so that we can recognize the creativity in all of us – we can use it to give shape and voice to our worst fears and traumas and losses and our most courageous and joyful moments. Creative arts psychotherapists offering music, drama and art therapies are an immensely precious yet scarce resource within mental health services.

It follows on that mental health professionals need to develop opportunities to explore and expand their capacity for responding creatively in the therapy room. See Appendix 7 for ideas for creative exercises for psychotherapists and psychotherapy trainees to practice tasks they may ask of their clients, and also to explore aspects of their own identity and origin and relationships, the narrative of their lives and expression of their inner and outer selves. Paul Daley (Daley, 2023) describes using culture and storytelling as the best ways to talk about historical trauma, in his article 'Pushed into humanity', in which he reports on classes in narrative medicine in Melbourne asking how learning about storytelling can make better doctors. 'Narrative medicine just has a way of opening a vein, somehow. And all this stuff just comes out that is deeply vulnerable but also very beautiful. You know, objectively, it's very beautiful.'

In this way, the process of arriving at the reformulation in CAT offers opportunities for novel connections as therapists engage with clients in the creation of their story as a 'meaning-full' narrative. Similarly, Dr Joao Luis Barreto Guimaraes in Porto, Portugal, teaches poetry to trainee doctors to encourage empathy for their patients. 'I get them to look at poems that talk about empathy, compassion, solidarity and similar humanistic values that doctors should strive for' (Balch, 2024)

Klein (1932) defined positive mental health as the capacity to be creative and to take up causes in our communities, while Carl Jung (1963) described his psychotic break as his 'creative illness'. Effective approaches to mental health treatment require the integration of conscious reasoning (such as identifying unhelpful cognitions) together with the receptivity of intuition and the activity of creativity. Creativity and curiosity are essentially both effective when harnessed as therapeutic tools and as healthy exits. William James, the father of modern psychology, feared that psychological practice was more concerned with the literal, abandoning the literary and the metaphorical. Sullivan (2017, p37), draws from William James's understanding that:

> '...the profound risk ... of the literary migrating to the fringes of mental health is that physiological and literal accounts of mental health problems will rely on literal correlates of personhood in their explanations... There is a dimension of the existential inner struggle within this literary metaphor that is core to humanistic understandings of the self.'

You cannot harness change without a vision, so as navigators of this very human expression, we must give ourselves permission to be creative and imaginative. (See Appendix 7 for ideas for creative tasks for psychotherapy trainees). CAT is a radically humane, social and systemic framework for ways of thinking about mental disorder from the premise that we are socially formed in relationship to others and the self (Ryle & Kerr, 2020). As the reformulation process offers an over-arching descriptive account of the person, the model integrates well with Compassion Focused Therapy (Gilbert, 2003), with Internal Family Systems (Gregory, Jenaway & Lee 2023) and with EMDR (Walker, 2024) as well as alongside the creative arts psychotherapies described in this book (Petratou Chapter 5, Compton Dickinson Chapter 13, this volume).

We can embody creative techniques within the CAT therapeutic process to enable emotional knowing and memory reconsolidation as exit strategies, to develop compassionate internal dialogues with the self as a future preventative process to stay relationally attuned to ourselves and our needs.

Acknowledgements

With thanks to Elsa and Daisy for their contributions to this book (pseudonyms used to protect confidentiality).

Chapter 2:
The neurobiological benefits of novelty and play

Suzanne Lyons and Yvonne J. Stevens

Ryle pointed to the future interest of CAT in neuroscience and comparative psychology but did not really explore this further himself. We are mindful that the tentative exploration of our neuropsychology and the corresponding neuroscience may quickly become as outdated as do our discoveries of the outer universe over time, dispel one theory for another.

Developments in CAT further explored in this volume by several authors (Lyons Chapter 4, Randall Chapter 10, Compton Dickinson Chapter 13) explain the CAT Multiple Self States Model of trauma through an understanding of memory and its emotional reprocessing, from the premise that multiple states are procedural survival strategies for managing unmanageable feelings and unmet need. These are recognized and contained in CAT through the collaborative therapeutic stance of the observing eye position.

Complex PTSD (Herman, 1992) can be viewed as a condition in which the body and mind have not recognized that a traumatic event has passed. The body's threat system continues to prepare for defensive fight or flight or a protective frozen or dissociated state. At the same time, PTSD can be seen as a failure of *mindful dual awareness*, which results in over-reliance on, and hypervigilance for, internal cues and symptoms, and an inability to recognize external signs in the present as being different from the past. One client needed to see the registration plates of modern cars in the car park to recognise that they were in this century and not some forty years ago when they were a vulnerable child. Therapy needs to enable the nervous system to recognize when trauma is over by encouraging emotional presence in the present moment, this is embodied in the emotional presence of the therapeutic relationship facilitated by the imaginative capacity to play.

Novelty, play and right-brain development

'In interaction between a normal infant and a happy and receptive caregiving companion the dual intrinsic motive formation systems of the two subjects are mutually supportive in rhythmic, sympathetic engagements which demonstrate **synchrony and turn-taking** *in utterances and clear flexible emotionally toned phrasing with affect attunement.'* (Aitken & Trevarthen, 1997 p.667).

Trevarthen describes the primacy of intersubjective synchronization in optimal playful interactions between infants and their caregivers to foster healthy neurobiological development. This includes, amongst other more physical effects such as synchronised heartbeat, the infant's and caregiver's facial movements, voice, tone, gaze, touch and gesture and the playfulness of turn-taking in these interactions creating a rhythmic reciprocity. Trevarthen found these interactions stimulated right brain to right brain synchronicity and importantly therefore the development of the right brain of the infant at a crucial time of growth. These intersubjective communications Trevarthen called 'protoconversations' which arise out of these experiences of to-and-fro intimate moments of playfulness, forming the infant's future positive foundation for relationality, musicality and creativity. Although Trevarthen's interest is in child development, his work also informs possible directions for using these understandings of neurobiology to address a poverty or a deprivation in the 'the capacity to play' which we may find in the therapy room, and also to remind us of the primacy of play in authentic human social interactions such as psychotherapy.

Marks-Tarlow (2017) suggested that '"novelty" is what the right-brain specializes in, and this is what is helpful in building new ways of being, and she has written extensively on the importance of creativity and play. In her book *Clinical Intuition in Psychotherapy* (2012) she said, 'to be fully present, authentic, and effective, therapists must continually tune into interpersonal novelty, to render psychotherapy an inherently creative enterprise'. She also explains how, 'Through play, we bypass ordinary defences connected with survival-level processes, e.g. fear and self-protection or anger and rejection'. She also included a description of working with figurines to help a client work through her childhood sexual abuse.

In *Play & Creativity in Psychotherapy* (2017) she focuses on the informal use of play during psychotherapy as it is orchestrated intuitively, and how the conscious or unconscious use of play cuts across all modalities and is a major source for implicit learning through inter-creativity or the 'intersubjective' space between therapist and client, and, in CAT terms, the internalization of helpful RRs, and therefore a significant contributor to therapeutic effectiveness.

Siegel (2012) explains the importance of non-competitive play and how it can encourage healthy neuroplastic growth as the:

> '...emphasis is on new and creative forms of interacting with oneself, others, and the world. Imagination is given free rein, interactions are novel and spontaneous, and the outcomes are not predictable or constrained by goal-directed actions. Being playful is healthy because it frees us in our relationships to be able to collaborate without judgment. With playfulness our minds can become vulnerable and take risks as we push the envelope to go beyond our usual ways of being and of doing, and our brains can try out new combinations of firing patterns.' (p37-5)

> 'Many of us have aspects of our lives – of being playful, of being creative, artistic, and spontaneous – that after childhood may have gone by the wayside. State integration reminds us of the importance of honouring each of these states and finding the ones that we treasure and nurturing their growth and presence in our lives. When we are fulfilled in this way, we fill ourselves with the vitality of integration.' (p41-12)

In a sense, we are trying to encourage a client to reconnect with their own sense of creativity to have more confidence in a healthier sense of self.

Creating playful spaces in CAT

Creative embodied therapeutic ways of working can be very effective in facilitating a playful safe place with the aim of identifying and working towards the integration of fragmented states and reducing the effects of trauma. This is further facilitated through a dialogical approach, or conversations between the different self-states represented by objects.

Within a CAT framework, using objects can also aid and enrich the co-creation of the CAT tools of family trees, reformulation, CAT letters, or maps, or to create a healthy island, i.e. a client's imagined future place, including who and what they would like in their life on this island. Another clinical resource is Petratou's (2019) *House of Self States (HOSS)* (see Appendix 4), which uses a creative integrative and a containing mapping approach. The therapeutic relationship created through a playful lens also potentially becomes a new embodied experience and part of the client's exits, as the invitation to 'play' provides safer exploration and potential new ways of being. Ogden (2018) defines creativity from a bodily perspective as 'challenging habitual responses in order to move, think and feel in new and unfamiliar ways – to seek out and grapple with the risks that enliven us by their unpredictability and expand our window of tolerance'.

Creating safe spaces for play

Winnicott (1971) thought that playing was the key to emotional and psychological well-being, for all ages, engendering spontaneity and engagement, and that therapy should offer a playful experience of creative, genuine discovery. He used the term 'Potential Space', suggesting a safe interpersonal place in which one can be spontaneously playful while at the same time feeling connected to others, and he proposed that:

> '...psychotherapy is done in the overlap of the two play areas, that of the patient and that of the therapist. If the therapist cannot play, then he is not suitable for the work. If the patient cannot play, then something needs to be done to enable the patient to be able to play, after which psychotherapy may begin. The reason why playing is essential is that it is in playing that the patient is being creative.' (p.39)

Cozolino (2016) suggest that 'successful therapists' learn to be 'amygdala whisperers' by activating networks of new learning in the hippocampus and prefrontal cortex to create a state of mind that enhances neuroplastic processes and increases the likelihood of positive change. The process of play is about active inhibition of the neural circuit that promotes fight/flight behaviours. Play functions as a neural exercise that improves the efficiency of the neural circuit that can instantaneously down-regulate fight/flight behaviours. Likewise, Porges' (2011) work on the 'Polyvagal theory' of emotion, identifies playfulness as a hybrid state of mobilization and the activation of the social engagement system, promoting 'a calmer physiological state, and the neuroception of safety', making the individual more open to interacting with others and less likely to go into a reactive state of fight–flight–freeze–faint.

Conclusion

It follows on that we should be mindful of the environments we create and provide for children to help or hinder their developmental capacity for neurobiological health, for ensuring that they develop healthy self-regulating neurophysiology that prepares them for their future intersubjective connectedness to the world and the people they encounter. Trevarthen (2012) describes this as a necessity as he recognises that children come into the world primed to socially relate:

> *If we are to protect young children, their bodies and their brains, from harm in the complex, busy and sometimes cruel world they come to live in, a world that has to satisfy artificial rituals and beliefs of an adult industrial and e-literate society, we will have to value more and give response to what children bring to human life, the eager spirit of their joyful projects beyond their seeking to survive as organisms, and especially what kind of company they expect from us, their parents, brothers and sisters, teachers and professional caregivers. It turns out a newborn infant person has clear expectations of human sense and is active in starting a personal quest for meaningful stories in good company.* (p.208).

In the next chapter, Paul Sullivan introduces us to the playful idea of the 'zone of playful proximal development'. Gregory, in *Reformulation* (2020), describes how creative exploration within CAT can introduce new relational ways of expanding one's zone of proximal development (ZPD) for both clients and therapists (Gregory, 2020) and, presaging much of the book's following chapters, Sullivan promotes the 'benefits of a playful exercise in the imagining of new metaphors of selfhood and mental health' (Sullivan, 2017, p37).

Chapter 3:
The zone of playful proximal development

Paul Sullivan

Introduction

In this chapter, I will interpret the zone of proximal development (ZPD) from the perspective of chronotope or time-space configuration. From here, I will explore the 'zone of playful proximal development' and contrast it with a zone of serious proximal development. At the heart of the playful, I suggest is the possibility of joint, spontaneous improvisation.

Improvisation is embedded in conversation, which is the form of interaction most typical of 'talking' therapies. Of course, there are socially acceptable scripts and mental schemas that are at our disposal when we know the destination we want the conversation to end up at, but the best conversations are ones to get lost in. A conversation that one is lost in is a non-transactional, non-instrumental conversation. A conversation that keeps on conversing after the other person has left. One that begets reflection and hope.

A disclaimer – I'm not a CAT therapist, but these kinds of conversations have been a regular feature for me at CAT conferences. For instance, I recall getting lost in conversation with Jason Hepple on Bakhtin and Michael Holquist's work and how principles of dialogue synergistically work with the CAT concept of the Reciprocal Role; Yvonne Stevens on existentialism, Laing and Winnicott, James and play; Carol Gregory on therapeutic creativity and Rob Lam on chronotopes, chronotypes (or time-space reconfigurations) in the therapeutic encounter, and Mikael Leiman on the concept of resurrection in the epiphanic. It is out of these fascinating conversations that the story I tell in this chapter involves a multi-voiced perspective on improvisation and the zone of playful proximal development as it may apply to CAT.

Zone of proximal development

Vygotsky's (1978) 'zone of proximal development', or ZPD, is best known as a model of learning in which, with the help of an expert, difficult tasks are pitched at a level slightly above the learner's current capability. If the task is too advanced, it becomes too frustrating and off-putting. If it is too easy, then boredom sets in. This ZPD is set in the wider framework of Vygotsky's discovery that development occurs first of all on a social, interpersonal level and subsequently on an intrapersonal, private level. We learn to speak to others first of all (egocentric speech) before subsequently to ourselves. We count first of all on our fingers before silently and privately. We 'internalize' the tools that we use socially.

Ryle (e.g. 2004) and Leiman (e.g. 2002) clearly articulate the relevance of Vygotsky's ZPD to Cognitive Analytic Therapy. Ryle draws attention to 'actual experience' as opposed to 'innate fantasy' in psychoanalysis in shaping early Reciprocal Roles between child and caregiver that are internalized. The therapist, Ryle (2004) suggests:

> 'Provides a corrective emotional relationship because the reformulation enables them to withstand the patients' seductions and assaults and avoid reinforcing the specific individual dysfunctional patterns that undermine everyday relationships. Both the person of the therapist as offering concerned accurate reflection and the conceptual tools created during reformulation can be internalised by the patient. The relationship evolves through the course of the therapy. After an initial cooperative and sometimes idealizing response, most patients will experience disappointment and will experience mixed or negative feelings reflecting past losses and hurts often accompanied by a return of their usual symptoms and behaviours. The acceptance and non-reciprocation of these, and support as previously avoided memories are accessed, is therapeutically powerful, offering a lived experience of new possibilities.' (p15)

There are two key internalizations – the person of the therapist and the conceptual tools of reformulation. In technical jargon, an ontology, or way of being, and an epistemology, or way of knowing, are fused in therapeutic encounter. But this internalization depends on the skill of both patient and therapist in navigating the zone of proximal development. Along the way, there could be frustration, regression of symptoms and ultimately a lived experience of new possibilities. This is clearly a fine art when neither party is quite certain of where the ZPD starts and ends – with the casualty being therapeutic encounter ending in failure.

While Ryle draws attention to the shared space of reflection and dialogue mediated by the reformulation tools of CAT, Leiman's (2002) concept of the epiphanic sign demonstrates another key aspect of internalization – which is the role of signs. As opposed to 'tools', signs are the meanings derived from actions or artefacts that are open to interpretation. For example, while a sweeping brush is a tool to sweep a floor, if left in a prominent position, it could be a sign that its someone else's turn to sweep the floor. Leiman makes the point that symptoms are meaning-laden 'signs' for interpretation – for both the patient and the therapist. Unlike Bateson (1972), Laing (1960) and Szasz (1960) who trailblazed this idea, Leiman draws attention to the socially grounded, interpersonal nature of signs. To get to this position, Leiman draws heavily on both Vygotsky and Bakhtin, via the work of John Shotter. Signs can resurrect past experiences and past selves. This aspect of the sign Leiman refers to as the 'epiphanic sign'. He gives the example of a client kicking leaves on an autumn day and connecting, via the leaves, to his past boyhood and living that boyhood. In this regard, signs from the past are participative in the present moment and are not just representational.

Epiphanic signs help make sense of phenomena such as 'transference' and 'countertransference'. The therapist is not just a therapist offering tools, but also potentially a 'sign' of another being, e.g. a lover or a parent. An epiphanic sign that resurrects this other or has echoes of the other. In this context, engaging effectively within the zone of proximal development is a challenge of reciprocal interpretation of epiphanic signs, with all their connotations, in a dialogical exchange. Internalization of the therapist's words is mediated by the voices of a network of others.

Another way of saying this in more technical terms is that 'signs' embody an axiological position. While 'ontology' means a way of being, and 'epistemology' a way of knowing, 'axiology' is a way of valuing and depends on a cultural and personal system of moral values. For example, a Nietzschean value system is structured around strategy, power and position; an Aristotelian value system is structured around community, character and friendship (MacIntyre, 1981). Signs, in a moral system, signal prohibition ('one ought not'), disappointment and guilt ('how could you?') and other moral injunctions that are embodied in the voices of others, resurrected in the therapeutic encounter. Internalization in the zone of proximal development entails finding a space for playing with the seriousness of axiology and re-evaluating habitual Reciprocal Roles in this space.

Differences between the public and private in the ZPD

Both Ryle and Leiman nicely draw attention to the relationship between the inter and intrapersonal as a boundary that is criss-crossed in a therapeutic and learning encounter, within the zone of proximal development. In this next section, however, I will sketch out some of the characteristics of the public and private world on either side of this boundary, with particular attention to values, or the axiological. This is inspired by Holquist's (2003) point that epistemology, ontology and axiology shape one another in dialogue. How we 'know' is coloured by our personal and cultural ethics and by who we are and who we are with.

The first key difference is that the public world is governed by rules of censorship while the private world has no censorship at all. At first, this may sound counter-intuitive considering the online world in particular. Censorship may seem antiquated in the public domain. People frequently freely express whatever it is they think, within and outside the rules of the law (such as incitement to hatred rules in the public domain) with apparently little regard for these rules of censorship. The kind of censorship I'm writing of here, however, is censorship calibrated to reputation rather than to a legal framework. In other words, epistemology (how we know) is refracted through 'ontology' or the kind of being we are or would like to be and the kinds of beings we want others to be. In this regard, a virulent misogynist needs to self-censor what they say in public, such as an appeal to gender equality, if it damages that reputation, while a liberal egalitarian will do the same in reverse.

In contrast, in the private world, reputation (as an aspect of ontology) is not a concern. A private thought cannot harm a public reputation. This is a key difference to classic psychoanalysis which sees the unconscious as the zone of censored thoughts in the private world, available only through dreams or free association or hypnosis. In a dialogical view, everything is available in consciousness. Experiences and thoughts may be pushed to the far edges of consciousness or lurk in the corners of consciousness but are 'triggered' or brought to the fore in different situations and offer a background 'context' for the text of what is thought and said.

William James (1890) makes the point that the 'stream of thought' operates quasi-independently of the self. Thoughts are born and perish in a continual succession. Without being tethered to reputation, the stream of thought is capable of presenting a very large range of ideas, desires, feelings, potential actions and unlikely fantasies, with little regard for any personal ethics. Indeed, some of these thoughts may be abhorrent or intrusive and distressing. The stream of thought is quasi-independent rather than fully independent from the self because, as we know from CAT, there are 'habits' of thinking tethered to new Reciprocal Roles. Habitual thought patterns lead to 'traps', 'dilemmas' and 'snags'.

The implications for working within a ZPD are that shifting Reciprocal Roles can open the self to new, more productive patterns of thinking, as a new ontology is created in therapy. For example, the creation of a secure Reciprocal Role facilitates a stream of secure thoughts. The tools available for this in CAT (such as reformulation) can be used for this. However, as I'll argue in the next section, the lack of censorship in the private world also allows a ZPD (zone of proximal playful development) space for improvisation in the task of building new Reciprocal Roles.

The second key difference between the public and private world is that the public world demands clear articulation of speech and an accountable, auditable link between the clarity of what is said and who is speaking. Incoherent speech is greeted with requests for clarity (as is incoherent writing, in the case of academic work). In the private world, speech is predicated or shortened (as Vygotsky discovered). Denotation of concepts is critically important in the public sphere but the connotation of concepts (the ripples of meaning into feeling) as grey and jumbled and incoherent is a characteristic of the private world. Clear denotation of signs within the private world is obscure and hidden even to self – just connotations, feelings and vagueness. With the help of others, the struggle to denote can be accomplished publicly, but may also fall apart.

In a therapy context, Warner's (1991; 1998) work on 'fragile processes' illustrates this quite well. Particularly vulnerable or traumatized patients may not be ready for even the gentlest of denotations as they struggle to articulate their feelings. This can lead to rage or detachment from the therapy process – as they struggle with confident ownership over their experience. Instead, simple empathetic mirroring of their experience to build trust is what the therapeutic encounter allows. As trust builds up, the boundary between the public and private world becomes more permeable (as any intimate relationship can testify). In terms of the ZPD, it is useful to know that fragile processes may mean that the work of reformulation is too advanced (a tool that is read as a sign of losing control, for instance) and more basic 'being with', empathy and mirroring is within the zone of proximal development). Hepple (2012) illustrates this beautifully in the context of group work and the metaphor of the 'witness and the judge' for victims of childhood abuse. Simply being there to witness private, secret stories and vindicate them (judge) as wrong is in itself therapeutic.

The third key difference (relevant here) is that the private world does not have temporal boundaries and is able to resurrect and imagine the presence of others (the epiphanic sign). As such, a mesalliance of different beings through different times can be put in dialogue with one another. While this can also happen in the public world (e.g. art worlds), temporal boundaries contain our interactions within specific times and places. These can still be replayed endlessly in private memory, or public interactions may be rehearsed privately in advance. These boundaries are permeable when, for example, a conversation evokes another conversation or when a therapist is read as a past parental figure.

This temporal difference means the worlds are also spatially quite distinct insofar as they can operate in contradiction to one another – as they do in hypocrisy, lies, irony and private mockery or in public despair at private thoughts. Divided worlds can also work in harmony. For instance, the CAT concept of the 'observing eye' enables recognition of harmful cycles and patterns in behaviour and the capacity to change them. The skill of private detachment in the observing eye is one that can be strengthened, like an arm muscle with exercise. Doing this therapeutically involves working through the zone of proximal development.

Conversely, in absorbing optimal flow experiences, the private and public worlds act in singularity. Mindfulness, meditation and relaxation exercises are typically considered as skills (tools) that can be used to create this experience of singularity. Again, this is a skill that can be practiced via the zone of proximal development. Table 3.1 below sums up some of these differences:

Chapter 3: The zone of playful proximal development

Table 3.1: Public and private worlds, and working on their boundaries through the ZPD

	Public	Private	Boundary	ZPD
Reputational censorship	Stage management of self and its reputation appropriate to its role.	Disreputable thoughts kept secret/censored from public view but available to consciousness.	The Freudian slip; free association; improvisation; 'triggers' that put disreputable secrets centre stage; sore-spots.	Creation of new roles that facilitate new habits of thinking without reputational censorship; changing dysfunctional but privately reputable roles to disreputable roles.
Articulation level	Clear for comprehension by others. Gricean maxims of communication.	Clear monologues but also unclear, ambiguous, 'half-thoughts' in the world of connotation, secret experiences, voices of others and triggering signs.	Intimate and trusting relationships where others are trusted to articulate what is meant based on intimate knowledge. Also vulnerable to bullying voices of others being internalized.	Creating trust and intimacy. Understanding and living with transference. Playing with connotations and 'being with' missteps.
Temporal boundaries	Public interactions in a defined place and time.	Temporally unbounded. Private fantasies, nostalgic memories, flashbacks, future anticipations, 'what ifs' acting in parallel with public interactions.	Private fantasies, paranoia, delusions can overwrite the moment to moment of an interaction.	Mindfulness and relaxation exercises to stay in the moment. The observing eye can be developed to recognize publicly harmful patterns

The zone of playful proximal development

While there are many different directions to go in with regard to the zone of proximal development and how it is embedded in CAT already (such as, for instance, the successes and failures of the ZPD, its link to psychoanalysis and cognition and negotiating the asymmetry of authority built into the ZPD), in this next section, I will focus on instead on the creativity and playfulness within the ZPD, as befits the theme of the book. In particular, I'm keen to add another adjective to the ZPD – 'playful' – the zone of playful proximal development. That is, development occurs via play. It is a zone between seriousness and official stories that are well rehearsed, and playfulness that is so irreverent to official ways of being that it is shocking and distressing to engage in it. Where the 'proximal' zone lies, in between these extremes, is what could be dubbed the 'zone of playful proximal development'.

In taking this direction, I'm inspired in particular by Bandlamudi's (2015) important work in which she dialogues with both Vygotsky and Bakhtin to draw attention to the role of the carnivalesque in providing a 'catalyst for development'. I quote: 'laughter reveals hidden truths, and some truths reveal themselves only to laughter' (p11).

It is these truths that begin to emerge in a 'zone of proximal playful development', particularly when they are uncomfortable, difficult truths. This playful zone can be contrasted with the zone of serious proximal development. Both are parts of the ZPD, on the boundary of intersubjectivity, between public and private worlds, but the 'playful' refers to the set of tools that aim to facilitate play, while the serious refers to tools that aim to directly progress therapeutic change (such as mapping Reciprocal Roles, reformulation, goodbye letters). These tools can work in tandem with one another or in dialogue with one another and indeed can have role reversals (playful activities can be done seriously and vice versa). Next, I focus on tools and games that facilitate play. At the end, I will briefly touch on playful and serious attitudes or approaches.

A very good example of the role of play in the ZPD comes from Winnicott's (1971) work: Playing and Reality. He describes the case of 'String', a seven-year-old boy who had a set of 'curious' symptoms such as a compulsion to lick things and people, to make compulsive throat noises, and, frighteningly, to threaten to cut people into pieces. Winnicott played a 'squiggle' game with the boy where he would impulsively draw a line and the boy would complete it:

> '*The squiggle game in this particular case led to a curious result. The boy's laziness immediately became evident, and also nearly everything I did was translated by him into something associated with string. Among his ten drawings there appeared the following:*
> *lasso*
> *whip*
> *crop*
> *a yo-yo string*
> *a string in a knot*
> *another crop*
> *another whip.*' (Winnicott, 1971, pp11-12)

Winnicott goes on to interpret the 'string' as a sign. In particular, a sign of the boy's desire to tether different objects and people together, for fear of losing them, which he was in the habit of doing. In the wider context of the boy's being separated from his mother while she was hospitalized for depression, this interpretation of the squiggle as a sign not of laziness but of separation anxiety seemed very insightful. Winnicott encouraged the boy's mother to discuss separations with him, which had a positive effect on him (but he did still have significant problems later in life).

Here, the game of impulsive line drawing was a tool that allowed the boy to discover epiphanic signs (the mother's separation) and to encourage him to reflect on it with his mother (in CAT, a reformulation map would be used). The boundary between the private world of difficult-to-articulate meanings and the public world of the game, where meanings can be read into signs, was skilfully navigated by Winnicott. The connotation was transformed to denotation, that could in turn help the boy to make sense of his own patterns. This is an example of proximal playful development using the social tool of the squiggle game to enhance the articulation level.

The next example I will give has more to do with using games as a tool that effaces the reputational barrier separating private and public worlds, rather than the articulation level. So, it's a non-therapy example. This will be Keith Johnston's seminal (1979) work *Impro: Improvisation and the Theatre*. Here, he describes the barriers to playful storytelling which include a focus on the 'right answer', on 'being original', on personality resistance – and how these barriers can be played around with and dissolved in joint games:

'If I ask someone to invent the first line of a short story ... he'll tense up and probably say "I can't think of one". He'll really act as if he's been asked for a good first line. Any first line is really as good as any other, but the student imagines that he's been asked to think up dozens of first lines, then imagine the type of stories they might give rise to, and then assess the stories to find the best one. This is why he looks appalled and mumbles "...oh...dor...urn...". Even if I ask some people for the first word of a short story they'll panic and claim that they "can't think of one", which is really amazing. The question baffles them because they can't see how to use it to display their "originality". A word like "the" or "once" isn't good enough for them. If I ask one student for the first word of a story and another for the second word, and another for the third word, and so on, then we could compose a story in this way... Anyone who tries to control the future of the story can only succeed in ruining it ... once you say whatever comes to mind, then it's as if the story is being told by some outside force.'

(Johnston, 1979, pp124-12)

Johnson (1979) perfectly describes the blocking role of reputational censorship in participating in a game. With the desire to be 'original', all different contenders for a word or a line to start a turn-taking story are discarded and the task becomes extraordinarily difficult and challenging. This is despite the fact that any first line is as good as any other. Instead, students feel they need to plan ahead and assess all the possible failed first lines before selecting the best first line.

To overcome this kind of censorship, Johnson sets out a number of theatre game techniques including verbalizing instantly without screening it; teaching people to recognize their first rejected choice and articulating it. For example, Johnston describes the encouragement to recognize and articulate the first thing that comes to mind, below, without worry:

'I ask a girl to say a word. She hesitates and says "Pig." "What was the first word you thought of?" "Pea." "Tell me a colour." Again, she hesitates. "Red." "What colour did you think of first?" "Pink." "Invent a name for a stone." "Ground." "What was the name you first thought of?" "Pebble." Normally the mind doesn't know that it's rejecting the first answers because they don't go into the long-term memory. If I didn't ask her immediately, she'd deny that she was substituting better words. "Why don't you tell me the first answers

that occur to you?" "They weren't significant." I suggest to her that she didn't say "Pea" because it suggested urination, that maybe she rejects pink because it reminds her of flesh. She agrees, and then says that she rejected "Pebble" because she didn't want to say three words beginning with "P". This girl isn't really slow, she doesn't need to hesitate. Teaching her to accept the first idea will make her seem far more inventive.' (Johnson 1979, pp 81-82).

Other techniques include teaching people to recognize when they are 'blocking' themselves or others in games, because, for instance, of high status and a desire to control (reputation), while other people do more 'accepting'. These Reciprocal Roles can be reversed through specific games that reverse these roles – e.g. one player blocks (the blocker), another accepts, but also through reflection. For Johnson, 'blocking' can be quite an aggressive action that destroys improvisation while accepting all offers (all possibilities) can lead to imaginative scenes in improvisation.

In a therapy context, it may occasionally seem that efforts to progress and make suggestions are in a Reciprocal Role dynamic of blocking. It may be a Reciprocal Role procedure that impacts different situations for the client. Discovering the pattern could be a good indication of where the boundaries are in a particular zone of proximal development. Drawing attention to the role (as a disreputable role that damages self-self and self-other interactions) as a means of recognizing it with the 'observing eye' may be possible unless fragile processes prevail. Moving out of this Reciprocal Role may take work and play with spontaneity and improvisation, but is important to allow new Reciprocal Roles, and concomitant patterns of thinking, to develop.

Finally, the third example refers to the temporal-spatial boundaries and the differences between bounded and unbounded temporality in public and private spaces. For this, I will draw on some of the work outlined by Stevens and Petratou (2024) on creativity in CAT. In this work, Stevens and Petratou outline the variety of resources, tools and signs that enable clients to move from a state of being unable to play to being able to play – to tolerate ambiguity and uncertainty, imaginatively experiment and re-tell stories. Intonation, props, music, art and self-authoring with the aid of books and diaries (e.g. Lessing's *The Golden Notebooks*) are outlined as ways in which fragmented self-states can be slowly integrated and how destructive Reciprocal Roles can be reorganized.

All of these examples demonstrate the skill of the therapists in overcoming the hardened boundaries between the client's public and private worlds to create more permeable boundaries by playing with connotations and facilitating intimacy beyond the stage management of reputation. What I will briefly dwell on, however, are some of the temporal breakthroughs (e.g. living in the moment; saturating the present with the past) and spatial breakthroughs (from public to private and vice versa). The first is the doubling up of the private and public via mirroring. Petratou's example of choreography is remarkably innovative:

> 'For example, with one client I encouraged her to improvise a movement to express her anxious, shamed self-state followed by another movement to represent a freeing release from this shame. She embodied this by shrinking her shoulders inwards, hunching them up and down and vocalising a harsh sound, followed by throwing open her arms, releasing her chest and accompanying this with a long, soothing outbreath. I mirrored her movements, backwards and forwards, and we created a choreography together.'

Improvisation from the client was mirrored by Petratou. This allows the client to see her own movements publicly expressed but overlain by Petratou's enactment. It is both an immersive bodily experience and an out-of-body experience (experiencing a reflection through another, facilitating reflection). There is, in the movement, an invitation to blur the boundaries of self and other, private and public. Petratou comments that this movement facilitated a co-regulation of difficult, split-off aspects of the self (anxiety and fear). Co-regulation across the private-public threshold in a fused present moment. Metaphorically speaking, Petratou demonstrates how to go 'swimming with chronotopes' (Potter, 2020) (chronotopes meaning time, space configurations) within the boundaries of a ZPD.

Secondly, Coombes (2022) makes the point that 'Trainees can learn how encouraging a client to bring an object from childhood to a therapy session could lead to a reparative dialogue with a wounded inner child state.' (See Chapter 8, this volume.)

In this activity, the past is brought to the present and re-accentuated in the present. Re-accentuation is when deeply held connotations are given new connotations or literally intoned by the accent of someone else. It's used politically, for instance when the pejorative word 'queer' is used as a marker of celebration – e.g. 'queer eye for the straight guy'. Or interpersonally when words of others are re-accentuated lovingly or perhaps sarcastically given 'air quotes'. In Coombes' suggested activity, an object from the past could be re-accentuated in the present. This activity allows the co-existence of past and present and has the potential to facilitate a re-accentuation of the object and the experiences that the object connotates.

It is fascinating to read the case stories of how creativity is very usefully embedded in CAT. This openness allows a play of time and private-public space and re-accentuation/re-integration that is not so evident in other approaches. Traditional CBT, for instance, appears to reverse engineer a desired future state to a present dysfunctional state; psychoanalysis seems to pick up the fantasies and fantastical pieces from the past, and humanistic therapy can dwell on the optimism for future potential. CAT, in contrast, allows a constant play of time and space in play, boundaries and thresholds in a participative dialogue. That is, at least, my reflective view from the outside.

Discussion

At the heart of Bakhtin's (e.g. 1981) concept of dialogue is the concept of 'becoming'. This suggests that we have the potential to 'become' something extra, different from a lifetime of the same old stories. What is less evident in Bakhtin's version of 'becoming' is the help we need along the way. How do we improvise a different story to fulfil our potential to 'become'? In this chapter, I have concentrated on Vygotsky's ZPD and the differences between the chronotope (or time-space value) of the private and the public worlds.

Skilful attunement to this zone shows that it is possible to be creative in games and to improvise new stories and reaccentuate old ones, even though it seems completely impossible at the outset. I lingered over different types of play in the previous section – as tools that allow a spatial-temporal crossing of the private and public world. All tools, however, can also be read as signs. These readings may be hostile or sympathetic and curious. Games may be rejected (by both therapist and client) and read as too frivolous and, conversely, conversations as too serious. Each zone of proximal playful development is particular to the person.

Coombes (2024) has outlined a number of suggestions that nicely show how the dance between the serious and the playful can be integrated into therapy. This includes between-session creative and imaginative homework, giving trainees the opportunities to become comfortable with spontaneity, embodiment, projection and role-play techniques and dialogue between self-states.

In terms of playfully mapping how these techniques make sense, I will finish with a final diagrammatic flourish to attempt to pinpoint the zone of playful proximal development. I appreciate that it's unusual to present new information in a discussion, but the intention is a diagrammatic re-accentuation of the key ideas above to help clarify them.

Figure 3.1: Mapping the zone of playful proximal development

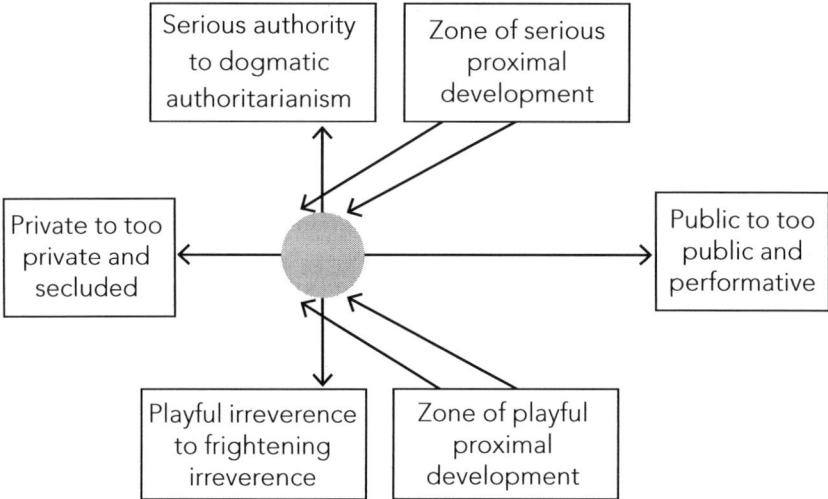

The circle above represents the zone of proximal development, while the areas outside this represent experiences that are both easily familiar and too challenging and self-destructive.

Let us start with the vertical hierarchy from frightening irreverence to dogmatic authoritarianism (and vice versa). The stream of thought can present us with intrusive, disturbing thoughts irreverent of our personal values and reputation. This can be private (would not confess to anyone) or public (e.g. inappropriate compulsions to shock). While these experiences can become open to some serious reflection in a therapeutic context, or with others, serious reflection can evolve into dogmatic authoritarianism, such as for instance an insistence on a particular interpretation or deep blocking of alternative ideas. Dogmatic authoritarianism in turn is vulnerable to parody, irony and irreverence.

On the more horizontal continuum between public and private worlds, they can be distanced from one another. This is what Laing (1960) refers to as the 'divided self', where public actions are performed robotically and the private world is too isolated to communicate with – although it can be, with great care, as Warner's work (1991; 1998) on fragile processes demonstrates.

The zone of proximal development is an intersubjective zone on the boundary between self and other/public and private. In this area, there is space for the internalization of new, productive tools, either through serious reflection, gentle authority of interpretation and serious activities, or through games and play and creative new expressions where the main objective is not success or failure, but instead is play, and the development of attitudes of play and seriousness that accompany these activities.

Above, I have labelled these as the zone of proximal playful development and the zone of proximal serious development. These labels, however, are just heuristics to help disentangle different Reciprocal Roles. In lived experience, activities become quite jumbled up with gestalt shifts as befits the dance between self-and-self and self-and-others. Improvising steps, being led and leading the dance, is probably a better metaphor for working well in the zone of proximal development.

Acknowledgements

Thanks to Yvonne Stevens, Lakshmi Bandlamudi and Min Yong for their reading, constructive help and suggestions of earlier drafts. Thanks also to Ken Russell for educating me in the art of improvisation and drawing attention to Johnson's work.

PART 2: Creative psychotherapy in practice

Reflections on a 16-session CAT therapy with a clinical psychology and CAT trainee

'Summarising' by Lynn

I find this very difficult … so much unravelling, contemplating, piecing together and attempting to assimilate into everyday life … with a fresh approach.

How DO I summarise 16 meetings?

What did we talk about?

A lifetime's relationship with cancer

Partly buried in the back of my mind … it took my Mother, will it come for me?

Then finding that I have to live with diagnosis, surgery, treatment, recovery

I really can't hide

Keep going alongside cancer, as I always did… somehow … it's OK … I'll get through it

I do

Knocked flat by my young son's long, drawn-out diagnosis … at only 22

We will get through it together… keep going

We do

BRCA1 discovery. I have to live with that too … what is it all about? Is it to be frightened of?

A small lull … dare I relax a bit?

No way… cancer is back with a deeply painful whack. My son in relapse

We will get through it together

Somehow we do

And All of the above occurred before I am about to get another diagnosis of cancer…

Proceed to minor operations to remove ALL my reproductive organs-a precautionary measure
Then, most recently, a secondary cancer... surgery, recovery, radiotherapy, recovery

Recovery? Yes... hopefully in remission forever
Will cancer kill me... end of lifetime
Recovery? Actually NO
Whatever, I have to carry on living with it

Then I am gifted the time to be heard and share my life's story
THIS is what we talked about.
I had been struggling with very low mood
I was debilitated by this.

I find it extremely hard to summarise or quantify the time I have spent with Ronja
I know that it has been absolutely invaluable
A revelation
A warm, comforting cardigan to wear when I need to

Ronja's reflection of the therapeutic journey that we undertook shines a bright light on how much we were able to form a kind of web of all the areas of my life, of my being
The web acts like a safety net that I can trust
And I am able to place into this web the new found respect I have for myself

The phrase 'honest compassionate communication' relating to myself has been life affirming
Thanking my body for faring so well throughout this cancer story...
Recognising the joy in my life, that I am still here to relish in it

Gratitude for the many weeks experience of CAT
I've been planting the CAT seedlings, nourishing them so that they take root in the soil of my life
If I can Mother these, then I can Mother myself
Such a great revelation at 69 years old

Printed with permission

Chapter 4:
Working with objects as a key to unlocking complex trauma

Suzanne Lyons

> *'There is no doubt that creativity is the most important human resource of all. Without creativity, there would be no progress, and we would be forever repeating the same patterns.'* – Edward de Bono

Introduction

In therapy, clients not only want to understand their difficulties and the patterns which maintain them, but by the end they want to feel differently about themselves and others. This is particularly the case for those with complex trauma. As Levine (2019) said:

> '…those roots are within the body, usually as fear and helplessness. Until that changes you can alter some of the thoughts but you're still fundamentally traumatised.'

This is perhaps why some clients will say, towards the end of a therapy, that they have gained insight, are thinking differently, and are using their exits beneficially, but they do not feel much different. It may be due to an underlying implicit embodied trauma that has not been tackled in therapy or has thwarted their potential progress.

Working with embodied creativity can enable us to engage an individual's dissociated, disowned, and implicit bodily held trauma from the outset, by recruiting both the therapist's and client's creativity and agency, and so enhancing the experience of the therapy.

This may be particularly beneficial for clients who have become emotionally cut off due to traumatic experiences. Words can sometimes get in the way, particularly for those clients who have repeated their story so many times that their words have become 'scripts' which they have learned to disconnect from, or who have actively avoided traumatic memories. By working creatively and engaging with implicit bodily held memories, it is as if we are going *under the radar* of their verbal scrutiny and well-practiced defences. Also, we may be more likely to bypass the inhibitory effect of shame which might otherwise cause clients to filter what they think and say to their therapists.

This chapter aims to provide practical suggestions, with some theoretical underpinnings, about how we can work relationally with that associated embodied trauma by using objects creatively and therapeutically, and how this can enhance both the therapeutic relationship and the traditional CAT tools. It includes an exploration of CAT theory in conjunction with an understanding of developmental trauma, and the importance of acquiring non-verbal therapeutic skills to help draw out implicit embodied trauma and memories, which by their nature are hard to access verbally.

Although the focus here is specifically on using objects therapeutically, this can be combined with other creative approaches within CAT. It has been said that the genius of CAT is that it is not just an integrated model but also an integrating one, where a rich tradition of creative approaches is welcomed and benefited from within the ACAT community.

My understanding and exploration of being creative in CAT developed through attending ACAT conference workshops and being inspired and encouraged to be more creative. Petratou (2019) and Wilde McCormick (2012) have also written informatively about the use of objects in CAT therapy. This chapter reflects my experiences through trying out some of these ideas in therapies I have provided, or have supervised, with thanks to the supervisees for their enthusiastic and generous sharing of their experiences and examples. In order to preserve confidentially for clients, their names and details have been changed.

The last few decades have seen new developments in the trauma literature and the work of Interpersonal Neurobiologists (IPNB), e.g. Siegel (2012; 2020) among others, and the importance of attending to and working with the physical embodiment of trauma in therapy. Eye Movement Desensitization Reprocessing (EMDR) has also elucidated the significance of this in recovery from trauma. ACAT CPD events have mirrored these developments in the therapy world through integration with CAT, Bristow (2006), Dower (2014),

Darongkamas *et al* (2016), Jenaway (2016), and Sheard (2017). These events have highlighted an awareness of the extent to which the effects of trauma are often implicitly held, often in disowned parts of the self; this sense of dissociated parts also fits with the CAT theory of multiple states.

The multiple states model, and using objects to work with 'parts'

Working therapeutically with small objects connects with the concept of the 'parts' of a fragmented self. Within CAT theory, Ryle (1997) writes about an understanding of working with fragmented parts, or multiple self-states (MSS) with the aim of moving towards an integration, and describes the importance of

> *'naming each state: Differentiating between the different states. Describing feelings, images, words associated with all states, including those largely dissociated. Beginning to recognise states. Linking states and relating to key figures and symptoms. All seem to be connected, not just chaos.'*

(See Appendix 2)

Psychotherapist Jean Knox (2011), writing about agency in psychotherapy and the neurobiology of self, engages with Bakhtin's (1973) ideas on dialogic selves, which CAT theory draws upon. She refers to Hermans' *et al* (1993) notion that 'each "me" has a speaking voice to represent its point of view vis-à-vis other characters and their voices in the polyphonic or dialogical self', and quotes Barresi (2002), who refers to Bakhtin's theory of how the 'self as constituted out of a "multitude of voice" each with its own quasi-independent perspective, in a dialogical relationship with each other.' Barresi quotes the idea of Hermans *et al* that 'Once embodied, there is a "voice", which creates utterances that can be meaningfully related to the utterances of another voice. It is only when an idea or thought is endowed with a voice and expressed as emanating from a personal position in relation to others that dialogical relations emerge.'

Connecting with these 'dialogical relations' is one of the aims of working creatively with a client and their chosen objects, which become imbued with aspects of themselves and significant others, where, for the client, each voice can be easily imagined. When these are laid out in front of a client, they can see the landscape and positioning of their parts, which can become interactive and dialogic, along a timeline if required. This invites the possibility of the 'observing eye' to find new perspectives and experiment with different positioning of themselves to their narrative, and working with their resources, including, if possible, their nurturing 'parts' for a healthier more integrated self.

Georgaca (2001), in this view of the self, envisaged it as a 'constellation of dialogically structured positions, each with their own world view and voice in relations of intersubjective exchange and dominance. The "I" moves between positions in an emotional landscape, depending on time, place, and situation, resulting in a multi-voiced self.'

The selected objects provide a bridge and a containing placeholder for a client's embodied emotions or states, and memories, enabling the client so they can then become the master of their own story. This can be worked on over different time periods and events within the client's life, with them having the power to physically move and orchestrate the characters of their story, creating dialogue and experimenting with previously forbidden emotions possibly such as anger.

Fragmentation through trauma, development of self-states, projective identification and dissociated selves as snags

When we invite clients to work therapeutically in this way, we are drawing on an ancient human ability to project their emotions into objects. Archaeological findings of talismans, for example, tell us that humans have been projecting powerful feelings into objects for millennia. These may include religious or magical powers intended to protect, heal, or harm individuals, or, as in childhood, transitional objects like teddy bears. When an object becomes imbued with a client's emotions, it can become immensely powerful. This can be particularly salient when helping clients process core pain. Marion Solomon, in her chapter on working with nesting dolls, from *Play & Creativity in Psychotherapy* (2017) describes how:

> '...our younger selves live deeply within our core. As adults, we may not be comfortable with this concept, or we may not understand the implicit parts of our history that affect our current experience of self and other. Shame and other feelings are mitigated through the use of the nesting dolls.'

Melanie Klein's work (1955) using creativity and small objects with children in psychotherapy, assisted in the development the theory of Object-relations, which underpins Ryle's (1991) creation of RRs within CAT. Using the theoretical concept of Reciprocal Role procedures (RRPs), we understand how a child will often survive difficult and unbearable emotional and/or physical trauma through developing, often unconsciously, strategies to manage emotional pain. This may be through cutting off from their distress, sometimes to the point of creating an internal structural dissociation, leading to disowned and dissociated states which make it difficult for them to understand themselves or relate to others. Ryle (1997) described his three-level CAT theory of the detrimental effects of complex trauma, leading to (1) restricted repertoire or distortion of the development of RRs, (2) disruption to connecting sequences leading to dissociation, and (3) limited capacity for self-reflection.

Responses to trauma are also dominated by the key survival elements of fight, flight, escape, freeze, submit, rescue/protect (of significant others) and attachment, with each self-state having a different embodied quality in some way linked to the trauma. The neuroscientist Panksepp (2012) has expanded this to 'Seven Primary Process, Emotions Action Systems', or (PAGS).

Clients who have experienced an overwhelming trauma, extreme shame, or terror of abandonment or abuse, often avoid being exposed to their feared memories, disowned emotions, or states. Fear of loss can sometimes also block therapeutic progress and can be a hidden snag, which has been a long-term survival strategy to *protect* the self from being overwhelmed or from experiencing its most dreaded feelings.

Working with objects can help identify a client's snags and allow for dialogue between feared states and the other objects; these may be disowned or dissociated parts of the self which carry pain, trauma, shame, hurt of feeling unloved, or acute fears. Asking clients to choose objects for these avoided parts also helps to make them more distinct, concrete and tangible for the client.

The work of Klein around 'splitting and projection' in Object Relations Theory has also been useful, for example, in helping clients to understand why they have wanted to keep caregivers as internalized 'Good Objects' and so have been left containing and holding the internalized 'Bad' themselves. In this case, we are often working therapeutically with physical objects to help the client unpick their processes around the fear of the loss of the 'Good object'.

Understanding implicit and explicit trauma memories, and embodied trauma states

In all therapies, we are frequently working with the effects of trauma, whether chronic 'low level', such as continual parental criticism of a child, or bullying, or more obvious events such as rape or physical assault. Siegel (2012) describes how traumatic experiences are often stored implicitly, creating difficulties in accessing and working on these therapeutically by verbal means alone:

> '**Explicit Memory:** *is coupled with an internal sensation of remembering. There are two forms: semantic (factual) and episodic (with repeated episodes being called autobiographical). The encoding or deposition of explicit memory requires focal, conscious attention. Without focal attention, or with the excessive release of the stress hormone cortisol, items are not encoded explicitly but are encoded implicitly.*'

> '**Implicit Memory:** *Involves parts of the brain that do not require conscious, focal attention during encoding or retrieval. Perceptions, emotions, bodily sensations, and behavioural response patterns are all examples of implicit layers of processing. Implicit memory in its non-integrated form lacks a sense that something is being recalled from the past.*'

> '**Implicit Knowing:** *The sense of an experience in the present or past within memory that is 'known' without words but is within conscious experience. Implicit is not the same as non-conscious but rather has the sense of an innate, preverbal knowing that is timeless in that it lacks a sense of the origins from which the knowing has arisen. Implicit knowing lacks an ecphoric sensation (e.g., smell, sight, sound) and can be a part of the retrieval of implicit memory, or it can be an ongoing meaning-making process in the present.*'

Where an experience is too traumatic, the memory will be held implicitly, more bodily than verbally. However, these implicit neural associations influence our feelings, thoughts, decision making and behavioural reactions, often without our knowing the origins of these from past experience. Part of the work of therapy is identifying and assisting the integration of these implicit memories into explicit and autobiographical memory, but this first requires accessing the implicit memories. For further explanation of these memory processes, see Siegel (2012), who describes how the right hemisphere dominates in early development towards holistic integration, through non-verbal reactions, visuospatial imagery, metaphoric meaning, context sensing, stress-response mediation, autobiographical memory and reflection, and an integrated map of the whole body. In contrast, the left hemisphere, which develops later, specializes in linear, linguistic, logical ways of being, and in cause-effect relationship seeking, and is more literal.

From this, one can infer that, within CAT, it is essential to recruit the body and the mind in an embodied way. Focusing predominantly on verbal and written forms of working alone, is unlikely to connect with potentially crucial implicitly held reactions which may be maintaining a client's RRPs, unless the bodily held trauma is made explicit through other processes. Sheard (2017), writing in *Reformulation*, talks extensively about the need within CAT for embodied working, saying that an embodied approach 'appears to "knit in" very well with CAT as well as challenging an implicit mind-body dualism and power relationship in both the theory and practice of CAT'.

In taking a more creative and embodied approach in our therapies, we aim to connect with and encourage the co-creativity of our clients and their self-agency, which can assist in addressing these power-dynamic issues and so also enable us to have greater awareness of our own and our client's embodied reactions. As many clients have felt powerless in their lives, there is something empowering for them in selecting an object to represent something feared or overwhelming, and then deciding where it will be placed in relation to other objects, or determining what will happen to it, and having power over the group or map of objects. This can lead to state shifts and insights through exploration and dialogic work between the objects which will inevitably reflect parts of the self.

Locked in patterns and unlocking through movement

Like other creative ways of working, we can quite rapidly tap into embodied traumas, and so it is helpful to have a plan of how to work with this for the client's maximum benefit, and so a better understanding of the neurobiology of processing trauma can be advantageous for the therapist.

Levine's (2012) work has facilitated an understanding of how having some physical control over something can assist in 'resolving' a trauma, he explains how the traumatized person needs to complete something physically in order to be released from the embodied trauma. He describes how trauma is 'locked' in the body, and it is in the body that it must be 'accessed and healed'. He argues that trauma is:

> 'fundamentally a highly activated, incomplete, biological response to threat, frozen in time.'

Individuals remain physiologically frozen in an 'unfinished' state of high biological readiness to react to the traumatic event, even long after it has passed, and that:

> 'self-protective and defence responses that were incomplete at the time of the incident (and lie dormant as potential energy) are frequently liberated through micro-movements, these are almost imperceptible and sometimes referred to as "pre-movements".'

Likewise, van der Kolk (2007) writes:

> 'Prone to action and deficient in words, these patients can often express their internal states more accurately in physical movements or pictures than in words. Utilising drawing and psychodrama may help them develop a language that is essential for effective communication and for the symbolic transformation that can occur in psychotherapy.'

Panksepp (2012) viewed emotion as intricately woven into the basic motivational drives that have evolved in mammals over millions of years. He has mapped seven different Primary Process, Emotions Action Systems or (PAGS), including Care, Seek, Lost, Play, Fear, Rage, Grief/Panic, finding that each of these has their own neurotransmitters and attendant motor activity. He states that:

> 'The primary-process emotions are all connected to movements, and the evidence now indicates that raw emotional feelings arise from the same ancient brain networks that control our instinctual emotional life... the facts indicate that these raw emotional feelings arise from the emotional action networks of the brain.'

These findings suggest that, when working on trauma with clients, it can be helpful to 'tune in' a client to any potential physical movement they may feel their body wishes to make; we can then help them find small, safe ways that they can respond to impulse or urge, e.g. for Flight it might be just moving their feet, getting up and walking around the room; if they feel frozen it might be to wiggle their toes; or if they feel the need to fight, throwing a cushion across the room or moving their hands or arms may help. It is surprising how, by asking the client 'What would your body like to do now?', they may instinctively know how to move to start releasing the trauma. Pat Ogden's work Trauma and the Body (2006; 2018) is also a useful resource for understanding more about a sensorimotor approach.

Clinical examples

Ann, a CAT therapist, described how, if a client chooses an object to represent a critical, overbearing, or overwhelming parent, she offers them a glass and invites them to cover the object to 'silence' them. Having done this, Ann will then encourage the client to 'observe' their internalized 'voice' with curiosity from a place of emotional safety, rather than overwhelm, 'Look, she's doing that thing again...', something her clients have expressed that they find revelational when next confronted with their overbearing parent. When in the therapy room, Ann described the power for the client in just lifting the glass momentarily and the sudden 'noise' in the therapy room bringing a realization of the enormity of their own experience. Ann said that she has often sensed the embodied transference from her clients from the relief of shutting out the projected voice of the parent, and the respite this brings them. Sometimes, the object and the glass have been moved by the client to the corner of the therapy room until the client has grown in self-confidence and is more able to respond to the critical voice, when the object may be brought nearer.

Ann also brought her experience of a client to supervision, whom she helped by providing a physical action in therapy to overcome her trauma. Janet, who was in her early 60s, had since childhood suffered severe abuse from her family, particularly from her father who was still abusive in his 90s. As a child, Janet's father wouldn't let her out of her bedroom; she even had to ask permission to go to the bathroom. She was often hungry, and he would put an apple outside her door to taunt her, as she was not allowed out and was forbidden from going to the kitchen. At the beginning of therapy, it was as if she was still locked in an embodied and paralysing fear of leaving her home. After discussing this in the session, Ann recreated and tuned Janet into this childhood scene, and using a ribbon to denote the bedroom boundary, together, hand in hand, they crossed over it to where the 'forbidden' apple lay waiting, where she could now freely eat it. Ann felt this seemingly simple joint activity had been a transformational moment in the therapy partly because in that moment Janet *had an ally and was not alone*. By the end of the therapy, Janet was going out and had even joined an evening class.

Another powerful example was Diana (forty-five years old), a client who used her creativity and movement to escape her embodied trauma, which had included feeling frozen during periods of extreme abuse. She was referred for CAT having experienced domestic violence (RR: Abusing – Abused), and after surviving a childhood where the rule was that 'emotions should not be expressed' (RRP: Dismissing, Suffocating, Cutting Off – Cut Off, Dismissed, Suffocated). During the therapy, Diana was given the opportunity to sculpt in a local stone quarry. Here, she explained to me that every time she hit the stone, she was letting out a bit more of her anger relating to her ex-partner who had tried to strangle her (this physical action of 'hitting the stone' can also be seen as a completion of the frozen trauma, previously trapped within in her body, as described by Levine above). This cathartic experience also harnessed her creativity as she sculpted a beautiful swimming fish, which became a sign between us, representing her reclaimed sense of self as the therapy came to an end.

Connection through transference

For the therapist, working with objects can become a vehicle or bridge for gaining a greater sense of a client, as they reveal more of themselves through their choices and explanations, but also through a more tangible sense of embodied transference and countertransference. This can happen when a client, in choosing an object, is connecting with their own implicit embodied resonation which can be sensed by the therapist as bodily felt transference and may intensify as the significance of the object is explored in more depth.

Within CAT, one way of accessing this felt sense of self is through the use of shared or co-created metaphor (see Turner, Chapter 7, this volume), and an object is essentially a physical metaphor, which is often central to CAT therapies and reformulation letters. In her book, Wilde McCormick (2012) describes:

'Working with images can help to create a safe and useful bridge between hidden memory with its often-overwhelming emotion, and consciousness. When the images are drawn, embodied, shaped, or experienced through objects, they become the mediators of a greater awareness. Someone who has never felt embodied and drawn themselves in outer space without a body can experiment slowly with starting the journey back into their body.'

How to be creative therapeutically with objects

In working with objects, the aim is to engage a client in this *playful* way, with each object holding a different position; to rediscover their silenced or buried voices, re-tell their story and identify parts of themselves and to develop conversations and voices between these parts of 'multiple intertwined narratives', working with spontaneous creativity to bring the experience to life and add ownership, allowing for different perspectives to be seen and leading to shifts in understanding.

From experience, using objects in therapy can be unexpectedly powerful, and so it is wise to establish grounding and stabilization techniques with clients beforehand.

Creating a collection of objects for use in therapy

It is possible to buy a 'job lot' of preowned toys or objects online, or charity shops are a good source. It is not advisable to use objects that have been owned by your own family members, particularly if they have strong memories for you, e.g. a much-loved object from a significant other's childhood.

The objects do not have to be a clear representation of something: the most used in my collection is a pair of black and white salt and pepper pots that are abstract figures and link in an embrace but are often used separately. An object can be as simple as a scarf: a black one has often been chosen to represent a difficult RR with parents. Objects are frequently chosen by clients to represent Reciprocal Roles, self-states, significant others, an ally, a nurturing figure, emotions or procedures.

The objects need to be contained in a box/boxes, a large bag or a small suitcase, the latter being useful if they need to be portable. I have found it helpful to keep similar objects in clear bags or nets, e.g., farm animals, and to have a bag to hold each client's objects as this speeds up the process since you do not have to hunt through to rediscover their chosen objects at the following session.

Suggestions for what to have in your box include:

- Animals, farm and jungle, insects.
- Soft toys: those from Winnie the Pooh (archetypical characters) are often popular.
- Iconic figures, e.g., Superman, Incredible Hulk, Action Man, Barbie, Pinocchio, a witch, a princess, a monster, a dragon, a knight, a soldier.
- Nesting dolls: gender-neutral ones such as those decorated with animals may be the best option.
- Faceless figures such as an artist's wooden mannequin, which can be bent into different poses (a faceless female jewellery stand is often chosen to depict a dismissive or neglecting mother).
- Weeping Buddha, often carved in wood.
- Stones and/or buttons.
- Scarves (in different colours).
- Ribbons/wool (when used creatively, amongst other purposes, these can be used as connecting lines, or denoting different time periods, like a timeline).
- Modelling dough, coloured pens and sticky notes: for recording dialogues between objects.
- Large pieces of neutral-coloured paper: it is useful to place objects on these so that they can capture further information including arrows, procedures and dialogue between objects or states, or as a surface on which to adhere sticky notes.

Using the client's own objects

If a client does not feel that your collection has the 'right' object for something, you can invite them to draw it, make it, or find one to bring in; this process itself can be insightful and revealing homework. You could also agree that an alternative object can be used as a placeholder until the 'right' one is found. Sometimes, a client may bring in a treasured item, e.g., one that represents a lost grandparent, or how they felt in relation to that significant other. Marks-Tarlow (2012) describes working with figurines a client brings to her session to help her process her childhood sexual abuse. For online therapies, the client can be asked to select their own objects, which is revealing in itself.

How to ask a client to select an object

The golden rule is never to suggest that a client might like to use a certain object to represent anything. When we are inviting a client to select an object by exploring our collection, we want to engage their creative, implicit embodied mind, not their semantic mind; we are not encouraging them to look for an obvious literal representation. We suggest that they do this without thinking about it too intently: they are searching for something which resonates with their felt sense of a characteristic of a person or a feeling. Most clients seem to be able to do this without too much difficulty, and some talk about an object 'calling to them'. Others may be resistant to connecting with their felt sense, a snag worth discussing in the session, and it may be that a 'Protector' part is asserting itself.

Occasionally, clients will pick one out and indicate that 'this' is of significance but not what they are currently looking for. If so, put it to one side and return to it later, as it often then reveals the role it has to play. Also, let the client know that they are free to change any object at any time if it does not feel right. They may also select more than one object for an individual. Objects can change over the client's timeline or during the course of therapy, reflecting therapeutic shifts.

Once they have selected an object, do not in any way attempt to interpret or make a judgement about what they have chosen, but just be curious, asking what it was about the object that drew them to it, why it feels right and how they feel in relation to it. Clients often express surprise at what they have chosen, and if we pay close attention, what they say about this is often informative. At the end of the session, ask your client to return the items to a separate bag or the container that holds the collection. These little objects are 'containing' very powerful emotions, so it is important that the client does this for themselves and closes the lid or fastens the bag. Try to ensure that the same objects will be available for the next session.

Recording the co-created relational groupings or maps

It is helpful for both the therapist, with the client's permission, and the client, to take photographs of the groupings of objects or maps. Many clients have camera phones, and these images can be used in a variety of ways between sessions. For the therapist, it is advisable to make a note of what each object represents for the client, and any embodied sensations or related emotions. At the next session, you may also be alerted to problems, if, for example, a client has no memory of this shared activity or what the objects represented, potentially indicating dissociation.

Enhancing the tools of CAT

What can objects represent?

In a session, the possibilities of what objects can be used for are limitless, but through a CAT-therapy lens, objects can be used to create or represent a family tree, or a CAT map; an individual object can signify one part of a Reciprocal Role, a specific person, a state, including disowned states, an emotion, a procedure, a snag, trap or dilemma, an illness, an abuser, an ally or nurturing figure, self-states, a trauma, an event, a place, a trigger, a client's resourceful parts or a healthy place, and positive feelings such as hope.

In this way, these can serve as a portable and interactive CAT map and can aid each of the three CAT stages of *Reformulation*, *Recognition* and *Revision*, through representing *procedures*, or a hoped-for or an actual exit, or through dialogue between these *embodied states* leading to better integration of self. These objects sometimes become transition objects between therapist and client.

Placement of objects

It can be insightful to watch how clients place their objects and to ask them how they feel about moving objects closer or further away from each other. It is respectful of the power dynamics to check out with the client whether it is alright with them for you to rearrange their objects if you feel it would be helpful in creating a CAT map or looking at a procedure around a state.

Creating a family tree with objects

Inviting clients to actively engage in creating their own family tree can tell us considerably more than just names and words. A simple way to start is to ask the client to draw their family, suggesting that matchstick figures are fine. The placement and size of the figures or pictures associated with them can lead to shared insights for the therapist and client alike. The addition of significant others, such as family friends, foster parents, teachers, past partners, etc, can also be helpful.

The client's selection of objects to represent themselves is significant in this process: it often works best to also have objects representing their vulnerable little child, teenage, functioning, and/or parental (if applicable) selves.

In relation to these self-objects, others can be selected for key people and elements to create the client's CAT map, this often gives an embodied sense of pertinent RRs. It may be that two or more objects are required to denote a person or their characteristics. For example, a client may say 'This object represents my son, but they can also be like this', while selecting another object.

Creating a Reciprocal Role map

The therapist can now move on to asking how their client felt in relation to each of their family members at different stages in their life and ask them to select other objects which resonate with those feelings, and delving down into the embodied sense of those feelings as they select each object, such as *how and where they feel it?* In doing so, an RR map is created, often with the addition of emotions, including the physically held quality of this: e.g. a volcano, or an Incredible Hulk figure may represent rage. As the therapy develops, objects can be selected and added for RRPs snags and parts that seem to be disowned, e.g. anger. As exits are developed, objects for these can also be added. As this could potentially involve an overwhelming number of objects, the skill of the CAT therapist is to pick out the pertinent ones, especially those linked with the states on the back of the CAT Psychotherapy file, which could also be a different place to start your use of objects with a client. Ask the client to select objects which reflect how they feel in any of the states, or any that you have noted as part of your assessment. Often through exploring these together, unique aspects of these will become apparent and these will end up with metaphorical names, which may encompass both the RR and the target problem procedure. Sometimes, the client will already have a name for this part, or you can encourage them to find one, e.g. what would they like to call their teenage state or a distressed 'little self'?

Reformulation letters: chosen objects provide a shorthand of metaphors to describe states, RRPs, TTPs

Working with objects in the first sessions of CAT provides a wealth of rich material and metaphors which a CAT therapist can use to compose their reformulation letter, and the client will understand how their choice of objects is being used to tell their story. It is likely to include a shared sense of the quality of their fear or trauma, which is holding them back or fuelling their destructive patterns.

Therapists working with children or people with learning disabilities have used photographs of the chosen objects in their reformulation and goodbye letters, with a beneficial effect. These letters have also then been used by clients as ways of communicating with family members, staff or related services.

Clinical example of starting to work with objects

Working with objects therapeutically can be another way of creating metaphors and deepening the therapeutic relationship. An example of this was shared during a supervision session with David, a CAT therapist, talking about his client, Paul, aged 34, during his third session. Previously, Paul had experienced quite a few other therapies for his difficulties, and in the six months before this CAT therapy he had been trying to make positive changes in his life but was feeling that he was going 'downhill' again and was overwhelmed and frustrated with himself.

Paul came into the session seeming downhearted about himself and lacking hope because he had relapsed. David offered him the opportunity to work with objects and was surprised by Paul's positive reaction to this and the way in which he engaged with them.

David's collection of objects included chess pieces. Paul selected a rook from these because it represented the way in which he saw himself, he felt he could only move in straight lines, backwards and forwards, reflecting the dilemma that David and Paul had already started to explore, an RRP of Controlled but Restricted or Out of Control and Giving up, and feeling bad about himself.

When David asked him how he would like to be instead, Paul selected the queen and said, 'Like this because it can go in any direction'. David explored this idea with Paul and together they saw how this had provided a different perspective for him and led to a discussion about how he too could be more like the queen rather than his habitual way of going between the two points of a dilemma, this allowed Paul to contemplate this possibility in a new way. In CAT terms, the rook represented the felt sense of his dilemma and the queen the beginning of a potential exit from this.

David and Paul went on to identify and explore several of Paul's states. These included feeling like a zombie, being overwhelmed, and he also described a self-destructive and an attacking state. He chose a figure of 'Shrek' to depict his sense of fear, and a Power Ranger to represent his goal of what he wanted to be like. He selected an archer to depict his Critical Self-State, because he said it was as if he was shooting arrows at himself, here he was making a connection between how he felt in himself and what the object signified to him in an embodied way.

In David's supervision session, we discussed how this experience of using objects had been beneficial for Paul in the session and had been similarly helpful for other clients, David's thoughts were:

- One of the uses of objects is that they can *contain* difficult emotions for clients, so supporting self-regulation, freeing the client to be more proactive in the creation of their diagrams or map with objects and words. Using objects in this way helps to externalize the client's difficulties, providing them with more space and distance, or in CAT terms, enhancing the observing eye, so enabling an individual a simultaneous overview and embodied sense of their emotions and patterns of relating, rather than being overwhelmed by them or ensnared by them.

- Working with objects can often have a more immediate impact on the therapist, making the transference more acute and embodied, and so is a particularly effective approach when the transference is otherwise feeling '*Cut Off*' or *flat*. For David, the chosen chess pieces gave him a more visceral connection with Paul's experience.

- As Paul was the one choosing the objects there was a greater sense of self-agency in this process which led to fresh insights and discussions for him. David also felt this activity had created a deeper therapeutic connection between them. He said Paul came into the room seemingly stuck in quite a hopeless self-state at the start of the session, where change seemed impossible. The objects seemed to quickly shift him out of this and broke the tension, the feeling in the room switched from stuck-ness to playfulness and was rich with possibilities. Through this shared creative playful exploration with the objects, Paul was 'laughing, joking and playful, he had switched to being more at ease, and more hopeful and energized', a more effective state for learning and change.

In supervision, Paul and David discussed the possibility that this kind of activity bypasses the habitual, more controlled, and verbal looping scripted part, so allowing for a different way of experiencing his difficulties and contemplating change.

Using objects to tune into embodied trauma or core pain – the 'dreaded' or 'despairing' object

Working with objects to tune into embodied trauma or core pain can sometimes help to get under the defences of a client's implicit protective procedures. One iconic object which is regularly chosen from my collection or brought into therapy by clients themselves is a wooden weeping Buddha, which is often used to denote a despairing place of immense sadness.

After a client has chosen an object for their 'dreaded place', we may be curious about why they have chosen that particular object, and when it feels clinically appropriate, we may ask the client where in their body they are feeling this 'dreaded' emotion and if anything else is coming up, and gently continue in this way for a while. The therapist may ask the client if the 'despairing object' would like to say anything to any of the other objects, or if any of the other objects may have something to say to the 'despairing object'.

There is often a powerful embodied transference with clients when sitting with them with our shared knowledge of why they are feeling like this. This sitting with emotions is a way of supporting someone to begin to find a procedural exit or have a different experience from that of avoiding and escaping from their core pain (e.g. RRP Cutting Off, Dissociating – Cut off,

Dissociated). It is often the essential work of therapy to be alongside a client and support them in with the overwhelming, unbearable feelings they feel and which they have buried in the past when was nobody there to validate or make sense for them. These could be emotions of sadness, grief, loss, abandonment, physical pain, feeling unloved, shame, powerlessness, or rage, but the selected object(s) help to hold and contain the emotion, which also provides a mutual focus for what is happening in the room.

Gestalt questions can be useful here, such as: where/ what are you feeling? If it were to have a shape/colour/sound/what would that be? Gendlin's (2003) 'Focusing techniques' can also be adapted to be helpful here. Other questions to a part could be: How long it has been acting in this role? When and why did it come into existence? How old is the part and how old does it think the client is?

Creating a dialogue between parts

As we aim for integration of a person's 'parts' or self-states, we encourage the client to ask questions about all their different parts and see how they feel about each other, particularly in relation to any unhelpful *procedures* that may be playing out, e.g. 'When your "Striving" part is active, how does your "Exhausted" part feel and what would they like to say to that Striver?' Empty-chair work, also used in Gestalt therapy, may be beneficial in this process, and objects may be placed on chairs to facilitate this, while movement also appears to be important to the efficacy of chair work. Pugh (2017) provides a description of this.

Including a nurturing figure, real or imaginary

We can help foster hope and a greater felt sense of self-compassion or a sense of a client reclaiming or 'rescuing' their younger or abused self by reconnecting with the healthier parts of themselves or rekindling memories of feeling loved, even if this was by a pet or grandparent who has died. Through encouraging clients to select objects representing positive relationships or voices for them, we are preparing for the moment in therapy when we need to bring compassion into their story or for a part. When the client is struggling to find compassion for themself, the therapist can then ask them what this positive object may say to them. Therefore, when a client is selecting objects, it is advisable to ask them to choose an object to represent an ally and/or a nurturing figure. Ideally, the object will represent somebody (or a pet) who has shown them kindness or care. If not a family member, it might be a teacher, friend, nurse or an imaginary character from a book or film, for example, or sometimes a favourite animal that they can tangibly imagine alongside them or acting on their behalf.

It can be helpful to practice this before doing any work that may be too challenging. Additionally, if the client is a parent who is capable of nurturing their children, or a pet, you could invite this RR or part in to provide comfort to their hurt 'little self'. You can also ask the client if they would like to move any of their objects closer to their despairing object(s), for support, and ask, 'Is there anything this part may need or want to do?'

A clinical example of how working with objects therapeutically can be cathartic

Sometimes, just the experience of choosing an object can unlock a traumatic response, as was the case with Becky.

Becky, a fifty-five-year-old, recently divorced mother, with a son in his early twenties, was referred due to suicidal thoughts. In her childhood, she had experienced a loving relationship with her maternal grandmother but had felt 'hated and rejected' by her mother. When we initially started working with objects, I asked her to select one for her little self and she chose a soft-bodied baby doll. Following this, she chose a faceless object to represent her mother and turned it away from the doll. When I asked her how the 'baby' was feeling in relation to the mother object, she picked up the doll, and, while holding it tightly, she cried and rocked for ten minutes. This was a transformational moment in the therapy which allowed Becky to reconnect with her 'little' embodied distressed self. In doing this, she was also able to bring in her own maternal self-role, thus connecting and integrating these two different parts of her, or self-states, and creating a greater ability for self-compassion. Unsurprisingly, the embodied transference in the room during this session was intensely powerful and it deepened our therapeutic relationship.

In this case, Becky, in the moment, implicitly embodied the RR of caring and loving that she had with her son and transferred it to the doll into which she had projected her little self and her associated core pain, and so was able to find compassion and the release of some of the embodied trauma of feeling hated by her mother. As she cried, she rocked, potentially releasing more of her embodied trauma through movement.

Summary

Working with objects can change the therapeutic dance, and potentially ameliorate embodied, implicitly held trauma for clients who may be overwhelmed or disconnected from their emotions or unable to leave space for dialogue with the therapist. When working with objects, clients may have a greater sense of empowerment as their projections are 'held' and contained in them, freeing the client to take a different perspective and use their observing eye in a novel way. This often gives them a sense of power over a previously negative sense of powerful others. This may particularly be the case for people with communication difficulties or dissociated states. It seems that, in general, being actively engaged in this interactive, creative process can lead to an increased sense of validation for clients and more equitable power during therapy, particularly when they begin to make connections and insights from their own explorations.

Being creative with objects within a compassionate and playful relationship can provide a safer and more advantageous neurological state for curious exploration and change. Using objects to facilitate the healing of complex trauma, hard-to-reach, or disowned parts, can provide a greater understanding and release of emotions such as rage, grief and fear, and the accompanying embodied feelings, particularly when the client makes movements or micro-movements when cued into the trauma. A client's chosen objects also assist the therapist in tuning into embodied transference, with the possibility of a deeper insight for both client and therapist. The dialogical process between objects facilitates identifying and managing snags that are often implicit.

This therapeutic approach provides the opportunity for novelty and gentle humour, which can enhance the therapeutic relationship leading to the development of new RRs, and neurological studies suggest that this combination of factors provides the optimum conditions for developing healthier ways of being, including a more integrated positive sense of self. An invitation to be curious and using objects exploratively can deepen and enrich a client's narrative, creating a bridge between the mind and the embodied states and assist the use of the CAT tools. Therapists often report finding that being creative in therapies makes these more distinct, alive and engaging, and so may diminish burnout.

'The left brain can help people analyse problems, spell out choices, or make conscious predictions about what might come next, only the right side carries the creative capacity for something entirely novel, spontaneous, or unpredictable to emerge. Herein lies the importance of interpersonal creativity ... of 'safe surprises' by which the therapist/patient pair can break through old stale patterns to stumble upon something new.' (Marks-Tarlow, 2017)

Chapter 5: Dramatherapy and playful relationality

Vicky Petratou

Introduction

Dramatherapy is an arts therapy that uses drama structures and other complementary creative therapeutic activities with the intention of helping clients to express, explore and reflect on problematic and psychologically challenging experiences. Its concepts and practices can helpfully contribute to both the theory and practice of Cognitive Analytic Therapy, by enriching it experientially and creatively (Petratou, 2007).

In this chapter, I will share some ways that such work has complemented my practice as a CAT psychotherapist and Dramatherapist. I will set out the kinds of Dramatherapy experiences, techniques and concepts that have been invaluable to reaching my clients and helping them to reconnect with their own creativity and sense of playfulness. I will discuss how some core Dramatherapy concepts (dramatic embodiment and projection, distance, space, story and roles) can invigorate the therapy process (Jones, 1996).
I will demonstrate how the practice of combining CAT and Dramatherapy insights can be useful to the process and progress of the work at all stages of therapy, including recognition, reformulation and revision. I will give examples of how such experiential processes can aid the exploration of the mapped problematic relational patterns and/or the self-states involved in ways that can help clients to notice them, embrace them and be in dialogue with them. In addition, I will discuss how Dramatherapy's active methods can facilitate the embodied development of meaningful therapeutic exits. Finally, I will reflect on some insights I gained through this work, in relation to how we can be helped with the noticing and naming of Reciprocal Roles in useful ways that can encourage clients' recognition of them when they are enacted in their lives.

CAT and Dramatherapy: a complementary relationship?

Anthony Ryle advocated the idea that as human beings we 'become' through ongoing communication and engagement with our internal and external worlds (Ryle, 2001). Our relational 'becoming' is theatrical and dramatic in nature, and in CAT we view selfhood as the various Reciprocal Roles we share with ourselves and the world. By always engaging in roles and meaning-making narratives (personal dramas), humans are not only theatre makers… they are theatre, as Augusto Boal (1995) suggested. By this token, we are all actors and spectators, observers and witnesses, a notion that is supported by both Dramatherapy and CAT. The view of the self not as a single separate unit (like the 'I am me' notion) but as a multi-voiced entity, which is continuously interacting with the changing environment, is advocated by both CAT and Dramatherapy (Stiles, 1997; Petratou, 2007). The CAT concept of Reciprocal Roles describes not only our selfhood but also the dramatic quality of our interactions, because it asserts that we are the outcome of the ongoing interplay of various internalising (in the present) and internalised (based in the past) relationships. Dramatherapy has a great deal to offer the practicing Cognitive Analytic Therapist, particularly in exploring how the client might relate to his internal and interpersonal world using creative and imaginative methods. For instance, creative reflective techniques used in CAT such as the Six-Part Story Method (See Appendix 5) and the House of Self States (HOSS) (see Appendix 4) have been informed and influenced by Dramatherapy (Lahad, 1992; Dent- Brown, 2024; Petratou, 2019).

Also, dramatic improvisations can help us to find out experientially how our roles are enacted and experienced and to discover new ways of relating/new ways of being who we could become. Creative dramatherapeutic methods can encourage playfulness, creativity, spontaneity, humour and vitality (Emunah, 1994; Boal 2006, Jones 2021). The use of key concepts within Dramatherapy, including embodiment, metaphor, projection, role, story and improvisation provide experiential means for encouraging clients to engage in a physical, emotional and reflective process (Jones, 1996; Landy 2009). This can help them to explore, expand and transform their Reciprocal Role procedures into something that involves the possibility of gaining freedom to be more flexible and responsive and able to make choices (Armstrong *et al*, 2016; Petratou, 2007; Stevens & Petratou, 2024).

Dramatherapy empathy and distancing

This is defined by Landy as the ways of separating oneself from the other, bringing oneself closer to the other, and generally maintaining the balance between the two states of separateness and closeness between two people (Landy, 1983). It can affect clients' lives on many different levels: interpersonal, mental, emotional and physical. In Dramatherapy, both the client and the therapist engage with varying levels of dramatic distancing to allow the client to meaningfully explore their lives without becoming overwhelmed. The therapist should act as a good container and guide to the client throughout any dramatherapeutic creative explorations used.

During the process of attending to clients' relative strengths and challenges/difficulties, the therapist needs to be flexible in experimenting with a variety of techniques and continuously observe the results and adjust their responses accordingly (Petratou, 1994). Those who are experienced in the use of the arts in psychotherapy know that a good measure of creativity and imagination is needed to adapt whatever method one chooses to use when working with a client's individual needs and abilities. Exploring relational emotional diversity/distance as a continuum, which ranges from relating with a high degree of emotional pre-occupation and emersion to complete emotional avoidance and disconnection, can be useful in choosing specific creative activities in therapy that could meet clients' particular ways of being with others. From the CAT literature, Jellema (2000) has suggested that clients who tend to avoid accessing feelings and those who have difficulties in thinking need a different approach (as cited in Ryle and Kerr (2002). This need for variation in approach, depending on the clients' habitual relational patterns, needs to be carefully considered within the theory and practice of CAT. Jellema (2003), in her review of attachment studies, stated that there is a clear difference between different clients' effective strategies, broadly defined along these lines:

- Preoccupied clients who tend to use more 'hyper-activating', affective strategies where attachment-related emotion is exaggerated.
- Dismissing clients, who tend to use 'deactivating' affective strategies where emotion is understated.

Jellema suggested that dismissive patterns are more common in Western societies than preoccupied patterns (Jellema, 2003). It could be argued that, originally, CAT, with its strong emphasis on verbal reflection and the logical conceptualization of relational patterns, might have been more aligned with a 'dismissive' pattern than a 'preoccupied' one. However, over the past 20 years, notions such as creativity, imagination and playfulness have begun to be more integrated into the language of CAT, both theoretically and practically, and it is now benefitting from developing a closer affiliation with the sensuous, emotional, sensory and imaginative elements of human life in order to promote a more integrated therapy. Dramatherapy is a creative therapy that can contribute fruitful reflective and experiential ways of encouraging this. Its concept of distance has a multidimensional nature and can be beneficial to both the theory and practice of CAT.

In Dramatherapy, the concept of 'distance' can be viewed in terms of an individual's relation to their feelings. Landy (1993) suggested that clients who have difficulty accessing feelings (i.e. who over-intellectualize their emotions) can be considered to have an 'over-distant' style of relating or 'dismissive' in Jellema's (2003) view. Those clients who struggle to contain their feelings because they find it difficult to think clearly about them can be described as being/having an 'under-distant' or 'preoccupied' style of relating in Jellema's (2003) view. Also with the increase of neurodivergent diagnoses in the UK such as autism, ADHD and dyslexia (Donaldson Trust, 2024), therapists may need to be more flexible, creative and able to develop a deeper awareness of how their clients relate, in terms of relational distancing that meets their needs. In addition to emotional distance, Dramatherapy draws on the concept of 'aesthetic distance' when referring to how closely the client might identify with a role that they may play in their life outside the therapy room – this means that the Dramatherapist will need to be mindful of aesthetic distance when engaging in therapeutic imaginative activities with their clients – carefully judging how close an activity might be to the client in terms of aesthetic distance so that a balance between under and over distancing can be struck. This is attained when the individual can engage emotionally without fear of being overwhelmed by their feelings and thinking without fear of losing the ability to respond in an emotionally attuned way (Landy, 1993).

This Dramatherapy concept of distance can be integrated usefully into the practice of CAT. For example, the process of developing the diagram/map is a more distancing (reflective) exercise rather than an empathic one as its emphasis is perspective and clarity in relation to the clients' experience of problematic and confusing relational patterns. The reformulation letter, on the other hand, because it is written in the second person and read aloud to clients, seems to be a more empathic and under-distant therapeutic tool in therapy. An example of a more 'distanced' writing-based activity is the third-person oriented self-characterization (Ryle, 1983), which is associated with a more Brechtian approach to writing which encourages a more distant stance, so that the client can reflect on what they are witnessing rather than empathizing with the characters involved.

Working with dramatic embodiment and improvisation

CAT theory suggests that the presence of early harsh and/or neglectful relationships in life can have a negative impact on a client's capacity for future role flexibility and integration. Such painful and disturbing experiences can distort our senses, how we respond to certain stimuli, and our ability to regulate our feelings in relation to these. In other words, early childhood trauma impacts the development of our body-selves and physical Reciprocal Roles. Dramatherapy theory and active creative methods can help CAT therapists and their clients to become familiar with and embrace how their bodies communicate through the quality of their sensory and expressive body-relational patterns. Jennings (2002) has studied the qualities of physical relating in the development of relational embodiment and has elaborated on highlighting some of the patterns that can be developed through aversive early childhood interactions with the primary carer. In CAT terms, these can be described (see below) in the form of Reciprocal Roles:

- Over-holding (always with) – overheld/fused – which can lead to anxiety and difficulties with separation.
- Under-holding (left alone, unattended for long periods) – which can lead to mistrustful and anxious feelings.
- Violating – violated and invaded (hurt, confused, fearful and anxious) which can lead to difficulties with blurred and confusing bodily and spatial boundaries.

If clients have physically felt overheld/underheld/violated, they may need reparatory embodied and playful therapeutic experiences to process the pain and confusion they feel in an embodied and creative way. For example, playful sensory activities with messy/sensory play (i.e., with music, dance, singing, breath, artwork, clay, Play-Doh or sand) can act as a grounding experience and help to facilitate empathy, engagement and re-connection.

Learning experience and social understanding is primarily based on our body (Jennings, 1990). This process happens as a 'myriad of experiences of giving to and receiving from, most often subtly expressed as micro-movements transmitted from on to the other' (Frank, 2023, p:21). If our bodies have been mistreated and neglected in our early relationships, it is recommended in Dramatherapy that extended physical play is needed to develop a more body-attentive experience. Developing a non-judgemental and compassionate bodily awareness requires a gradual, gentle approach (Levine, 2015). The concepts of embodiment, body boundaries and rhythm need to be considered when thinking about our interactions with others, particularly if we have experienced these distortions to embodied development in childhood. How do we communicate with our bodies as therapists in CAT? How do we work with the negative impact our clients' experiences have had on their bodies? Re-regulating the rhythm of breath through playful mirroring and breathing exercises can be a good first step towards helping clients to re-attune with their bodies and the bodies of others.

By paying attention to non-verbal communication and its dynamics and involving the body in dramatic activity/movement within the therapy process, Dramatherapy practice has shown that taking different body identities can have a transformative effect, resulting in the client gaining new perspectives and increased insight as well as promoting more permissive and integrated ways of relating to their own bodies, and in their interactions with others. As Jones (1996) stated, physically participating in a dramatic activity, the body and the mind are jointly engaged in discovery. Wilshire (1982) in referring to the mimetic/mirroring movement said that we can learn about our own bodies by being bodily engaged with another's, leading to 'mimetic engagement'. In therapy, the therapist would need to engage actively with the 'doing with', by mirroring the dramatic movement improvisation and help the client to engage with his emotional states in a more embodied way. For example, one client who was exploring his tendency to continuously strive to attain additional senior leadership positions at work realized, when engaging with a short dramatic movement improvisation, that 'it's like I always have the "effort-switch on" and this time I allowed myself to experiment with switching it off for a change… and I feel more free…'

Embodying difficult self-states dramatically through a gesture or a meaningful movement and then improvising another movement that the body is drawn to afterwards, and repeating this sequence together with the therapist, can be a validating and transformative experience that can help clients to improvise dramatic movements of relief and release. In a client-led mirrored-movement exercise, one woman began with two movements – one to represent 'hiding' and another to represent 'confidence' – and then, with guidance, as we moved together, followed this with another movement that expressed what her body really wanted to do, which was to sway left and right in a rhymical way while bending her knees. This opened up in her a sense of acknowledgement, transformation and liberation from feeling rigid. Reflecting afterwards on this short, playful movement sequence, she said:

> *'The choreographed covering of my face (in shame?), then opening out my arms wide and releasing the tension in my chest... then bending my knees ever so slightly and "dancing"... this movement I found... its as if it releases me from myself – or the false images and narratives I have created of myself. All that's left is to find an old "discotheque" (do they even exist anymore?) and have the guts to invite my partner to step on to the dance floor.'*

Co-creating improvised, expressive movement in this way and trying to match the client's rhythms and emotional states is an act of embodied dialogue as it activates a sense of co-discovery and expands communication and trust. This is a key principle of 'doing with' the client, and it runs throughout Dramatherapy and CAT. I suggest that it should be possible for CAT therapists to expand their role-taking and take on a more embodied and flexible approach, in which additional roles such as storyteller, facilitator or co-actor, varying in their degrees of emotional/aesthetic distance from the client, may be taken (Petratou, 2007). Facilitating meaningful, playful and expressive enactments allows the client to see, tolerate and contain their emotional state and begin to safely 'reveal rather than conceal' it (Anderson-Warren & Grainger, 2000, p: 85). Embodiment work can be used to help clients to 'inhabit' their bodies more effectively and taking different body identities can have a transformative effect, resulting in the client gaining increased insights into how their own body interacts with others.

Integrating these methods into a CAT approach means that we can explore our clients' painful relational patterns in imaginative and playful ways, and this often leads to clients discovering exits to their entrenched Reciprocal Role procedures quite spontaneously, which can be a very beautiful experience when it happens. It can help us to move away from an over-reliance on verbal discussion with our clients, because a lot of communication, connection and embodied involvement between people is experienced non-verbally. We need to provide space for experimental play (a play space, or stage) for dramatic projection, story work, dramatic embodiment and role-playing. Such spaces have great therapeutic value in addressing and working with conflictual/entrapping patterns and self-states. They can illuminate subtexts and underlying themes, and unacknowledged physical experiences (disembodiment) which might otherwise be concealed by verbal description. Too much attention to verbal modes of reflection can drive the process into becoming a disembodying, and overly cognitive experience. It is useful to consider how we, both client and therapist, can disengage or disembody ourselves from our emotional experience and seek to re-engage and revitalize the body. As we have seen, this can be very effectively achieved through dramatic embodiment work using expressive movement, mirroring and working with sensory material such as clay. Engaging actively in providing empathically adjusted bodily gesture, vocal intonation and facial expression can help clients to feel safer (ventral vagal response) and encourage reciprocal social interaction through right-brain to right-brain emotional attunement – playful activity (such as Dramatherapy embodied, imaginative and at times humorous methods) can activate the social engagement system, allowing a wider range of emotional expression and nurturing a sense of contentment and well-being (Schore, 2019).

Finally, Dramatherapy and other therapies like EMDR pay attention to helping their clients to ground their bodies before they engage in exploring traumatic narratives. I think that CAT can benefit from offering some grounding experiences to clients through imaginative and physical resourcing, not just during the revision process, but also in the early part of the work. Helping the client to develop their grounding and containing capacity while they are processing painful past and present experiences during the reformulation process could be a good addition to the model of CAT.

Role-playing fictional characters and/or personification

Role play as a therapeutic activity isn't exclusive to the arts therapies; as a technique, it has been used by many different modalities. But the arts therapy tradition has a lot it can offer to therapists wanting to use role play in their practice, and as an arts therapy with a particular emphasis on 'dramatic expression', Dramatherapy is well positioned to inspire, influence and model how it can best be employed in the therapeutic space. One of the ways that Dramatherapy can enrich the process of role play is by helping CAT therapists to pay attention to enrolling and de-rolling processes. For example, whenever we engage with role-work it is important to warm up physically in order to release any rigidity that the client may have in their body, before they are asked to begin embodying their character's physical qualities or self-states within the role-play activity. Similarly, it is important to cool down/de-role when we come out of the character at the end of the role enactment and various theatre techniques can help with this process (Bloch *et al*, 1995). Role reversal is another very powerful activity that can help clients to empathize and develop their mentalizing skills. When we consider introducing this technique, we need to consider when and how – in terms of what kind of preparation and scaffolding is needed – this is introduced into the therapeutic work. For example, if the client is feeling very angry with the other person it is often impossible to allow themselves to embody or access how the other might be feeling, so planning and pacing, in partnership with the client, is vital.

This core Dramatherapy process of role play can be helpful in guiding clients towards integrating polarized antagonistic roles (the two poles of a dilemma or two self-states that are antagonistic and not in dialogue) and/or discovering new roles. The dramatic dialogue technique (for details, see Petratou, 2007) was devised as a Dramatherapy method to facilitate a creative experience of dialogue between self-states that don't often 'listen' to one another. In this process at the revision part of therapy, two self-states are identified and given some aesthetic distance by creating them as fictional characters and putting on costumes, using props or using projective means to represent these states in the form of objects, masks etc. If the client finds it difficult to embody the chosen dramatized roles, then we just work at the projective level by personifying them in the form of chosen projective objects. If the client is able to embody these roles, then we can start with them being projected and then move to role play, or we can go straight to embodied role play. When working with role play, we need to attend to an enrolling and de-rolling process. Once the characters are enrolled, we ask each of them to speak to the other (who is portrayed by a chosen object) about their experiences, what they want to happen and how they can make this possible. I have presented a list below that has some guidelines/ questions that can facilitate listening, negotiation and conflict resolution. These are questions that the therapist can use to facilitate the dialogue. These can also be written on paper – in individual work, I prefer to do this because it seems to help the client to feel safe, contained and held enough to engage with this challenging but helpful process:

- What do you think is/was going on (between these different self-states/ characters)?
- What do you think about it?
- What do you feel about it?
- What would you like to happen?
- What small thing can you do to help this happen?
- What small thing can the other do to help this future wish to happen?

This is not an exhaustive list and some additional supportive questions might be asked if needed, but one needs to be careful not to overwhelm the client. Once both parts have taken their turns, the client de-roles from both characters and creates a constellation (small relational sculpture using objects to illustrate the interaction) on a cushion of the two roles in dialogue together. The client takes a picture of this constellation as a useful reminder of the encounter. Sometimes, the client might want to create two constellations, one representing how they felt before the dialogue and one how they felt after the dialogue. Following this process, we both step back and the client shares their reflections on this 'dramatic dialogue' process.

Often, clients choose a dominating and dismissive state/role and a powerless, silenced state/role to bring to dramatic dialogue. Creating metaphoric names or characters for these states and making a dramatic 'make-believe' space with clarity and respect for it, is very important in helping the client to develop enough aesthetic distance to be able to engage with these painful states in a meaningful and containing way.

In this role-play situation the therapist's role is initially to be an active facilitator and guide, then a witness, and then a co-reflector. This process can't be manualized because the therapist needs to be attentive to the needs of the client in the here and now. Some adaptations or changes can be made but the important thing is to follow the order of warm-up (enrolling), dramatic dialogue (main activity) and cooling down (de-rolling, photographing, and post-action reflective process). These three levels of action are key to the effective use of the creative means and structures to make this activity meaningful and attuning to the client. I have used this activity in a simpler format for online sessions as well, and the clients have found it equally useful. However, because we don't have access to the therapy props of my clinic when we are online, I ask clients to choose two props from their home that we enrol into specific costume elements of the client's role (these can be scarves, hats, sunglasses etc), and then de-role the character and associated props at the end.

On one such occasion, the client brought into the play space the dialogue of two contradictory parts of herself: the Wild Woman (often seen as naïve by the Judge) and the Judge (often seen as dismissive by the Wild Woman). Once the activity was over, the client felt less stuck, more liberated, and more able to accept some difficult choices in her current life. Because this activity is facilitated by the therapist, both parts felt listened to, as there is no space for interruptions. This process helped her to negotiate between these two parts and to clearly notice and accept each other's negative impact as well as their strengths and gifts. In this way, Dramatherapy offers helpful, creative experiences that can facilitate the development of fresh awareness and help us to expand our relational communication (Cassidy *et al*, 2017). Following this activity, I sometimes ask clients to write a short reflective piece on their experience. Box 5.1 illustrates the dramatic dialogue of a client who created two characters to portray the dilemma of two of her self-states: Stella – fiercely independent, unattached and adventurous – and Penelope, who was committed, comfortable and confident in her relationship with her partner.

Box 5.1: Client's own words reflecting on the Dramatic Dialogue activity

'Stella and Penelope'

Theme one: Case example of Dramatic Dialogue

Stella is the free-spirited, independent and powerful woman who keeps her cards close to her chest. She is strong on her own. She likes how she is on her own.

Penelope is in a committed relationship, comfortable and confident with her partner. She is strong with him. She likes herself, how she is with him.

I have two scarves. Scarf 1 (black & red) is Stella; scarf 2 (colourful) is Penelope.

Wearing Stella's scarf, I speak to Penelope. The Penelope scarf is lying on a cushion next to me. I tell her how I envy her and want what she has, but I am scared that it will tie me down to a one-dimensional woman. I speak to her nicely, but also with frustration. I tell her, 'Come on, let's go out, let's see what we can become together.'

When I put on Penelope's scarf, I change my body composition slightly, and turn my back to the scarf that is Stella, lying on a cushion behind me. I can't stand to think of Stella, I didn't want to talk to her before, because if and when I do, I feel like I can't be Penelope. I want what Stella has, but I feel like it clashes with Penelope. Penelope in the perfect relationship, committed, totally happy in sharing her existence and her life with someone so intimately. Talking to Stella as Penelope gives me the courage to see them both, as they already exist within me as [the name of the client]. It makes me sympathize with both, and recognize that even though they clash, somehow, they both exist within me, and to allow them to talk can help me reflect on them calmly. How I can join them or see where their limitations meet and what their desires are. I can be both and be okay with that, or at least move with that.

Having those two roles communicate with one another gave me the distance to observe with curiosity, not judgement or even sympathy in the beginning. By the end, I could sympathize with them. I feel like it's helped me flesh out feelings and thoughts that I didn't dare to before, or didn't know how to without panic, and judgement.

After sharing her reflections, the client made some additional comments which illuminated how this creative dramatic activity had been helpful to her.

- Trusting the therapist: 'I trust you in this exercise and think that it could help me in an unpredictable way'.
- Trying something new: 'It's easy to fall into a habitual way of thinking about things that leads to the same place of thought. Give it a go and see what happens.'
- Respecting the process: 'What helped me feel less awkward was seeing you deliver this as a serious exercise, just as serious as any other technique/question, so I committed to it as such'.

Story making

Stories and characters within them can become good sources for meaning-making, empathic development and inspiring therapeutic exits. Ryle and Kerr (2002, 2020) and more recently Kerr and Beard (2024) have encouraged the use of arts therapies' methods, especially during the revision stage of therapy if things feel stuck. However, for many years in my therapy work, introducing arts experiences has been beneficial at all stages of CAT therapy (Petratou, 2007). During the reformulation stage, story making and storytelling can enrich the process of therapy and help the client to be more participatory i.e. using the Six-Part Story Method (Dent-Brown 2024; Appendix 5), or sharing a fairy/folk tale or a mythical story that has a meaningful connection with the person's experience (Gersie and King, 1990). Another way of introducing storytelling in the initial phase of therapy is to invite the client to write a life story or significant life experience as if it were a fairy tale, and then core themes of this story can be included in the reformation letter, which is then read aloud, or even role-played with the client. In the recognition phase, stories can help generate useful metaphoric reminders to help with identifying self-states or problematic patterns, such as the pleasing trap (see example below). Experimenting with rescripting various endings to these stories can also be very helpful in the revision stage of CAT.

We can use myths, fairy tales and stories from films and books in different ways depending on the individual needs of clients. The timing of this activity needs to be considered; the stories can be brought by therapists, chosen to be relevant to what the client is going through, or they can be introduced by the client by encouraging them to share stories that they have remembered or created themselves. One way to explore a story is to ask clients to choose meaningful scenes/themes which hold some significance for them and then to reflect on them, enact them, draw them or write a poem about them.

Engaging with a meaningful story becomes the vehicle which can carry and contain our clients' complex and at times painful and confusing life experiences at an aesthetic distance, in ways that they are comfortable working with. The therapist can ask questions about what happens in the story, or how the characters of the story act, which can be helpful in clarifying the details, but also serves as a means of empathizing and co-creating ideas for therapeutic change between client and therapist. Here are two examples of the kind of stories I have used in my clinical work.

You don't need my help? I'll help you anyway!

Brief stories or dramatic moments can be taken from various sources including books, theatre, film and TV. TV characters and stories can be very accessible because many people are already aware of them (especially from popular sit-coms and soap operas). One of my favourite 'therapeutic' TV characters is Mrs Doyle from the Irish sitcom 'Father Ted', who seems to have been perpetually caught up in what CAT would define as the 'pleasing trap'. One specific characteristic of Mrs Doyle is that she repeatedly offers to make cups of tea for people she is interacting with, and 'refuses to take no for an answer', making tea for them whether they want tea or not. In my work with one client, this character helped us to see how difficult it sometimes is to let go of the compulsion to please others. It also helped us to realize that 'tea' is not always welcome, and that forcing someone to receive it even if they don't want it doesn't guarantee that the intended impact of 'pleasing others' will always be received in the way that it is intended. The client realized that trying to please can also be quite intrusive and dismissive (you will have my tea, even if you don't want it!). In Reciprocal Role terms, Mrs Doyle's understanding of this interaction is 'pleasing to pleased', but for the recipient of the unwanted cup of tea, the Reciprocal Role would have been more experienced as 'forcing to forced' – not as positive an experience as Mrs Doyle (or the client) would have imagined!

This example is a useful illustration of how it is often more useful therapeutically to look at the 'impacted' side of the Reciprocal Role first, rather than the 'impacting' side, as this usually gives us a clue as to whether the client might need to consider introducing change into how they relate with others or not. For example, if I asked Mrs Doyle what was going on between her and Father Ted with regards to the cups of tea, she might tell me 'I'm being kind to him because he loves the tea I make him' ('impacting' position, the top part of the Reciprocal Role). But if I asked Father Ted how he feels about having multiple cups of tea made for him whether he wants them or not, he might tell me that he feels stressed and irritated by Mrs Doyle's 'well-meaning intentions' (the 'impacted' position). With one client, looking at her 'internal Mrs Doyle' helped us to engage compassionately with her compulsively pleasing tendency, and to also notice not only how it could be creating tension between her and others, but also to recognize that, as compulsions often are, it was actually quite difficult to switch off. Using the Reciprocal Roles being played out between Mrs Doyle and Father Ted is a good example of how drawing from the stories of fictional characters, which allows for some dramatic aesthetic therapeutic distance, can be helpful in recognizing something with the client that would have been quite difficult to address or discuss in any other way.

In addition to stories from literature, or popular media as mentioned above, I may share therapeutic short stories and anecdotes with clients, and at other times we create stories together, from images that the client relates to, or perhaps inspired by therapy cards (i.e. OH, Cope) and postcards. Sharing and creating stories that remind us of the effects and consequences of particular interactions between characters can give us insight into a client's own relational patterns, allowing them to embrace, explore and own, their unique tendencies. These stories can be developed into drawings, improvised scenes, acted by both client and therapist, or with the therapist taking the role of actor and the client witnessing this. These exchanges can produce what Stern (2004) referred to as 'now moments' in therapy, which can often be full of relational co-presence.

Procrustes: doing the 'right' thing in the wrong way...

When working with a client who had experienced a lot of neglect and physical abuse in his early life, we recognized that he was often taking a protector role towards his friends and his children. The client thought that he was in a 'protecting-to-protected' Reciprocal Role with these important people in his life. While we were working with this, I told him a story inspired by the mythical character of Procrustes, who loved inviting travellers to stay at his home for the night. However, Procrustes was obsessed with making sure that the bed he gave them was a perfect fit, and in order to ensure this he would cut their legs off to fit his bed if they were too tall or stretch their body to fit the bed if they were too short.

Procrustes, a character from Classical Greek Mythology, has more in common with Mrs Doyle than one might think, as his need to look after people in a way that suited his way of pleasing others (the perfect cup of tea or the perfect bed) can end up with unintended and unwanted (even traumatic) consequences. When telling this gory and dramatic tale, I try to share it in an animated way, which helps both me and the client to relate to it. I have found that it helps clients realize that others can often have quite different needs to them and that some things that we might find positive and useful can often not actually meet the needs and wants of others.

Listening and relating to this story helped this client to realise that the Reciprocal Role that he was engaging with was often experienced by those affected more as controlling/controlled than protecting/protected. In our work together, the image of Procrustes became a key reminder of how this controlling/controlled relational pattern could take over their life.

Conclusion

Dramatherapy processes can help clients to 're-parent', 'befriend' and promote dialogue between their different self-states. Through the playful interaction that Dramatherapy processes provide, we can help clients to engage and explore experientially the intentions, process and impact of problematic Reciprocal Roles, traps, dilemmas, snags and unbearable core pain, in transformative ways. There are multiple ways of relating within the same relationship – we can experiment with those and learn from them. Dramatherapy activities can help us to develop our awareness of the negative 'impacting' parts of our Reciprocal Roles – those abusing, neglecting and overbearing parts (even those which have 'good or protective' intentions) and grow our ability for compassion towards the 'impacted part' of the Reciprocal Roles.

Dramatic embodiment and creative projective experiences can contribute to clients developing fresh awareness, which can facilitate change/exits. These exits are not fixed solutions in themselves but signposts of ongoing recovery – they are there to be rediscovered over and over in life at times of increased stress or tiredness when habitual patterns may re-emerge. We need to be interested in our internalised reciprocal roles and reciprocal role procedures. We need to de-shame them in order to explore them and begin to resource ourselves with more awareness about relational action and impact. As we have found with Mrs Doyle and Procrustes, many of those 'impacting' parts of our RRs often come with perfectly good intentions – the Priest would like a nice cup of tea, my guests would love a bed that fits them perfectly – but intention doesn't always have the impact that we want it to.

The use of an aesthetic play space and the carefully considered creative processes employed within it (i.e., the use of dramatic embodiment, improvision, poetry, story making, puppetry and other dramatic projective tools) can be usefully incorporated into CAT. The goal here is to promote in our clients a sense of experimentation and the possibility of playful re-explorations of previous conflict to access a meaningful integration of their different self-states (Petratou, 2007). Dramatherapy can help individuals to shift and expand themselves by developing their capacity to improvise and play and to reconnect with their bodies. We all can benefit from creative transitional spaces and experiences throughout our lives in order to re-engage with the world when harsh experiences crush our ability to be present and responsive 'in' the moment.

Chapter 6:
Beyond your wildest dreams

Sophie Rushbrook and Nicola Coulter

Introduction

Dreams are an integral part of our existence. They enable us to process daily disturbances and improve emotional decoding of brain networks (Walker, 2018, p207 and 216). We all dream, whether we remember doing so or not. Being deprived of Rapid Eye Movement (REM), the phase of sleep during which dreams occur, can be catastrophic for both mental and physical well-being, (Naiman, 2017). Interest in dreams goes back millennia, from the ancient Egyptians to Joseph and his coat of many colours in the Bible, through Shakespeare and Freud, to the present day and the interest of dreams in the therapeutic space.

The dreamwork technique described in this chapter is one of several methods designed to work with dream material therapeutically. It is adapted from Gestalt therapy (Fritz Perls, 1969; 1973) and can be used to create a metaphorical understanding for the therapeutic material, reduce repetitive traumatic nightmares and enhance the therapeutic relationship. A clinical case is presented in this chapter to illustrate all the steps in the process to enable the reader to grasp the simplicity and depth of the technique, providing an additional tool to tap the rich seam of material from this imaginative theatre production of the unconscious mind. Adaptations beyond the realm of the dreamwork technique are introduced to pique interest and expand the experimental reach of this technique for the reader, complementing the therapist's own imagination, style and creativity.

Tony Ryle developed Cognitive Analytic Therapy (CAT) as an integrative model, and while this dreamwork can be used in a standalone way or within different therapies, it facilitates the three CAT stages of reformulation, recognition and revision.

Theoretical background

Sigmund Freud (2010) transformed our understanding of dreams, describing them as the road to the unconscious. He believed each dream to be meaningful, representing repressed desires and motivations stemming from infantile wishes, often sexual in nature. Desires that could not be expressed or experienced consciously due to the constraints of societal judgements could be satisfied through latent meaning hidden under the manifest content of the dream.

Carl Jung also explored how dreams symbolically offered understanding, but, unlike Freud, who proposed that dreams were repressed and unknown unless interpreted, Jung perceived that they revealed archetypal images and were a means for the unconscious mind to communicate directly with the conscious one, revealing more to the dreamer than they concealed.

Fritz Perls, the founder of Gestalt therapy, further developed Freud's idea, from understanding dreams as the road to the unconscious to being the road to integration. He agreed with Jung and Freud that the content of the dream was linked to aspects of the person's psyche but, rather than seeking to discover the hidden unfulfilled desires or archetypes, his endeavour was to enable the dreamer to find their own route of discovery. Perls postulated that dreams could be used to link the mind and the body through embodying the dream material and experiencing the emotional content of the dream. He proposed that this enabled access to conscious awareness rather than merely thinking of the dream.

While Tony Ryle did not pay great attention to dreams per se, his integrative model encourages the use of creative techniques. The awareness of Reciprocal Roles, in particular disavowed roles, can be challenging to access through talking alone. Embodying and experiencing the metaphor of the dream facilitates conscious awareness in a simple way, revealing the depth and breadth of the different parts of the self at play.

Conceptualization of the dreamwork

There are some basic assumptions that need to be adopted when learning this dreamwork technique for effective practice to follow.

The dream belongs to the dreamer. It is created by the dreamer and represents who they are. While we are on a voyage of discovery together with the client, we are not the authors or experts of their dreams; rather, we are facilitators of the dreamwork process. It is crucial that the interpretation of the dream is the dreamer's prerogative, not that of the therapist. The therapist's role is to model a stance of calm curiosity in the dream exploration. The process is collaborative and continually flexible, with the therapist always attending and attuning to the client's willingness to participate.

Every element of the dream represents a different part of the dreamer and there are no unwelcome parts of the dreamer or elements of the dream. All dream material is valuable as each element has the potential to offer an important portal into varied and possibly disavowed parts of ourselves. Since all elements of the dream are welcomed with equal interest, fear can give way to curiosity. What is not feared no longer represents danger. The dream provides an opportunity for the dreamer to safely traverse the dreaming landscape via metaphor and this creates an experimental playground for exploration of fears and desires of the body and mind. With an intention to always work towards integration, dreamwork primarily functions in a self-to-self frame. Later, through exploring with another (in the first instance the therapist), it can include self-to-other and other-to-self reciprocations, moving from internal to external dialogue.

The dream is a metaphor. It *can* be a representation of reality, but it is still *not* reality. Dreaming about being in a car crash is not being in a car crash, even if this is something that has happened previously. It is a dream car crash with a dream car, a dream road, and a dream-self. It may be a representation of an actual crash or may represent a sense of feeling out of control, for example, being crushed in a situation at work. Even remembering the dream is different from being in the dream when asleep. Past and future events are not currently in existence. The dreamwork focuses on the client's conscious experience now, to allow their mind to capture with imagination, the different elements of the dream in the service of greater knowledge and integration of parts of self.

The context of dream telling and dreamwork influences the process and outcome. For example, the same dream may be different when told on another occasion or in a different context or to a different person. Dreams, including repetitive dreams, often change over time as the dreamer's relationship and emotional response to the dream alters with exploration and awareness realized through the dreamwork. Insights from dreamwork serve as therapeutic links providing an understanding for past and current relationship patterns and experiences.

The mechanism of this progression to change through embodied dreamwork can be formulated as revision in CAT work in terms of movement from existing role reciprocations identified during the reformulation phase to adaptive ones. For example [Withholding – Cut Off] giving way to [Loving and Caring – Loved and Cared For]. Similarly, revision may be evident as the dreamer's relationship to the therapist changes during the dreamwork process. The client may experience support rather than judgement as the therapist offers an adaptive relational experience for them, which may also be generalised in their relationship to their dream. Perhaps, for example, [Judging – Judged] moving to [Interested and Curious – Valued and Seen].

Over time, as the dreamer is guided through the dreamwork process, the model can offer a technique that the client may apply to themselves independently after treatment. As they explore dreams as an opportunity to gain new insight, they are also guided to understand the underpinnings of the technique. Clients report continued and effective independent practice of this technique and note that it has transformed their relationship with their dreams and nightmares.

Dreamwork outline: step-by-step guide with case illustration

Step 1: Provide orientation and obtain consent

Orientation is important to establish that the client is willing and consenting to the process of dreamwork. Orientation should be kept brief, taking no more than a minute or two, as lengthy discussions about dreamwork can interfere with effectiveness and it risks becoming an intellectual exercise rather than an experiential exploration.

Working towards consent involves balancing the tension between permission seeking and communicating confidence, avoiding conveying distrust in either the process or the client's ability to deal with it. Assuming a light, matter-of-fact tone will encourage a sense of trust and safety. The emotional tone of the dream content or reflections may also be uncomfortable at times. Establish the client's willingness to continue in the spirit of exploration and learning. Sometimes we might ask: *Are we good to continue here?* The key is to pace the work flexibly in attunement with the client.

Therapist: *Dreams work behind the scenes to help us process our daily disturbances. They can give us rich information which can help us* understand ourselves better and can be interesting to explore. We can look at your dream in a different way, which may seem a bit unusual, but it's an experience which can help you to make sense of your own dream. Would you like to give it a try?

Step 2: Describe the dream

Once the client demonstrates a willingness to give this a try, invite them to describe their dream, or a fragment of a dream, in as much detail as possible. Notice the emotional tone, the mood and atmosphere. As the client is describing their dream experience, transcribe their words as well as you are able without interrupting their flow of speech. As you are transcribing, underline words which represent elements of the dream which later may be embodied by the client in Step 3.

Therapist: *Tell me about your dream with as much detail as you remember it and I will write it down.*

Sarah: *In the dream, I'm with my two daughters on an adventurous journey but not in a nice way. We go to a cave which is unpleasant and dank like a swamp. I realized that you could get drips on you, which were contaminating, and you could die. I got some drips on my leg. It was awful because we knew that I was going to die. Also, we realized that if the girls stayed here, they could die too. We realized that they were going to have to leave me behind. I said, 'Right girls, you are going to have to leave me here'. I felt brave, I knew what needed to happen and I was going to stay. But the next part of the dream was me pleading with them as I didn't want to be left on my own, it was a horrible place, and I didn't want to die on my own. I lost all of my bravery, and I was pleading with them, 'You can't leave me, I've got to come with you, you have to take me with you'. I remember Sam saying, 'Oh yes, we have got to take Mum'. Jackie just said, 'No, she is right, we have to leave her, or we are all going to die'. I was upset that Jackie could be so matter of fact. That's what I can remember.*

Therapist (looking for the emotion): *How are you feeling during the dream?*

Sarah: *Anxious and unsettled, we were trying to get somewhere, home I think, I didn't know where we were, it was such a struggle and then the contamination started and that was really upsetting, it was all going wrong. As wrong as it could be.*

Therapist: *Anything else you want to say about this, for instance, what are the colours like? Smells? Sensations?*

Sarah: *Gloomy, dark – not nice.*

Therapist: *Anything else in this place?*

Sarah: *No, damp, dark, rocky, gloomy.*

Step 3: Embody, 'become' an object or figure in the dream

Select an element, an object or a figure from the script to explore. Often, this will be the first one that is mentioned in the account of the dream. Otherwise, a choice can be made regarding emotional intensity, while holding in mind the client's openness and ability to engage. Regarding the therapist's decision process in this case study, Sarah spoke about the cave first, so this element is an obvious first choice to embody. It wouldn't necessarily be helpful to *start* with the drips, because they are likely to be the most emotionally intense element and may represent the 'danger/monster' in the dream. Typically, progression to exploring the 'monster' in the dreamwork over time depends upon the therapeutic relationship and the client's zone of proximal development (ZPD). Once the client has some familiarity and ease with the technique, it is valuable to incorporate the most emotionally charged elements. Avoiding this difficult work implies that not all parts of the client are welcome and would remain disavowed. Furthermore, one might assume an element is the 'monster', but it doesn't necessarily turn out to be so; for example, the drips may have a positive intent and want to get close to dream-Sarah or be caring in some way. This information may only be discovered once the clients have embodied the element in question.

Ask the client to *be* the selected dream element, and to feel and speak from this position. Demonstrate curiosity in exploring the dream through manner and voice tone. The therapist needs to stay out of the way as much as possible, while listening and observing intently, holding the client secure in the present during the process.

It is important to follow the protocol and be disciplined to stay in the dream process. Clients might move out of the present tense, or even out of the dream material. It is common to need to remind the client to stay in the present tense as if it is happening now inviting them to experientially drop into the dream.

Therapist: *I'm going to ask you to **be** a part of the dream now as if you are in the dream now. Can you speak from the present tense, and I will* *continue to write it down. Try to stay in that part as much as possible. I will help you if need be. So, you have mentioned the cave. Could you be the cave? Like this, as the cave ... I AM ...*

Sarah as the cave: *I am the cave,* ***it's*** *large and* ***it*** *is gloomy ...*

Therapist (smiling warmly): *So, I am large, I am gloomy ...* (gently bringing Sarah to the first person and embodying the dream element, while inviting her to finish the sentence).

Sarah as the cave: *Yes, I am large, I am gloomy, I am dark, damp, and I'm a shell, there's nothing living in me. Sometimes there is life inside, but it is just passing through, no one wants to stay there in me ... I am feeling quite upset now.*

Therapist: *Is the cave upset, or are you, Sarah, upset hearing yourself as the cave?*

Sarah: *That was me.*

Therapist: *Is there anything else you would like to say as the cave? Continue exploring until the client has no more material to offer.*

Step 4: Explore how different objects or figures relate to one another

Greater depth of personal understanding can be accessed through embodying the different elements of the dream and communicating between different dream elements. As the client is embodying one element of the dream, ask them what their sense is, in relation to other elements of the dream from this position. For example: *How do you* (as the cave) *feel/think about the drips/Sarah/the children? What do you want to communicate to ... the drips/Sarah/Jackie/Sam?*

Remember that the dreamer is also an element of the dream, so we can enquire how they feel about the dream-self. Sometimes it can be helpful to refer to the dream characters as 'dream X', in this case 'dream-Sarah', as this can maintain clarity that we are exploring the dream elements, not reality.

Therapist: *So, how do you feel about dream-Sarah and the girls being within you?* (Speaking to her as the cave.)

Sarah as the cave: *I feel sorry for them because it is really sad what is happening to them, a no-win situation, I see the push-pull going on for* them. It is quite nice for me though to have someone passing through, I have such a timeless existence here. I don't have anything to do, it's just rocks, it's the same all the time.

Therapist: *How do you feel towards the drips and how they are landing on Sarah?*

Sarah as the cave: *Well, there are these contaminating drips, I don't really know about these drips, I don't know where they come from, if they are part of me or if they are outside of me. I think they are unkind to Sarah.*

Step 5: Repeat the process for embodying different elements in the dream

Repeat step 3 and 4 as many times as necessary and as time allows. You can work on a fragment of a dream or use all the material occurring in the dream.

Therapist: *OK, so now, can you be the drip?* (Said with good eye contact in a warm and matter-of-fact style – conveying that it is not frightening to explore this.)

Sarah as the drip: *OK, I am the drip … I have dropped on Sarah's leg, I've got her, I was trying to drop on her and I'm pleased about that, and I will now be able to get in her system. I will own her. That doesn't feel very nice, I don't feel very proud of myself. It's quite nasty.*

Therapist: *So, as the drip, do you feel nasty or is there a part of you perceiving the drip to be nasty?*

Sarah as the drip: *I'm not nasty, I just need to get what I want. It feels nasty as if I am afraid of being judged but I just need dream-Sarah to stay with me. I'm not trying to be nasty.*

Therapist: *How do you feel (as the drip) about dream-Sarah having to separate from her girls?*

Sarah as the drip: *I feel dispassionate about it, tough luck really, their problem. I'm determined and it's lonely on my own. I want her to stay with me.*

Step 6: Invite sense-making

Offer the client a chance to consider and comment on how the areas that have been explored within the dream resonate with their life now or with anything in therapy, maybe considering the relational processes previously noticed in the therapy.

Therapist: *How does this resonate in your life now?*

Sarah: *Well, I am conscious of the fact that my daughters are leaving home, and I am feeling bereft. I guess, I have a sense that I want to own them, to keep them close. On the other hand, I also want them to spread their wings and move on into their adult lives. So, this is reflected in the dream. Part of me wants to let them go and part of me wants them to stay.*

Therapist: *Does it resonate with anything we are doing in therapy?*

Sarah: *It makes me think about how I can feel bereft when I feel separated from others and how equally I can cope by cutting myself off from them to manage my feelings – like how I felt when you talked to me about the end of this therapy.*

Step 7: Review the client's experience of the process

While reviewing is a useful part of this process, it is important to resist the urge to review sooner than step 7 as this disrupts the flow and risks moving into interpreting and analysing rather than embodying and experiencing.

Offer an opportunity for the client to reflect and comment on their experience of taking part in this dreamwork technique.

Therapist: *What was your experience of the dreamwork today?*

Sarah: *I remember one part where I felt really emotional, and I had a very powerful connection. Because we have worked on a dream before, it was easier this time to get into the character of different elements, I found that while I was doing it, I began thinking about my relationship with myself. I started wondering, when I was describing, about different parts of me and how they relate to one another.*

Step 8: Invite conclusions

Make final conclusions together about what has been learned or understood by the client from this experience.

Therapist: *What strikes you from today?*

Sarah: *It's made me want to think more about these many distinct parts of me, one that is brave and one that can be very vulnerable and needy (as dream-Sarah). Also, as the girls, I realize that their responses to me are not about them but about me. So, part of me is sensible and practical (as Jackie) and knows that tough decisions need to be made, and that other* *parts of me (Sam) feel compassion and a sense of duty – like them, I can stay and sacrifice myself and my own needs. Equally, as the cave, I can be very lonely and empty which feels dank, gloomy, dull and depressing. What was interesting was that as the drips I felt mean, and I didn't care about dream-Sarah. So, part of me can be very cold and feels cruel to myself and to others, I recognize it in myself, I just don't like to admit it.*

Therapist: *Ah, interesting how this awareness is developing and how you can see these different parts that are presenting for you and how they interact with each other.*

Step 9: Share therapeutic observations

The therapist will inevitably make their own sense of what the dreamer is revealing. The challenge is to avoid imposing this on the client. At the very end there may be time and space to share one's experience of being the listener, but this is always done with caution. Since the ownership of the understanding belongs to the dreamer, if the client says it doesn't resonate, then the therapist would accept this. If the therapist imposes their interpretation, however insightful, this betrays the premise of the work and risks invalidating and disrespecting the client.

Therapist: *I was also thinking, as you were describing this, how you often you put others first but at a cost to yourself. We have spoken to the 'shoulds' and how it feels unkind for you to not comply. My sense of you is that you are prepared to be matter of fact, like Jackie in the dream, and even share your disgust of yourself and of others, like your experience of the drip, but it is harder to reveal your neediness of important relationships, to ask people to help you. Does that in any way resonate with you?*

Sarah: *Yes, that makes sense to me. I definitely struggle to be vulnerable; I don't like to feel needy. I feel weak but also reliant on others. I feel like it is tricky to be needy or to rely on others.*

Therapist: *Yes, that is interesting and helpful to be aware of.*

Client: *it is even difficult to admit to you*

Therapist: *I was also thinking about you with your elderly neighbour. How you are very generous and kind to him but there are times when you feel encroached upon.*

Sarah: *Yes, that's true, sometimes, this feels bad to say, but it feels like he is like the drip, trying to keep me close. I feel resentful and want to get away,* *but I stay to be 'good' and bury my feelings of resentment. I kind of keep them hidden in the cave!*

Step 10: Return the dream to the dreamer

At the end of the process, it is respectful to return the dream to the dreamer. The script written by the therapist is given to them, representing their ownership of it.

Troubleshooting

There may be times when it feels like the dream technique is not working, especially when learning. Taking the time to review and reflect on what may be getting in the way can be helpful; being open to asking questions of ourselves without giving up on the technique is recommended as difficulties encountered early on can most often be easily resolved. Some ideas and suggestions have been added below to assist in the readers troubleshooting process once practice in the model is underway.

Attend mindfully to creating a space where therapeutic work can occur within the relationship while observing tolerable limits (ZPD) for both therapist and client. If the therapist feels anxious, this will interfere with attunement and no doubt reduce the sense of ease in the environment for both parties. Enthusiastic therapists may jump in too soon, the client may not have developed an established relationship with the therapist and is perhaps not yet familiar with the therapist's style and the nature of the therapy. If a client brings a dream in very early sessions, the therapist may choose to simply introduce dreamwork to the client and defer engagement in the process until the client is ready.

Sequencing during the dreamwork is important to consider. Introduce the technique in a way that invites curiosity in the client towards their dreams and dreaming experience; offer a sense of interest rather than trepidation towards the dream. The choice of dream element to embody is important and can influence the effectiveness of the process. It is usual to take them in order but there may be reason to deviate from that should the client need to. The aim is always to do as much as we can but as little as we need to.

Since the therapist chooses which element to explore, it will be helpful to be aware of elements we may be avoiding asking the client to embody. We need to be mindful of our decisions regarding which of the elements we are asking them to embody. *What are we interested in? What are we excited about? What is our experience of hearing the dream? What is being enacted with the client and us in this moment? Is it possible we are avoiding addressing any element?* Try to remember that we are seeking to gain awareness from all aspects, the sunshine, and the shadow.

We want to address the 'monster' in the dream, however it would not necessarily be the *first* element of the dream to embody, as this may risk activating the client's threat system making it more difficult for them to remain embodied in that element of the dream. It is important to mindfully consider whether they are ready to embody that element. Important elements will return in other dreams and, although it is not helpful to avoid these in their entirety, timing and client willingness will always be significant. For instance, if someone has been raped and experienced dreams about being raped, it would not be helpful for them to be introduced to the dreamwork by immediately embodying the dream-rapist. However, with a good therapeutic relationship, and confidence in the dream process, it is important for the dream-rapist to be embodied in time, so that the client can access those abusing parts that may be enacted intrapersonally; self-to-self. Embodiment of the abusing part can reveal its intention. The intention could be anything, for example, from wanting to hurt dream-self to wanting to get close to dream-self or feeling pushed away. When we communicate that these are all elements of the dream and there is nothing to fear, it was dreamt, it did not happen in that moment, and it is not happening in this, we invite a new relationship with the dream and with themselves to emerge.

Ideally, the therapist learns this technique experientially, gaining familiarity and trust in the model themselves, and learning from their own dream exploration that embodying the less-palatable aspects of the dream can be interesting and a valuable route to discovering new information about oneself.

Depending on the therapeutic background or temperament of the therapist, it might be tempting to interpret or ask a lot of questions. This will certainly impact the flexibility and the flow of dreamwork and act as an interference rather than an intended assistance. Sometimes there is an impatience for the work to make sense and for the client to find it useful, which all adds pressure and takes away from the experience of self-discovery that this technique affords. The challenge is to be patient and remain compassionately curious. We are there as if to facilitate the flow of the river, not to change its course. The therapist's role is to remain warmly neutral; conveying a sense of approval may be communicated as leading the client's direction of exploration, and conveying disapproval may be seen as blocking it.

Clients may struggle with the metaphorical concepts and respond concretely, receiving the metaphor literally. While we still might attempt dreamwork with these clients, we would be prepared to drop it as an intervention if the process of delivering it became an unhelpful re-enactment.

Should a client dislike the experience of the dreamwork, is suspicious, or doesn't find it useful, then it may be important to move the focus to exploring the therapeutic process and looking to identify enactments in the room, for example: *What was that like to do that with me? What showed up with you? With us? Where are we/you on your map?* Sometimes the *experience* of delivering the technique can be the most valuable endeavour and careful attention to this can yield awareness of expressions of Procedural or Reciprocal Role enactments in the therapeutic encounter.

Adaptations of the dreamwork

One of the joys of this work is how it can be applied in different ways, not just in working with dreams. Embodiment provides an invitation to explore creatively and playfully, in a visceral way. Once a client is familiar with this through the dreamwork, it is easy to switch into other embodied explorations, perhaps only briefly yet often yielding poignant insights for the client. Some examples of this from our own practice are described below.

Exploring the self through a selected imaginal object

For example:

Therapist: *Tell me, if you were an animal, what would you be?*

Client: *I would be a monkey.*

Therapist: *Can you **be** that monkey in their habitat?*

Client as a monkey: *I am swinging through the trees.*

Therapist: *What is around you?*

Client as a monkey: *The jungle, a tiger.*

Therapist: *What is it like to be in the jungle? How do you feel about the tiger? Now can you be the tiger? What are you like? How do you (as the tiger) feel about the monkey?*

Extending the Six-Part Story Method

For those familiar with the Six-Part Story Method (Dent-Brown, 2011; see Appendix 5), we have extended the method to embody elements of the client's created story. Invite the client to *be* the different elements in the story, the habitat, the tools, the obstacles etc, and then to explore how the different elements feel and relate to each other. This extends the metaphor and yields further meaning.

Art

The client could bring in drawings or be invited to draw something. For example, you could ask them to draw a house and them in it and notice how they draw it and embody different aspects.

Therapist: *Can you be the house?*

Client as the house: *I am big, with big windows, with empty rooms.*

Therapist: *What does that feel like to you as the house?*

Client as the house: *I feel bold but a little lost.*

Therapist: *How does this resonate with you? You said, as the house, that you were bold, lost…?*

Be an object in your life

Invite a client to share an object that they treasure or, indeed, that they don't like, for instance their car or house. Invite them to embody that object. In the case of a client who is very proud of their car:

Therapist: *Can you be your car?*

Client as the car: *I am fast, I am expensive, I am red.*

Therapist: *So, is there a part of you who feels fast, expensive, and red? What does that mean to you? What does that tell you about the qualities that you value? Is there anything here to be interested in? How does that resonate with how you feel about your life?*

Be the disorder

For example, invite embodiment of a disorder.

Therapist: *Can you be the anorexia nervosa and speak from there?*

Client as the anorexia nervosa: *I have control.*

Therapist: *How do you feel about Gill* [Gill is the client here]*?*

Client as the anorexia nervosa: *I fear for her, and I want to protect her.*

Therapist: *How do you protect Gill?*

Be an element of the disorder/problem

For example, invite the client to embody the vomit:

Client as the vomit: *I am being pushed out and rejected.*

Therapist: *How do you feel about James* [James is the client here]*?*

Client as the vomit: *He wants to get rid of me.*

Therapist: *Does this resonate with you in any way?*

Client: *I felt like my dad always wanted to get rid of me. And I felt I must be disgusting, there was something wrong with me. I feel like I am disgusting like the vomit and don't deserve to stay.*

Body dysmorphia

Like being the disorder, be the body part that is unloved:

Therapist: *Can you be the legs?*

Client as the legs: *I am the legs, I am unloved, rejected, frightened etc... I am alone, nobody wants me.*

Using client's turn of phrase

Pick up examples of how the client uses language, for example:

Client: *I feel like I am sinking, like there is a heavy weight on me.*

Therapist: *Can you be the weight for a moment?*

Client as the weight: *I am strong, I am pushing Julie down in the water.*

Therapist: *How do you feel towards Julie?*

Client as the weight: *She is weak, she makes mistakes, she needs to be kept down and hidden.*

Therapist: *Can you be the water?*

Client as the water: *I'm holding her, I want to support her.*

Therapist: *How do you feel about the weight?*

Client as the water: *I'm angry with it, it's hurting Julie.*

Review:

Therapist: *Does this make sense to you in any way? Is there a part of you that wants to support you and another part of you that feels you should be kept down and hidden?*

These are just some of many ways to creatively use the principles of this technique. Once the client is familiar with the idea, it is often easy to bring in the technique naturally and flexibly as and when an opportunity arises.

Conclusion

This dreamwork technique offers an opportunity for collaborative, creative and often playful access to imaginal material that may be outside of our client's understanding or conscious awareness. Together, there is an opportunity to explore procedural patterns of relating, while maintaining a safe distance from the trauma of lived experience.

Dreamwork invites visceral re-experiencing of the dream, while ownership and interpretation respectfully remain with the dreamer. The client's embodied relationship with the dream may change from emotional disturbance to curiosity and insight. Disavowed material may become available, and the richness of the dream's metaphors can deepen therapeutic understanding. The technique is easily learned by the therapist and can potentially be taught to the client.

Future developments of this technique can be extended to several different adaptations so that the principles can be applied rapidly and briefly to capture the essence of a moment, such as a turn of phrase, pain or even a feeling of being stuck. We are limited only by our imagination and our willingness to explore with playful curiosity.

Sophie and Nicola have written about this dreamwork technique in *Reformulation* and presented the technique at conferences as well as for UK training events. They have been using and adapting this technique for over twenty-five years.

Chapter 7:
Enabling change through metaphor and imagery

James Turner

Introduction

This chapter is intended to explore and inform readers on the use of metaphor and pictorial metaphor as part of the therapeutic encounter. The technique, arising from clinical practice, has been extensively researched and evaluated and appears to have salience for the work we do (Turner, 2011; 2014). In CAT, metaphor is a recognized clinical focus and there is a growing body of research into the use of metaphor and creative approaches to therapy which this chapter is informed by.

In my CAT clinic, I started to listen out more to capture metaphoric images as they arose in my clients' dialogue. Catching metaphors as part of the conversation prevents lost meaning as the conversation develops, (Törneke, 2017) and exploration of the metaphor enables discovery of more information as it is live in the discussion (Bayne & Thompson, 2000). One day, I started to draw these caught metaphors on a piece of A4 paper using rudimentary representative drawings and a limited colour palette (highlighting pens). With further reading, it seems as if I was intuitively following steps suggest by Kopp (2013), who suggests that paying attention to metaphor was enabling, listening out for the metaphor, and asking what images or picture comes to mind. Kopp (2013) sees the client's imagery as central, but I also find that the therapist's imagery of the client's metaphor is valid.

I would like to reassure colleagues that this working on the pictorial metaphor is not art psychotherapy, but an attempt to support the work of CAT therapists with their clients to enable the change process. I am mindful of Potter's work on mapping on a CAT diagram, how the client's words drive the pen and hover over the page. It is thus with the pictorial metaphor, a memorable image that is captured, that is emotive and can become a central theme to the dialogue. The image is grounded in the client's understanding and therapist's understanding, explored and developed together, and comes to represent complex emotional aspects of the care as well as hoped for or exit positions.

I recall a dialogue with Tony Ryle in which I discussed the development of this work on pictorial metaphor, and he replied, 'CAT is what works, if pictures work then use them'. This seemed a fair proposition for an integrated therapy, to build on the usefulness of metaphor as part of CAT work, but then to extend this with a deliberate focus on the imagery that emerges around a metaphor, drawing it, checking this out with the client, and using these central themes to support the process of change.

Context and supporting theory

Metaphors have been an essential feature of human communication since time immemorial (Barker, 1985), being mental constructs that shape our thinking about the world and reality (Saban, 2006). Metaphor is considered an indispensable structure of human understanding through which we figuratively comprehend our world (Hermans, 2003). Lakoff and Johnson (1980) write that we are not simply given our world, but it is constructed through the way we make meaning of our perceptions and thoughts. Lakoff and Turner (2009) suggest that conscious knowledge is commonly understood through metaphor: 'knowing is seeing, when we see something in a new way, we know it in a new way' (cited Siegelman, 1993, p5).

Metaphor, it is argued, is a primary or first-order development of the mind. Metaphor not only enables language to develop; it is also through metaphor that we come to understand the world (Siegelman, 1993), and we more than likely use metaphor when discussing experiences of high emotion (Fainsilber & Ortony 1987). Potts and Semino (2019) view metaphor in health and illness as significant and idiosyncratic; likewise Charles and Felton (2020) perceive them as representing inner states. Metaphors appear to have several functions:

- **Understanding a history:** Witztum *et al* (1988) describe metaphor as a 'kernel statement' expressing something essential so the mind can manage complex concepts (Serig, 2008). Metaphors provide a language of flexibility (Billow, 1977) linking complicated thoughts, feelings and emotions, simplifying these complex emotional strands into a memorable event, at the same time reducing the infinite possibilities available to the mind.

- **Exploring emotions:** McMullen (2008) notes parallels in both metaphor and emotion as well as metaphor and the conceptual. We use metaphor intuitively and unconsciously to understand the mind, emotions, and all other abstract concepts (Eynon, 2002) in so far as the metaphor enables us to understand unembodied things.

- **Expressing the inexpressible:** Metaphors, through understanding one thing in relation to another, by focusing on similarities and analogies between the two phenomena, are considered instruments of discovery (Saban, 2006). Their value lies when the metaphor is interwoven into a story, as if it mirrors the patient's situation, reframes meaning and suggests methods for resolution (Heiney, 1995). Metaphor 'condenses complex and even opposite feelings, needs, wishes, fears and experiences, it does so with great economy and apparent simplicity' (Fraser, 1998, p142).

- **As a shorthand:** Serig (2008) notes that metaphors can unearth buried affect and provide insight by making the past present and the unconscious conscious. Strong (1989) noticed metaphors of the 'greatest significance are those expressed without consciousness … are part of the patient's language, or in dynamic terms "outcroppings of the unconscious"' (p203); as if, working with metaphors brings a heightened consciousness and involvement in and with the metaphor (Siegelman, 1993).

- **Vivid description:** Metaphors can seemingly be used to get to, explore and understand a person's inner, psychodynamic representations of the world (Domino *et al*, 1992), they can reduce defensiveness and provide 'aha' moments, leading to insight and change (Pernicano, 2010) and may play a substantial role in identifying how patients cope psychologically with their illness (Spall *et al*, 2001). Metaphors work on an interactive level, having a shared language, creating meaning within a literal system; both the speaker and listener must understand the current meaning and at the same time have referent appreciation based upon their existing understanding of the phenomena in which the metaphor is applied (McIntosh, 2010).

- **Supporting the therapeutic relationship:** The relationship's foundation rests on a successful alliance whose quality depends on the extent the patient and therapist agree on tasks, achieve goals and the quality of the bond developing between them (Keijser *et al*, 2000). Kok *et al* (2011) found that the poetic nature of metaphor can create a therapeutic relationship with patients as space was created within language to allow new construction of meanings to generate changes while Gibbs (2019) noted metaphor as an active enactment in relationships and the environment. As metaphors arise, are noted and used, they become educational tools, extending and broadening the boundaries of beliefs about thinking (Abbatielo, 2006) and the imaginal and metaphoric forms of cognition' (Kopp, 1995, p133).

- **Visualizing exits:** Strong (1989) notes that the use of and acceptance of metaphor as a genuine form of patients' experience and communication could provide counsellors with a viable medium for effecting change. Metaphor can help make meaning of the problems of living through their expression (Barker & Buchanan-Barker, 2005). Battino (2002) notes, 'if you work within your patients own metaphoric imagination, then you are closer to their internal being' (ibid, p22).

Pictorial metaphor (PM)

Images and imagery are all around us and are worthy of exploration. The CAT diagram picture enables the creative mind to see problem procedures. The pictorial method is the study of the self's spatial and temporal dimensions as an adjunct to narrative. Metaphors, deriving from the imagination and dialogic nature of the individual, the dialogue that occurs within, between, and without, can be expressed in pictures and such visual metaphors can be noticed (Dent & Rosenberg, 1990).

In CAT, the diagram pictorially summarizes the patient's problems, how they were developed and how they are maintained, similar to a case conceptualization (Freeman & Dattilio, 1992) where schemas, behaviours, thoughts and actions are understood in the individual's psychological context. Acting as a mind map, the CAT diagram allows the therapist to integrate and organize a formulation in an easily adaptable way (Williams *et al*, 1997). The literature suggested that an image-laden metaphor represented as a picture is not such an inferential leap as a means to explore a patient's problem procedures and information, and allowing an active focus; in fact, it can become a central summary of the case (Williams *et al*, 1997).

Metaphors have been noted to be empathetic and resonant (Black, 1998) and their art representations have inherent strength, producing alternative perspectives for both the patient and observer (Riley, 2004). Aldrich (1968) considers metaphor as a fusion (or function) of the object and interpretation whereby a created object holds metaphoric understanding. Freeman and Dattilio (1992) discuss a sketch made by the therapist to represent the core problem and Lacroix *et al* (2011) note that bringing an image to conscious awareness can alleviate conflict through the therapeutic relationship.

Using art techniques suggests that change happens because of the transference of verbal information into visual form offering an alternative means of meeting need (Gentile, 1997). The picture is bringing the metaphoric image back to life (Witztum *et al*, 1988) which can lead the patient to developing transformational plans for life, plans to change, if you like, arising from the developing imagery, transforming mental representations (Francis *et al*, 2011).

Metaphors are considered to reflect and activate pre-existing conceptual mappings in long-term memory (Glucksberg & Keysar, 1990). Wilkinson (2010) notes, that long-term emotional memories can be affected positively through the process of therapy and that art representation of metaphor can be psychologically enabling. Metaphor helps to change perspective, provide a bridge between thought and feeling and provide a consistent language in therapy helping significant events be recalled through the use of metaphor (Stott *et al*, 2010). This bridge between thought and feeling is well documented (Kopp, 1995; Strong, 1989).

CAT therapists and pictorial metaphor

The therapist is already familiar with constructing a picture in the form of a diagram (Ryle & Kerr, 2020). The diagram is an enabler, as is the pictorial metaphor (PM); they can become a memorable image, can come to mind to create a full stop, a pause even, in a patient's behaviour, an 'aha' moment (Siegelman, 1993), and open other possibilities for action. The PM is akin to a mind map in a pictorial form, one way of quickly accessing key experiences. In creating a pictorial mind map, metaphor such as this can be quickly updated and amended as new resonant images emerge between the client and therapist.

CAT therapists, in the author's facilitated pictorial metaphor workshops, had used clip art on the diagram and linked images to the map and had renewed interest in using metaphoric pictures subsequently. Verbal and pictorial metaphors being linked to the diagram held the highest level of agreement across the statements that were rated by the author's Delphi research. Clearly this is an important aspect of working within the CAT model and applying this PM technique to processes already in place. It would seem fair to say that if the metaphor did not relate, then one would suggest that it may be the wrong metaphor. As the metaphor should be jointly arrived at through collaborative understanding, it should therefore be representative, as McIntosh (2010) notes.

Therapist metaphors

Barker (1996) observes that family therapists may offer metaphors for strategic direction while Searle (1985) reinforces the importance of meaning in metaphor; it is always the speaker's meaning that is important. Martin *et al* (1992) noted that patients tended to recall therapists' intentional metaphors approximately two-thirds of the time, especially when these metaphors were developed collaboratively and used repetitively.

One of the early concerns expressed by participants was the therapist drawing the metaphoric picture and indeed the therapist offering a metaphor. What is important is the collaborative co-construction of the PM. Results of my research supported therapists offering metaphor, in fact, Martin *et al* (1992) reinforce the therapist noticing and offering metaphor which was a distinguishing aspect of their research. Training materials and a self-assessment developing out of the emerging data were tested in practice on CAT groups as well as snowballing groups as the researcher put his theories out into the public domain. The important aspect of the therapist drawing is the checking for fit and co-constructed way the metaphor comes to be on the page.

Experience of using PM

Following an extensive Delphi and action research study, ten important factors for using the PM emerged, as shown in Table 7.1.

Table 7.1: Top ten coded statements/events

Shared understanding
Client-derived
Locate to model
Therapeutic alliance
Collaborative
Willingness to work with metaphor
Simplicity
Work within ZPD
Ongoing
Non-judgemental

The most important factor was to gain a *shared understanding* of the metaphor because metaphors that are taken for granted and not explored can lead to misunderstandings. Therefore, if one hears a metaphor that seems to have salience for the patient's situation, it is useful to clarify the meaning rather than just accept it and move on. Responder's comments (in italics) have noted the importance of a shared understanding and shared language between them to '*deepen joint understanding*'. As well as *understanding* of metaphor, the therapists '*empathy and understanding*' for each patient was noted.

Client-derived material is the bedrock of the therapeutic encounter. Sometimes this is in the form of a history, a story, a set of immediate emotions and sometimes as metaphor images. Responders noted the ability of metaphor to 'combine and express complex and often contradictory issues', 'capturing complexity and enrich description' while 'providing a bridge between "thought and feeling"'. Client-derived metaphors were viewed as most significant, but it was supported for therapists to offer a metaphor if it felt appropriate. When a client or therapist introduces a live metaphor, as it emerges, it allows the client to shape his or her own conscious experience, thus new meanings and new sensations are experienced (Fraser, 1998). The usefulness of metaphor in managing emotions, and using them as part of an ongoing therapy, is that they have a way of 'changing perspective from a locked pattern of thought' by 'translating actual experiences into a pattern that can be generalized and applied to both past, present and future'.

Locate to model applies to the integrated model where the research was initially formulated. The use of metaphors would be incorporated into the stages of the model of reformulation, recognition, and revision. This is important because this is '*a*' metaphor technique as part of established encounter work not '*the*' metaphor model.

The importance of the therapeutic relationship, in the ability of metaphors to extend and develop the relationship, while supporting collaboration emerged. Metaphors built a 'shared language' while 'aiding the clients understanding of the therapeutic process'. Using metaphor helped to set achievable goals and 'get to previously untouchable or unmentionable' emotions. Responders suggested that therapeutic collaboration was supported through the process of listening and focusing on the client's experiences and recognizing that metaphors are part of a client's identity and are a 'powerful means by which the therapist can communicate with him/her'.

A focus on and willingness to explore the client's meaning of a metaphor was noted to support collaborative relationship. Whereby an element of creativity in the encounter appeared to aid recognition of client problems. What seems important is the nature of metaphors linking 'the creative exploration of the client's sense of self and may reconnect the client to a new sense of self' and 'so by engaging with them the therapist is getting close to a client's emotional self'.

One metaphor at a time, 'keep it simple', was supported and as you can see in Figure 7.2, the image is rudimentary but was jointly explored with the young person and emerged from the dialogue between them. Equally, this case study expresses the usefulness of working in a clients ZPD as well as being non-judgemental in the development of the art. This was especially important when using the image as a pictorial metaphor as many responders noted they had pejorative experiences of artmaking from school. What helps here is that the therapist is the art-maker in this model, making the initial drawing, but confirming with the client at all stages whether it was representative of their 'image'.

The results of the Delphi research were considered transferable to other therapeutic approaches for testing, so the researcher explored the approach further with CAT therapists and with a group of counsellors and with a sample of bereavement counsellors. The Action Research philosophy of the research supported data being collected from a range of samples, as the individuals have a depth and breadth of experience and still represent heterogeneous and homogenous groups (Parahoo, 1997). The remainder of this article will outline findings from bereavement counsellor groups.

Descriptive case studies

With the clients' permissions granted, I will present four case studies demonstrating the use and practice of the PM method.

Case study 1

By means of stepping into pictorial metaphor, I am providing here an example of a pictorial metaphor from a non-CAT clinic experience, as I see the value of metaphor and PM in bereavement work and have worked extensively with CRUSE bereavement counselling service, developing an understanding of the value of PM with them. The case study illustrates the wider use of PM as well as the depth of meaning of one event in a person's life and how pictorial metaphor can capture it.

This is a very personal story of helping my daughter explore her responses to grief. Niemeyer's work often guides me here, the sense that bereavement is a narrative, not a set of stages. After the sudden death of her grandmother, 'Dad' she said through her tears, 'it's like I have been given a jigsaw but there's a bit missing, as if I have a hole in my heart that will never heal'. My own heart ached for her, but we explored and discussed how of course her loss is an absence, but over time, while her missing piece of jigsaw would remain, the hole would in fact become smaller.

Figure 7.1: 'A hole in my heart'

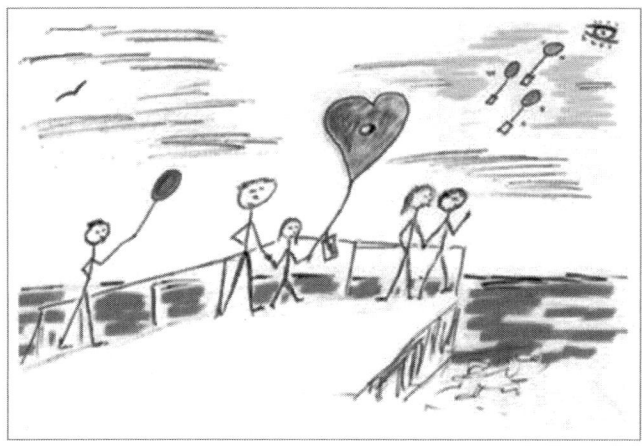

We began to explore this imagery and metaphor as meaning making and as part of her developing understanding. She described how her loss was like a hole in her heart and how she wanted to have a goodbye event to mark Nana's passing. Between us we created an image of a balloon ceremony to say goodbye, where we would write a note to her 'Nana' and release these to the heavens. As she spoke, I drew. You can see the parts of the jigsaw being the people in the drawing; the place is significant as it is where her Nana lived. One balloon, heart-shaped with a hole, is held by her, as she is holding my hand, and some are released with the notes of farewell. In the top right-hand corner is the CAT eye, observing but also experiencing. She found this picture genuinely enabling.

Case study 2

Mark (a pseudonym) is a middle-aged company director/owner who had a motorcycle accident causing a degree of brain trauma. He came to therapy to help manage his recovery as well as to look through a CAT lens at his premorbid coping mechanisms. The accident left him feeling angry, with feelings of worthlessness. As well as exploring the impact of his accident on his activities of daily living, we explored his past and Reciprocal Role procedures systematically. This sat well with him as an engineer, as he saw CAT as 'a method with a procedure… I wanted to gain a set of actions for continuing future use'.

You can see on his picture several images. One is a representation of the accident crashing into a barrier. He commented: 'The investigations during my therapy lead to some important points. Knowing these and their background allows me to act accordingly when situations arise. Jim summarized these points with a picture.'

Again, the drawing starts with an eye, as seen in the top left corner. Then drawing the crash seemed important, as it was a significant event and it helped us to see its impact – how it had changed his world somewhat, as shown by the question mark. He reported that he was tired a lot of the time, anxious about performing to the high level he was used to, and felt he was letting people down. A reflection of a Reciprocal Role of 'criticizing to criticized' is indicated by the pointed hand with the word 'critical' written on it. He noted: 'A glance at the picture reminds me of all the major points and the relevant thought behind them. It summarizes the important findings that I need to keep fresh, clear and forward in my mind.'

The images of the chequered step with the compassionate holding hand arose as we discussed ways for him to stop and check in with his thoughts recognize his patterns, akin to a check step in a castle, that stops the person and gives them time to think. This enabled him to put some actions into his weekly routine to aid his recovery, like afternoon naps, as well as to generally be compassionate towards himself. The image in the top right being a spotlight on his roles of 'confident self (expectant) to worthless self (performing)'. He noted: 'The picture gives me a precise, practical view of the therapy, why it was required and the outcomes it produced.'

What I find interesting here is the impression of CAT as practical and how the picture reminds him of both the major points (in his reformulation) but also the thoughts behind them. I am also thinking of the comment that the picture summarizes points that are 'fresh and clear in my mind', an important reflection. I am informed by Paul Gilbert's (2009) 'compassionate mind' work at the moment and found with this client that it was very important to help him become more compassionate with himself, hence the 'supporting hand'.

Figure 7.2: Mark's drawing

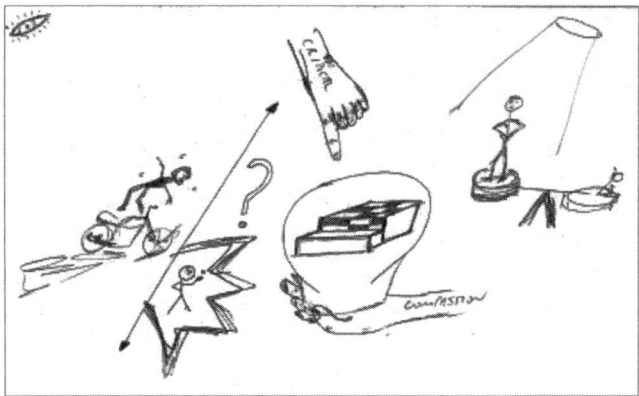

Case study 3

Joseph is a young man with an anxiety disorder and some traits of obsessive-compulsive disorder.

As his story and as therapy emerged, we began to map his metaphors. They seemed to speak of the meaning of his world and experience within it, as well as the process of change in therapy. I seem to draw from left to right, as we in Western cultures tend to write. This enables space on the page to have a flow to the images, as they initially emerge between us to speak of warded-off and difficult places, and then move across the page to images of the preferred position of change. I always start the blank page with drawing an eye in either the top left or right-hand corner (the I-thou). I also draw an eye on the diagram which provides a bridge between the two, as if the metaphoric representations in art also represent the problem procedures identified in the diagram.

With Joseph, the first metaphor we drew was the clock, bowl, thermometer and vortex. The clock was an indication of the anxious days passing, the bowl with him inside expresses how he feels every day, as if swimming through soup, the thermometer shows how his anxiety can rise like heat (it has FFF on it denoting fight, flight and freeze in response to anxiety), and the vortex represents his catastrophic thinking. You can see small dominoes in the vortex being suggestive of the way thoughts can fall into another thought, as dominoes if they are placed in a sequence can fall onto the next one and so on. As he noted in his goodbye letter: 'As I progressed through the therapy process, I identified some images that described my overcoming of this initial "swimming through" and these were depicted by Jim and positioned at the 'other end of the vortex'.

As we progressed through therapy, we drew further images onto his diagram that reflected the work we were doing and how he changed over time, perhaps even towards a hoped-for position. The hoped-for position is akin to Zatloukal *et al*'s (2019) work, whereby metaphor can act as a process to map preferred futures. In this respect, the heart, wind cloud and moving clock in the bottom left represent our relationship, how he described the therapeutic encounter as holding and progressive, time on the move. On the right-hand side of the vortex you can see a question mark and star constellations, representing hoped-for new beginnings and opportunities, and a fish, Dory from 'Finding Nemo', a DreamWorks film, where the fish Dory appears to have an ability to seize opportunities while at the same time being anxious. Joseph wrote: 'The image of the fish, for example, came from the idea of a fish that is able to keep on swimming, regardless of difficulties it encounters.'

A final important image was that of a path upon which walks an explorer, leaning against a palm tree. This was a hoped-for and felt position, as if he was prepared. He used to come to session with a small bag with various objects in it, so we metaphorically added to this bag the changes he had felt and worked on in therapy. He noted:

'The image of an explorer emerged towards the end of the sessions in an answer to a question from Jim as to how I now perceived myself, having gone through the process of therapy; in this case I perceived myself as being ready to venture into the potentially exciting realm of the unknown, complete with a 'toolkit' that I could use in order to examine and help any psychological problems that I found flaring up in myself.'

Figure 7.3: Joseph's drawing

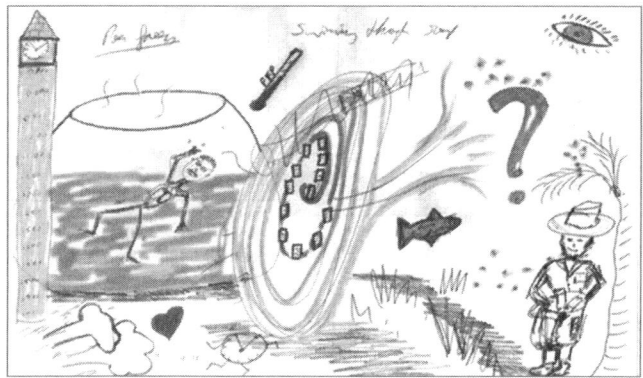

Case study 4

Charlie (a pseudonym) works in student health and has a PhD as well as multiple other skills. She came to therapy stressed and anxious about work and some relational difficulties she was experiencing with her close family. She had previous therapies, but these had not helped enough, and she felt were 'a waste of time', so she was sceptical of CAT. As her history emerged, she spoke of a metaphor of anger as a bomb, the ACME bomb that we then drew on her page. This was related to a 'criticizing to criticized' RRP. She noted the anger as being linked to where 'criticism and unhelpful comments from my mother and sister were something I grew up with from an early age, only I was never able to see them as such before'. The image helped to see how central these were, as she noted: 'I still feel the sense of anger is somewhat positive. It's a realization that it is not my fault, that I have not been treated right, and that I do deserve better. I didn't have this knowledge before.'

The person standing at the water's edge, holding a chest, is significant as this is where she came to an 'ah-ha' moment on the beach one day: 'My first breakthrough came at the beach, in the sea of all places... I suddenly realized I had to look much closer and a lot further in the past to find the root cause [of her upset].'

The other images on the page are change-related, a small (sad-looking) and larger (happier-looking) matryoshka, the smaller one recognizing the young person she was and the larger one how she feels now, happier and more prepared for the future. These images are supported by a person with a bag and tools, as if 'I have tools in my backpack to get me there'.

The flags 'rising above' also denote change and some core exits, one flag 'the real whopper…all illuminating breakthrough' with "good enough" written on, reminds the client that 'good enough is achievable, perfect does not have an upper limit'. She wrote: 'from this realization then came my flags: F*** it, "it is what it is" and the most important one, "I can only do what I can do" … all perfectly obvious from a rational point of view'.

These comments she made in her goodbye letter and appear to show the resonance of the flags in expressing the thoughts and emotions she shared in sessions, and how the images can represent painful emotions but also hoped-for changes and strategies for change.

Figure 7.4: Charlie's drawing

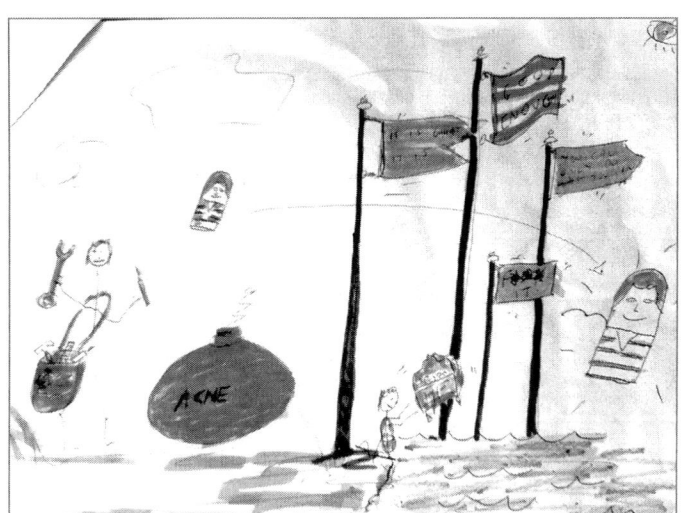

Limitations

Not every client and every encounter raise opportunities for the representation of metaphor in a picture and there are times when one has to abandon working in this way, or when this way of working does not sit well with the client. I recall one client who was quite determined not to have a picture when I suggested we draw something together. S, I stopped drawing, therapy progressed as per the CAT model with our attention on metaphors as part of the therapeutic work.

Likewise, some people (therapists) are cautious as they have perceived ideas about art and art making, but while this work uses images as representations, I don't see it as art or art therapy, but as a way of enabling the encounter. As you can see from the case examples, the drawings are quite rudimentary – they don't have an artist's skill, but they do represent the metaphor. Each image is checked out for congruence as they develop with the client, asking what colours to use, and whether the image resonates (and if it doesn't, I change it so that it does).

Choosing and using a metaphor can be spontaneously derived from either the client's or the therapist's dialogue. However, therapist-derived metaphors are contentious and may speak of the power imbalances between and client and a therapist, whereby the therapist may be seen as the 'expert'. Therefore, co-constructed and dialogic therapies, being mindful of these vicissitudes, should guard against this potential by always coming to a shared understanding of metaphor. This leads to participation that is inherently collaborative and the 'push and pull' of the relationship is more visible (Potter, 2010). Often therapists 'lead' encounters, so why not 'lead' in drawing? What is important is to 'check out' as one draws that the image is 'OK' for the client and to engage them in its further development. Questions might include: 'Is it ok if I sketch out the image that has come to mind? Does it look like this? What else is on the page? Are there any colours that are important? What might change look like? These are all helpful in exploring the image.

Summary

I hope that this chapter has been useful and that you feel there is enough detail here for you to have a go at drawing with your clients the metaphors that arise between you in session. My clients and I have genuinely found this an enabling process, one that appears to enhance the CAT model and provides a visual representation of core pain, central themes and preferred positions. The pictures appear to be another transitional object as part of CAT. I have been privileged to notice and complete hundreds of pictorial metaphor pictures with clients. Some have been complex, others less so, but it is about what works for each individual. Don't feel the need to have a very complex image, just something that resonates and works.

Chapter 8:
Relational dialogues with the inner child

Louise Yorke

> 'The baby inside. This was a totally new theme to me before this therapy.'
>
> (Goodbye Letter to Tony Ryle: Ryle, 1990, p. 52)

Introduction

When lives are affected by complexity, therapy can be transformative. Inner-child work is described here as a trauma-focused tool that can inform relational dialogues in CAT to improve therapeutic outcomes.

The door to the inner child, CAT and me

The first door that opened onto the world of the inner child was in the house where I lived. Like many children, I felt somewhat mystified by the world and my role in it. At some point, another door opened and in walked Dibs (Axline, 1964). In real life, Dibs was a troubled five-year-old boy. After a year of play therapy, where his feelings and family relationships were explored, a door opened that enabled Dibs to achieve his potential. Axline had recognized that, when he was given 'what was needed', namely, a new way of relating involving noticing, exploring, connecting and recognizing, Dibs was able to express his feelings and interact socially.

Years later, still reflecting on life's mysteries, I walked through another door, holding the scroll of a doctoral psychologist. Having learned of the link between childhood and adult development, I should not have been surprised by who I met upon stepping inside the clinic room. There, albeit in another guise, in another story, in the lives and relationships of others, was Dibs. And so it was that the child's needs for healthy relationships led me to CAT and to develop within it a relational approach to working with the inner child.

Historical foundations of inner-child work

Throughout history, a key element of psychological practice has been to process and understand traumatic experiences. Pioneers Charcot and Janet recognized 'that merely uncovering memories was not enough; they needed to be modified and transformed, i.e., placed in their proper context and reconstructed into neutral or meaningful narratives' (van der Kolk & van der Hart, 1989, p1538). Informed by the studies of Josef Breuer, Freud (1962, p33) acknowledged that there could be 'a return to health' once traumatic memories had been recalled and processed.

Freud's contemporary (Jung, 1902, p293) also recognized that there was a relationship between historical trauma and the present, citing 'traumatic neuroses, where the illness stands in reciprocal relationship to the injuriousness of the cause'. Jung describes how the child-self, or '*puer Archetype*' (Jung, 1951, p8284), as if frozen in time, has the capacity to affect the life of the adult-self. Later, Winnicott (1958, p238) identified the necessary and positive impact of a relationally attuned 'good-enough' parent, who could give the child what they needed, to enable the development of secure attachment, independence and associated trauma-moderating relational capacities.

Recent developments in inner-child work

Ultimately, these early psychological conceptualizations of trauma form a pathway to inner-child work, which recognizes that psychological problems are resolved by connection with and processing of the trauma and its impact on inner aspects of self. The child-self has become a recognized focus for resolving trauma (Axline, 1964). Working from the 1970s in the established Jungian tradition of journaling, art therapist Lucia Capacchione (1991; 2015; 2017) used words and images to access the inner child and enable left and right-brain dialogue as a means of integrating and overcoming traumatic memories. In the following years, inner-child approaches proliferated, with each model integrating different theories, for example: phases of childhood development (Bradshaw, 1990); Transactional Analysis, Cognitive Behaviour Therapy and Neurolinguistic Programming (Parks, 1990; 1994); Emotion-Focused Therapy, developmental theory and structured inner-child work (Taylor, 1991).

More recently, the importance of being in dialogue with the patient's inner world has become a mainstay of trauma-informed therapies (ISSTD, 2011; van der Kolk, 2014). The most recognized of these can involve forms of imagery processing and rescripting, for example: Eye Movement Desensitization and Reprocessing (EMDR, Shapiro 2001), Trauma-Focused Cognitive Behaviour Therapy (Smucker & Dancu, 1999; Ehlers & Clark, 2000), Internal Family Systems (Schwartz, 1995; West, 2021). Some approaches specifically include inner-child work as the focus of imagery rescripting, for example, in combination with cognitive behaviour therapy (Hestbech, 2018). Furthermore, it has been shown that processing and rescripting traumatic childhood imagery has outcomes consistent with EMDR (Boterhaven de Haan *et al* (2020). Imagery rescripting has also been shown to be effective as a stand-alone treatment for post-traumatic stress disorder and associated emotions, such as anger, shame and guilt (Raabe *et al*, 2022), when compared with psychoeducation and emotion regulation skills.

The inner child in socio-cultural narratives
From Buddhism to TikTok

The inner child is also recognized in socio-cultural intergenerational narratives from Buddhism to TikTok. To cite the Buddhist monk, author, activist and mindfulness teacher Thich Nhat Hanh (2011):

> *'When we think of listening with compassion, we usually think of listening to someone else. But we must also listen to the wounded child inside of us...go back and tenderly embrace the wounded child. Our ancestors may not have known how to care for their wounded child within, so they have transmitted their wounded child to us. Our practice is to end this cycle.'*

On TikTok, Such (2023) notes:

> *'If we didn't get a need met in childhood then this version of us will act out as that self even if we are twenty, thirty, forty years old... the only way to overcome that is to heal our inner child and give that child-self what they needed ... to move forward as adults.'*

Television

The inner child also makes an appearance in a range of documentary and drama series. On reality television, after swimming in ice-cold water, the participant, Chelcee Grimes, reported an unusual experience:

> 'I think my inner child, you know that scared five-year-old young girl who lost her dad, I just seen her, I met her again in the water so.... Hmmmm... yeah... it was just, I think I was just releasing some emotion that I still had there... I might cry a bit more, but I think I'll go back home, um... just lighter... yeah.' (Freeze the Fear with Wim Hof, 2022, Series 1, Episode 6, 12:46).

Another reality show follows Joey Essex who describes his therapeutic journey:

> 'I took a step back and I thought I was that little boy again, it's a bit weird. I felt a bit sad inside. That place, it's always been there, I've never looked into it, I've never processed it... I've realized running away from memories ain't done me any favours at all.' (20:30)

> 'Therapy has made me think a lot about what I need to do to make me happy and one of those things is reconnecting with my past.' (Joey Essex, 'Grief and Me', 2021, 44:16)

Television drama also acknowledges the inner child. In 'Silent Witness' (2004), when the pathologist's long-lost son speaks to her, he evokes the inner child:

> 'It's like there's a two-year-old guy, right, and he's in there [pointing to stomach], and there's a wee five-year-old guy in there beside him, and then there's this the nine-year-old guy and he's ... I mean, he's really panicking. He's really freaked out. He doesn't know what... Then all of a sudden, he's a completely messed up fifteen-year-old, right, and then... And now I'm like a thirty-year-old man... And all I've ever wanted is for you to love me.' (42:53)

The increasing availability of narratives involving the inner child extends awareness of the relational origins and relational means to revise trauma, which aligns specifically with CAT.

CAT and working with traumatic experiences

As an integrative approach, CAT brings a relational theory, framework, language and method as a means to change unhelpful ways of relating that have traumatic origins. The concept of the inner child is consistent with CAT and its organizing principle, the Reciprocal Role procedure (RRP), which links the child and adult in developmental relationship (Ryle, 1985, p3). CAT addresses trauma through its three stages, Reformulation, Recognition and Revision, where unhelpful ways of relating are described, mapped and revised (Ryle & Kerr, 2020, p21). Despite Ryle (1990, p100) designing a model to address relational trauma, the question is often asked of the supervisor, 'Would trauma therapy be helpful after CAT?' When indicated, relational inner-child work offers an accessible within-CAT answer to that question.

Integrating trauma-focused models to CAT

CAT supports the use of a range of models and tools to address the consequences of problematic relational events. As Ryle and Kerr (2020, p55-56) note, 'techniques to work through and process current or historical experience' can include 'no-send' letters, behavioural experiments, empty-chair work, creative or body therapies, or more formal processing'. These interventions, particularly for those with dissociation, aim at 'improved integration, self-reflection, executive function' and better relating with self and others.

In recent years, approaches used in CAT to process distress include EMDR (Jenaway, 2016), Internal Family Systems (Lee *et al*, 2022), empty-chair work from the Gestalt tradition (Perls, 1973). Such approaches have an evidence base and efficacy. Although these methods are valid interventions within CAT, they often require additional time in training and may distract from the CAT relational focus and timeframes. By contrast, relational inner-child work offers an accessible and relationally consistent method that can make use of skills and techniques within the repertoire of the psychotherapeutically trained clinician.

Historical applications of inner-child work to CAT

The potential for CAT and inner-child work has been described by Akande (2007, p6-7):

> 'Most clients can understand and envisage a process whereby roles may be parent or child derived. I often suggest that we need to evoke

that inner child and listen to what s/he is still struggling with. Most clients believe that they do have an inner child. However, many also have difficulty listening to that inner child.'

Akande describes how, after connecting with the inner child, the client wrote in their goodbye letter about 'the intense sense of loneliness' that had been carried by the inner child. A significant change was noticed following connection with the child: 'Once he had listened to his inner child and felt more connected to him, the whole self was then ready to be connected to the outside world.'

The need for a description of inner-child work in CAT

When writing about CAT and trauma, Pollock (2001, p89) recognizes how imagery rescripting in parent-child scenarios can be beneficial to the recognition of complexity in relationships. This can inform understanding of self and others and revise the impact of trauma. In such scenarios, Landreth (2012, p14) suggests that:

'Play is the child's symbolic language of self-expression and can reveal (a) what the child has experienced; (b) reactions to what was experienced; (c) feelings about what was experienced; (d) what the child wishes, wants, or needs; and (e) the child's perception of self.'

Pollock (2001, p87) also advises caution when using imagery techniques, particularly if survivors are asked to contemplate the abusive parent as being loving and caring. Rather than reliving abusive relationships and experiences, exercises using inner-child work with CAT focus on the child-self, the relationships with self and others they needed and how to revise narratives in ways consistent with trauma-informed working.

The theoretical and practice-based foundations for inner-child work are evident in the psychological literature; these are used in therapies, including CAT, to address psychological distress. However, within CAT, there has been no detailed description of using brief dialogical processing of traumatic events or relationships with the key actors from the reciprocal relationship (the child and adult), in dialogue with the inner child.

Overview of inner-child work in CAT

The inner-child technique is used following the Reformulation phase. The two-step model involves reimagining and rescripting traumatic events to revise problematic embodied experiences. The scenarios make use of a multisensory approach using discussion, drawing, mapping, thoughts, memories, emotions, sensations and movement.

The first step involves facilitating a connection between the child and adult-self. During the second step, problematic events which have involved the child-self and relevant others are processed. By these means, mapped unhelpful Reciprocal Roles and procedures are revised to create exits as new ways of relating. By connecting inner and outer aspects of self, the approach facilitates change, central to the revision of trauma. As van der Kolk (2014, p283) describes:

> 'Beneath the surface of the protective parts of trauma survivors there exists an undamaged essence, a Self that is confident, curious, and calm, a Self that has been sheltered from destruction ... to ensure survival.'

The method allows complex relational events to be processed, and the benefits generalized, within the relatively short time frame of sixteen- or twenty-four-session CAT. Inner-child work has also been used to good effect in eight-session CAT by clinicians familiar with the technique. Once the model and method are internalized through therapy, these approaches can be used once sessions have ended, to support therapeutic gains.

Working with neurodiversity

Intellectual ability is no guarantee of emotional availability or capacity. Given this, and subject to assessment and personalization, inner-child approaches can be used across the range of intellectual ability and neurodiversity. In fact, drawings and images can reduce the information-processing load for those with cognitive impairment. Visual methods can be tailored to the needs of the individual. Images can be sourced, for example from magazines, or picture cards can be used. Pictures do not need to be complex; often a stick image can have considerable power when a scene is described. Cognitive or memory impairment need not inhibit the recollection of key events and feelings which support inner-child work. Similarly, as the scenarios rely on events that have happened or were hoped for, difficulty with abstract concepts is not necessarily an obstacle to this type of work.

Online therapy

Inner-child work can take place online to good effect. As is relevant to all online therapy, there is a requirement that the discussion will not be overheard, and the context is safe. Scenarios can still be drawn and held up on the screen. In some cases, the therapist can draw the image as it is described. However, online scenarios may rely on verbal descriptions of events. After the exercise, follow the usual protocol for reflection and discussion of feelings, noticing exits, mapping, debriefing, self-care and setting between-session activities.

Application of inner-child work in CAT

CAT is recognized for its wide-ranging trans-diagnostic application. Similarly, the inner-child technique can be used across the lifespan as listed in, but not limited to, the areas below:

- Addiction
- Child and family
- End of life and bereavement
- Forensic
- Gender and identity
- Learning disability
- Mental health
- Personality disorders
- Physical health

Three key stages of the inner-child technique in CAT – Prepare, Process, Progress

Prepare: Begin CAT in the usual manner. During the Reformulation phase, as is good practice in any therapy, identify coping skills (e.g. DBT skills, family support) and suitability for and interest in revising unhelpful patterns learned from childhood. Accessible reading such as West's Internal Family Systems-informed picture book (2021) can develop the client's understanding of parts of self, or self-states that can result from trauma.

Process: During sessions five to fourteen, in sixteen-session CAT, the inner-child technique is used, alongside other trauma-informed methods, as indicated, to process and revise experiences that have been traumatic or problematic, in the sense that they have led to unhelpful ways of relating i.e. problematic Reciprocal Role procedures (RRPs).

Progress: During sessions five to sixteen, the progress phase involves mapping, discussion and practice of new ways of relating. These exits, generated by the inner-child work, are summarized in the goodbye letter.

Summary
Step one:
1. Describe and draw or use a photograph of the child-self alone in a trauma-free context.
2. The adult-self is drawn, or they 'climb into the photograph' to meet their child-self.
3. What does the child need? If this is not known, ask if the child-self needs a hug.
4. How do the connected child and adult feel and act? Describe exits e.g. Loving-Loved.
5. End the scenario. Reflect and map new ways of relating. Describe how the exits may have affected the child's and the adult's life and may affect their future.
6. Remind the client to look after self and notice thoughts and feelings between sessions. In the next session, check the impact of the exercise and continue with mapping and reflection.

Step two:
7. Subsequently, use scenarios from Reformulation or in-session discussion, which illustrate problematic or traumatic RRPs between the child-self and key people: parents, siblings, teachers, peers.
8. Draw and describe the scenario in outline, then rescript with what the child actually needed.
9. Reflect during and after scenario. Map new ways of relating as exits and consider their impact.
10. One scenario per session: preparation, active processing five to fifteen minutes, reflection, mapping.

Introducing inner-child work

The concept of inner-child work is introduced at the start of therapy. It can be helpful to acknowledge that such techniques are used in a number of therapies to process complex feelings and events. The processing work typically lasts between five and fifteen minutes within a created scenario; the rest of the session is spent setting up and reflecting on the exercise. The practice takes place with the person in therapy actively voicing and discussing thoughts and feelings, both as the child-self and the other person(s) in the scenario. The therapist prompts and supports with tone of voice, suggestions or movement to enhance involvement with the scenario. Such exercises have led to a reduction in distress for the child- and adult-self and a greater understanding of relationships and problematic experiences. There is an option to stop at any point or to use grounding techniques, although in practice these are rarely required.

Options for introducing inner-child work: Introduce the method as suits the context.

- 'We have noticed that unhelpful ways of relating that started in childhood are still happening. To process and understand those feelings, it can be helpful to connect with your child-self and the events that were happening at the time. The aim is to reduce the frequency and impact of repeating unhelpful patterns.'

- As the therapy unfolds, a less formal introduction can be used: 'It sounds as if that child was unhappy, and it might be helpful to connect with them to hear what they have to say and to find out what they needed instead.' The procedure is then described as the stages are implemented.

When inner-child work is avoided as a new experience: Feedback from people in therapy suggests that inner child exercises can be helpful and, although often unfamiliar, can be readily accessed with positive outcomes. There may need to be some reassurance. This exercise does not focus on drawing skills but uses drawing to bring the recollection to mind more vividly. However, if the client does not want to draw, the therapist can do it, as the client describes the context. Alternatively, the scenario can rely on spoken description. Sometimes, inner-child work is avoided because of the potential for embarrassment when undertaking a new and potentially shame-inducing discussion of emotions and experiences. In these circumstances, validate these feelings and acknowledge that, while the work might appear unusual or feel initially uncomfortable, it may be beneficial to experience its effect before making a final decision.

Another means of supporting engagement with this work is to suggest internet research regarding the inner child. This can be a helpful exit to enable engagement with the work, as the peer-support, popular media and psychological literature are accessible and recognize the value of dialogue with the inner child. The research can take place in-session or as homework, to suit the clinical context.

When inner-child work is avoided due to dislike of the inner child:
In therapy, clients often want to avoid thinking about the past, with the child-self being blamed for negative experiences. At these times, their neglecting, criticizing ways of relating from childhood have been internalized. By connecting with the child and comforting them, trauma can be processed and integrated to reduce the distress felt by the child- and adult-self. Noticing reciprocal relationships from the reformulation letter and map can be beneficial. These illustrate the intergenerational and historical origins of current problems and are often sufficient indication for use of the inner-child technique. Alternative trauma-processing techniques can also be selected, as informed by Reformulation and the evidence base, for use instead of or alongside inner-child work.

Some individuals may want to destroy their inner child. Having internalized danger in childhood, they consider the child-self and adult-self dangerous and to be avoided. Again, at these times, recognize how these ways of relating are consistent with mapped unhelpful RRPs, and consider the potential roles of fear and shame in maintaining avoidance of certain parts of self. In these contexts, the non-judgemental observing eye has an important role.

It can also be advantageous for the therapeutic dyad to consider how to respond to a child who has experienced profound abuse; this typically involves the child being comforted. However, as comforting may not be a familiar way of relating for the client, attempts to do this might initially feel unsettling for them.

These discussions provide a rationale for inner-child work. In essence, the work may not always be easy but it offers the opportunity to process and alter the response to complex experiences.

When the technique is beyond current zone of proximal development:
Just as Ryle (1990) discusses the importance of hope in reformulation, inner-child work is offered in the spirit of non-judgemental hope for the resolution of trauma. However, although such work can benefit those who have experienced trauma (Raabe *et al*, 2022), when assessing for inner-child work, it should be considered that not everyone is at the stage in therapy where they can find this way of working helpful. Despite supporting the need for inner-child work, there may also be an understandable reticence or inability to engage with the work, for example contact with the image cannot be sustained during the exercise. Such reactions can occur at a time of crisis or dissociation, when there are no coping skills, strategies or support, or the client expresses dislikes their child-self. When difficulties occur while planning or during scenarios, there are several options to consider: persevere together in therapy; notice and name reasons for current difficulties; discuss in supervision; agree to try another approach. This could involve other trauma-processing techniques or use of CAT but with a focus on current relationships.

Starting inner-child work
Step one: bringing the child-self into the scenario
The first step involves the child-self and adult-self meeting. An image of the infant self or young child is brought to mind. Draw or use a photograph of the child, alone in a safe, non-traumatic situation. Talk through the drawing or photograph in sufficient detail for the scenario to be clear for the therapeutic dyad. Questions you might ask include, 'Where were you? What were you doing? What were you wearing? What colour was it? What was the room like? How did you feel?' This exercise is completed as a dialogue and connection between the adult- and child-self, rather than an exploration of the internal world of the person in therapy; there is therefore no need to invite the client to close their eyes as part of this practice, unless they ask to.

First connection
Choosing a safe scenario: When abuse has been part of the client's life, it can be challenging to find a location for the scenario that is not linked with trauma or associated feelings. For some, a bedroom will be a safe place, for others it will be a location that evokes distress. If it becomes clear that the image chosen is connected with trauma, for example, a

conversation starts about abuse or dissociation occurs, stop, reset and change the location of the image to a place where the child feels safest. Acknowledge that traumatic events can be addressed as the therapy continues, but that the first connection session is just to connect the adult- and child-self in a safe way.

Bringing the adult into the scenario: The adult-self is then drawn or imagined in the photograph to bring them into the image. The therapist can learn much from the drawing process, for example, is the pressure of the pen or pencil hard or soft? Is there self-criticism as the exercise is completed? Questions may also be asked during the scenario such as is the adult-self near or far away? Do they need to move closer to the child? If a photograph of the child-self is used in this exercise, ask the adult-self to 'climb into' the photograph to connect with the child.

Questions: Once both child- and adult-self are in the image, ask 'What happens next? What does the child-self need now?' Often the response is 'A hug', at which point, ask the adult-self if they can hug their younger self. It may be necessary for the therapist to move their arms as if to hug a child and to suggest, 'Perhaps the child needs a hug?' This suggestion is predicated on the reformulation, where, typically, the child-self has experienced some sadness or trauma. If the client doesn't express the need for a hug, remember that the child-self is still likely to need that comfort, but they may not be willing to endure it, given the potential historical absence of love and care in their life. If the adult does not recognize the need to hug their child-self, it may be helpful for the therapeutic dyad to consider more generally how distressed children often find solace when hugged, and then this can then be applied to the child-self in therapy.

Example: The child is alone in their room. The adult-self comes into the image. The therapist hears the adult say, 'The child leaned into my arms' and that, when hugged, they feel 'Lovely, safe, warm'. Your questions can extend the experience here, for example by asking 'Is the child snuggled in?' Although the primary aim of the first connection is for a physical connection or containment, the child- and adult-self can reflect together on feelings evoked by their connection experience: 'Does the child want to say anything to the adult about being connected? Does the adult want to say anything to the child about being connected to them?' End the scenario by agreement. Reflect and map exits.

Every scenario has the potential to generate an emotional impact between sessions. In this context, writing down feelings, self-care, talking with trusted others and using exits from the map are recommended – there will be an opportunity to discuss the effect of the scenario in the next session.

Tips:

- This exercise aims to generate a reparative relational experience, one that offers an opportunity to begin altering the inner child's and adult's negative sense of self. When reflecting during the exercise, aim to hear the child first. This values, gives voice to, and brings into dialogue, a possibly long-silenced part of self.

- The situation the child finds themselves in may be made safe during the scenario. However, it can be unhelpful if the adult-self suggests that they take the child-self far away from the situation in the scenario. Simply removing the child from the situation in the scenario, or key actors such as a neglectful or abusive parent, may represent a fantasy or compensatory strategy, for example rescuing, but it is not a healthy exit, and may mean that the opportunity to process past events is lost.

- Connecting with the young child-self is an important exercise, even for those whose overt trauma may not have taken place until later in life.

Managing discomfort during the exercise: If the child-self does not feel comfortable when they connect with their adult-self, discuss how they are feeling. Are these feelings consistent with mapped patterns? Can the adult-self recollect positive elements of the child with which they can connect? Can the adult connect with their inner child's vulnerability and comfort them?

Tips:

- If the child-self cannot be hugged by the adult, consider whether there are other means of connecting. For example, if they are on a beach, can they make sandcastles or walk together?

- If it has not been easy for the adult to connect with the child, or there is no apparent emotional connection between them, make use of the non-judgemental capacity of the Observing Eye to notice and validate the understandable difficulty in making a connection. Although not the hoped-for outcome, this lack of connection can inform the therapy and, in this sense, is welcomed as it indicates the nature of the current relationship between the adult and the child.

- The adult-self's responses to connecting with their child-self may include relief and happiness. However, feelings of sadness, anger or frustration may also be reported. At these times, exits such as accepting and having self-compassion, given historical traumatic experiences and current associated feelings, are valid responses.

- When the client dislikes the inner child, it can be helpful to talk about and draw an image representing these feelings. At the end of therapy, even if inner-child work has not taken place, it can be helpful to draw a second image to represent the relationship with the inner child. Very often, such images reveal the progress made in the self-to-self relationship – for example, in the first image the inner child is far away from the adult-self, while the second image shows the child hand in hand with the adult-self.

Step two: processing scenarios

Future sessions involve processing any number of scenarios. There are two primary methods: the child-self and the adult-self together, and the child-self and others together.

Scenario options

The child-self and the adult together: Together with the client, choose a scenario and set up in the usual way through drawing and discussion. The adult- and child-self discuss the associated unhelpful RRPs and identify, discuss and role play what the child needed but did not receive. This means that exits are identified and the adult- and child-self consider how the new ways of relating could have affected their life, had they been in place since childhood. The adult considers how they might apply the identified relational exits to their current circumstances and what impact this may have. This inner-child imagery extends and amplifies the usual application of CAT in recognizing and revising RRPs to find, map, internalize and practice exits.

The child-self and others together: Use of the inner child and the adult self in scenarios is consistent with much of the inner-child literature. Relational dialogues with the inner child address the relationship other-to-self as well as the self-to-self relationship. Therefore, in the scenarios that follow, the initial adult-and-child connection, the adult-self does not appear. The scenarios involve the child-self with people (parent, friend, sibling or other) who are linked to traumatic events in the child's life. The child is then asked what they needed from the person or people to revise the event. The change is then imagined by the adult in therapy, who then has dialogues between the child-self and the other person in the scenario, with some prompting and observation from the therapist. New ways of relating are identified and their emotional and physical impact are considered during and after the scenario and are then mapped as relational exits. Processing traumatic events with the child-self and others together further extends CAT by enabling healthy dialogue between the child and the key actors who have had a significant but often problematic role in their life.

Scenario selection

Some therapists use a hierarchy to rate the distress of specific scenarios, starting with the least distressing. Other therapists, while mindful of not addressing the most challenging topic as a first scenario, work with what is brought to therapy or the image the client identifies that week. Current events and associated RRPs or target problem procedures (TPPs) can be linked with childhood, e.g. 'Was there a time when you had this feeling when you were a child? or, 'When did that first happen?' By whatever means scenarios are identified, it can be helpful to take a developmental approach, starting with those when the child was very young.

Avoiding enactments: A number of example scenarios are provided below. Even when a client describes a seemingly minor event, or if the event was not discussed during reformulation, it is likely that it has had a traumatic impact. No matter how inconsequential some examples may initially appear, for example knocking over a vase, there is potential for the therapeutic dyad to repeat dismissing or neglecting enactments if scenarios raised are not processed in therapy.

Scenarios

Generalization: The processing of these experiences by the client has the capacity to reduce their general distress in ways that sometimes appear disproportionate given seeming insignificance of the situation being discussed. As a consequence, this sometimes reduces the need to process multiple traumatic experiences in therapy.

Meeting the child's needs: As long as the requests in scenarios are appropriate and not harmful to self or others, the adult-self should grant what the child needs and that they have asked for. This means the child hears a welcome response from the 'parent that they needed', showing that they are listening to them and will act in ways that support healthy relating. Opportunities can follow, such as the parent thanking the child for speaking and starting a conversation about their needs and the relationship between them.

Enabling the child-self to speak: In most cases, the client's child-self will be able to speak to others in the scenario. If the child finds this difficult, however, the adult-self can enter the scenario and speak the child's words for them. The adult-self is usually able to do this, however, if this is not the case, the therapist can come into the scenario to support the child – always in dialogue, asking the child what they need and want the therapist to say. Before this method is used, consider whether the adult-self or the therapist, in speaking for the child, may be enacting rescuing or controlling roles.

Scenario examples: with the child-self and others
Scenario 1: The merry-go-round of anxiety

A family were sitting on a merry-go-round that was spinning at speed. One child enjoyed the experience, the other, who is now in therapy, feared they were being ridiculed by the father and sibling for being anxious and felt overwhelmed and tearful. This situation represented patterns in relationships since childhood. The therapist asked: 'What was needed for the situation to be OK, enjoyable?' The response is: 'That the merry-go-round would turn more slowly'. This was then imagined in therapy, with the child-self asking the parent if they could slow down, a request that was implemented and discussed. In such scenarios, the parent has an opportunity to apologize and to let the child know that they will welcome them talking about their feelings. The therapist can encourage the sensation of slower movement by gently rocking and speaking slowly, with a calm voice. The slower sensation is noticed by the child who feels 'pleased and more comfortable', having voiced their needs and experienced a positive response.

This exercise can facilitate confidence in subsequently speaking up in family and work settings, help the client to recognize that communication, actions and feelings can be changed for the better.

Scenario 2: The meaning of a hug

When care has been lacking, the child may bring a longed-for scenario to therapy, such as a parent hugging the child-self. The client (or the therapist if the client is unwilling) draws an image of a parent hugging a child. Emotions and sensations are explored as the drawing is completed. Conversations between the child and the parent, who responds as the healthy parent the child needed, can take place: 'Why were hugs avoided? Why were feelings not spoken about? What was the impact of not hugging for them and the children they now have?' Feelings can then be discussed with the intention of exploring and revising them during the exercise, which can have a positive impact on the client's sense of self in past, current and future relationships.

This exercise can generate a range of feelings, for example, of being loved and having compassion for self and others. These new ways of relating can occur even if the parent is no longer alive and the relationship involved misunderstanding and conflict.

Scenario 3: From addiction to connection

A more extended scenario can involve the child discussing traumatic events in the home, for example parental addiction. There may have been inconsistent care, neglect and abuse, and the client may have been given responsibilities beyond their years, e.g. caring for an intoxicated parent. In therapy, the adult draws or describes the scenario and talks about what the child-self needed. Often, the child knows what they needed, having thought about it on many occasions. If required, the therapist can prompt them by asking questions: 'You have come home from school and are at the door of your house. What did the child need to happen?' The child-self can then describe how the parent opens the door, asks about the child's day and makes dinner. The child explores what food they would have liked to eat, gaining a considerable sense of satisfaction from knowing that, unusually, they will have both a cooked meal and a menu choice. Afterwards, the parent and child spend time together engaging in a range of activities as fits the individual context, until the parent reminds them it is time for bed. As the scenario progresses, the therapist can ask questions, such as: 'What happened next? What did it feel like when this was happening?' The child-self describes the impact of the loving family scenario that they needed, such as being able to sleep well that night and wake up happy to go to school, rather than in their usual fearful way.

Such scenarios as this can enable the child-self to feel safe and loved in a setting where they are able to play and engage in activities that were not previously possible. The adult-self in therapy is then able to recognize and take steps to revise the impact of neglect, which may include a lack of trust and feelings of anger in their relationship with self and others.

Scenario 4: The dialogue with grief

In this scenario, the client is given an opportunity to hold a conversation with an object of grief. Often, this will be with a parent or loved one. A common scenario may involve a child-self meeting and talking with a parent who had died when they were an infant. In the discussion, the child is both able to get to know and to say goodbye to the deceased parent. The child-self can speak to the parent about how their death has affected them. This may include conflicted feelings, for example, both love towards them and anger with them for leaving. The child also has a chance to ask questions of the parent they have brought into the scenario. They can hear that they were loved by the parent, who has an opportunity to talk and reflect on the past and future with their child.

Letter-writing and reading in this context can also support relational dialogues. Letters may not have the same direct impact as the spoken 'in-person' scenario. However, they can meet the child's needs in terms of the zone of proximal development (Vygotsky, 1978), or open up what is possible for the child within the therapeutic dyad at that moment. Letters can also be kept and used for future reference.

Scenario 5: Speaking up about abuse

In situations where the client has experienced physical and sexual abuse, scenarios are discussed and agreed upon. Where appropriate, conversations might take place with the abuser or others, such as a person who lived in the family, for example a parent who did not stop the abuse. In accordance with many trauma-focused therapeutic approaches, the aim is to process preoccupying thoughts and feelings rather than re-experiencing the traumatic event in detail. The technique supports dialogue using scenarios or letters. By reflecting on what the child needed, the client's thoughts and feelings can be expressed, and they can recognize and revise the impact of traumatic events. This scenario, with role-playing facilitated by the therapeutic dyad, can lead to change in ways consistent with the Bakhtinian concepts of the witness and the judge (Hepple, 2006, p25). Here, the relationship with the inner child extends the reparative function of the therapeutic relationship:

> 'Once transformation has happened, the past, present and future world can never be the same again. This is, I think, the core component of change in psychotherapy. It is not so much internalization of the therapist but, through the therapeutic relationship, new ways of relating to future others are now a possibility.'

Ending the scenario and reflecting on its relational impact

An inner child scenario typically lasts for a single therapy session. The therapeutic dyad orchestrates the scenario, as previously described. They agree when the scenario has reached a conclusion. Sometimes the comment is made: '*I don't want to leave the child*'. At this point, it can be noted that the child-self has always been present but is now recognized. This means the child and adult-self can be in dialogue whenever they choose. Just as CAT's relational model is internalized, so it is with the concept of the inner child. Connecting with the inner child to manage distress can be supportive throughout therapy and also once formal sessions have come to an end.

The exercise can have a significant benefit, generating relational exits such as: 'noticing and speaking up to seen and heard'; 'loving to loved'; 'holding boundaries to safe and contained'. Reflections on exercises have included: '*Now I see my child-self I realize that others have a child-self and that, like me, they also deserve love*'. This technique can both improve an understanding of self and others, reduce associated risks and generate opportunities.

At times the emotional impact of inner-child work is delayed or may be considered unhelpful but is then recognized at the next session as having had a positive impact. At other times the exercise is not felt to be helpful, and this opinion is not revised. Here it can be worthwhile to reflect in supervision on the Reformulation and the technique used to support efficacy in future scenarios. However, where inner-child work is not beneficial, other trauma-focused techniques can be used. Therapy may also focus on RRPs in the present, make links with the past and develop relational exits, in the usual manner of CAT, rather than processing past events.

Mapping relational dialogues

Mapping is key to the relational dialogues with the inner-child approach in CAT and is thoroughly described in Potter (2020). Inner-child work in CAT can make use of multiple mapping methods including in-the-moment or 'messy' mapping, as well as template maps (see Appendix 6). The template format, which can be hand-drawn or produced electronically, facilitates consistency, clarity and a common mapping language for clients and clinicians. When using a template, individualization and personalization in mapping are encouraged through the use of images and quotes.

How scenarios can impact the future

The inner-child technique can be extended if needed. After a scenario has been explored, exits can be discussed and role-played as movies or future templates in ways similar to techniques in EMDR (Shapiro, 2001). The impact of identified exits can be discussed, such as: 'How would relationships be different in light of new ways of relating?' The new ways of relating and their impact can be written down as a letter. For example, the parent the child needed may say: 'If I had been consistently caring, you may have trusted and had confidence in relationships, rather than seeking approval. We could have spoken together so that you would have had the confidence to speak about your feelings, rather than fearing you would be rejected and abandoned if you talked about your needs'.

The letter can be written from the perspective of the client, e.g. 'I could have...', or of the parent the child needed, 'You could have...'. When the letter with a number of examples is complete, it can be read aloud in session by either the therapist or the client.

The dual focus – the inner and outer self

In focusing on the inner child, this chapter may appear to overvalue the internal world. However, it is the processing of inner distress that enables the integration of the child and adult-self and thereby of inner and interpersonal aspects of life that have been affected by trauma (van der Kolk, 2014, p283). Applying exits to effect change is a core aspect of CAT. Talking about exits arising from scenarios and how they impact emotions, activities and relationships likewise supports the connection between the inner and outer self to inform life beyond trauma. Frameworks such as the Good Lives Model (Ward, 2002) can also be used to focus reformulation and exit-based discussions about multiple elements of the internal and external world, e.g. social, spiritual and physical ways of relating.

Therapist perspectives on using inner-child work in CAT

The development of CAT-focused inner-child work

Inner-child work and associated relational dialogues within CAT enable the revision of traumatic experiences. The method involves Reciprocal Role procedures being lifted from the map, processed and put back on the map as exits. The development of inner-child work in CAT has been informed by the literature, life experiences, observations, outcomes and comments arising from therapy sessions. Feedback from colleagues (Iszard *et al*, 2022), has also shaped this approach. As with any therapeutic technique, inner-child work in CAT is likely to be further developed by those who use it within their practice and will be informed by the developing evidence base.

From Iszard *et al*, 2022:

'Inner-child work is consistent with trauma models. It provides a helpful relational framework for reprocessing early life trauma and identifying resulting enactments, which repeat both intra- and inter- personally, either at the parent-derived or the child-derived pole of the Reciprocal Role. As an experiential way of engaging the self-to-self and self–to-other Reciprocal Roles discussed in CAT, inner-child work helps clients recognize the emotional parts of themselves and find ways to soothe or address rather than ignoring them. This helps clients name which parts of the current difficulties they face that they might have some agency to change.'

'The inner child method has been an invaluable tool for scaffolding reflection, recognition, and expression, both as a process that brings to light the suffering that is unseen and unnamed, and in supporting expression of emotions that have remained disavowed, often to preserve the attachment relationship, albeit unhealthy, with a caregiver.'

'Inner-child work is a gradual process and a two-way venture shared between client and therapist, but also between the client's child-self and adult-self. It has been a valuable approach which facilitates sharing and awareness. It brings words and images to places that have until now been hidden, or cut-off, through a compassionate and non-judgemental process in which the "I" can see "me".'

'The model has many strengths, including increasing awareness and understanding of survival patterns and how they first emerged, and encouraging healthy emotional expression in a corrective and containing therapeutic relationship that doesn't repeat the harmful relational patterns of the past; it provides an empathetic bridge between child and adult selves which can support integration and healthy self-to-self relating.'

Therapist feedback on client perspectives

'Clients have said that inner-child work has provided them with a release of uncomfortable emotions, has helped them make sense of distressing experiences and process traumatic memories, so that they are no longer haunted by them.'

'Clients have described an experience of connecting the dots between their current ways of coping and early life experiences, or of making connection with their child selves before traumatic events happened in a way that feels reparative. In their goodbye letters clients have said that they realized why connection with the inner child was so important; it helped them to connect with a part of themselves that they had not realized had maintained, and yet could also change, their distress.'

Therapist feedback on learning inner-child work

'The approach is best learned through training and experiential role play, or at the very least the supervisor giving clear examples of what could be done or said.'

'Additional experience and training in emotion regulation, imagery, grounding and psychoeducation around trauma can be helpful as well as planning, support and exploration of the technique through supervision.'

Therapist feedback on challenges to working using inner-child work

'At first the model can initially feel unorthodox and not obviously part of the CAT model:'

'The method can initially be challenging to apply in practice, particularly with clients with impoverished life experiences and dissociation, or clients who genuinely don't know how to address themselves in positive and helpful ways; for example, some clients do not know what to do with a crying child, or struggle with imagery and experiential exercises. It can be difficult to avoid enactments as an inexperienced practitioner, particularly rescuing and shame-triggered dissociative enactments. Some find it really powerful and integrating. However, when the child is hated, the client can often feel very ambivalent about the work.'

'The chapter contains quite a few examples of getting around difficult scenarios and roadblocks which might come up; I would say that it's not always been easy to set up. Much like other trauma work, clients can put up defences against doing it and it is easy to fall into avoidance if you don't feel confident about its potential efficacy. Working within the ZPD, mapping and more traditional recognition and revision work alongside inner-child work will be important in building reflective capacity and in recognition and revision of target problem procedures.'

Therapist summary on the integration of inner-child work within CAT

'This approach is particularly synergistic with every phase of the CAT model. It supports Reformulation, recognition, and revision of TPPs as healthy exits. It also adds experiential depth to the therapeutic work and facilitates the expression of emotions, integration of different self-states and trauma processing. It also provides a reparative relational experience between client and therapist. Experiential work is not always easy but it's probably the most effective strategy. I view it as particularly important for clients who find it hard to access emotions, although this is also the group most likely to avoid the work. This way of working is particularly synergistic with relational approaches and adds a new dimension to the CAT model. It has become a core part of my practice as a CAT therapist.'

Supervision of inner-child work

Beginnings and endings are important in life, just as they are in therapy, and so it is with this concluding section on supervision of inner-child work within CAT.

Supervision is vital when working with the inner child. Familiarity with the model can be supported by role play with, for example, the supervisee as the therapist and the supervisor as a person connecting with their inner child. Weekly supervision is part of training in CAT. Supervision should also take place regularly when the therapist is learning and using the inner child model to process, map, monitor and refine techniques in a method which is part therapy and part theatre.

Outcomes are informed by knowledge of the literature, model adherence, ongoing reading, reflection on enactments, the capacity for creativity and an understanding and application of both the 'C' and 'A' in CAT. Key to the work is the supervisor's and therapist's relationship and shared confidence to apply theory and integrate techniques. This enables a structured and safe step into the narrative informed by the world of the inner child.

Chapter 9:
Innovative approaches within a learning disability service

Sarah Nicholas and 'Col'

Introduction

Working as a therapist in a service for people with learning disabilities, I am acutely aware that individuals with cognitive challenges frequently experience disempowerment and inequalities in society (Fletcher 2016). This has led me to reflect on the potential for power imbalances in therapy and the importance of adjusting my clinical practice to ensure therapy is a collaborative process. I also recognise my responsibility in tailoring therapy to be inclusive of neurodiversity. Within my service this has required consideration of how I can adapt therapy to provide opportunities for people who may not have access to the words needed to express their world. I have therefore explored and utilised creative approaches to engage people in meaningful therapeutic conversations that can help make sense of their problems within the context of their own life stories (Lloyd & Clayton, 2013).

Cognitive Analytic Therapy (CAT) requires therapeutic space that allows the exploration of the relational experience of the individual both inside and outside the room (Hepple, 2010). CAT provides opportunities for the use of creativity to capture the relational world of the individual, but this needs to be managed while ensuring that the therapy still adheres to the CAT model (Lloyd & Clayton, 2013). Adopting creative tools in CAT needs additional consideration from the therapist, as well as robust support through supervision, to ensure that the therapy does not get lost in translation. During my CAT training, I was fortunate to have the supervision of Suzanne Lyons who encouraged and developed my confidence in bringing creativity into my CAT practice. In this chapter, I shall explore the use of innovative approaches, with illustrations from a CAT case I have worked with as a trainee under her guidance.

This case describes the use of CAT with Col, a man with learning disabilities and a forensic history. For the purposes of anonymity, names and client-identifying information have been changed. Written consent was obtained from the client to share his anonymized information, details of the CAT process, maps and letters.

In using therapeutic approaches with people with learning disabilities, it is essential to consider the wider societal context and how this may have impacted on the person's life experiences and emotional well-being (Lloyd & Clayton, 2013). As Col has a complex combination of inter-relational and social difficulties, CAT was selected as it provides a relational and versatile therapeutic model.

Referral

Col was referred for CAT by his care coordinator who has worked with him for many years. He is a man in his twenties with a diagnosed learning disability. Col has traumas from multiple experiences of neglect, instability and abuse during his childhood. As a teenager, he was detained after assaulting children in his local community. Initially, he was placed in Young Offenders Institution. Col was discharged from the young offenders' unit eight years ago and now lives in the community under twenty-four-hour supervision. His care coordinator reported concerns regarding Col's pervasive low mood, social isolation and low self-esteem.

Assessment

At our first meeting, Col appeared nervous and said he was worried about the appointment. Col reported not sleeping well the previous night because of this. When I inquired about his unease, Col explained that, while in the young offenders' unit, he had been made to attend an offenders' treatment programme. He said he had found this really upsetting. Col was reticent to say why, other than it made him feel worse. I mapped out with Col how he was feeling about our meeting. This mapping in the moment enabled us to shift the focus away from his painful past to having a conversation in the present (Potter, 2010). The side-by-side mapping (Potter, 2016) also began the process of building a therapeutic alliance, which is at the heart of CAT.

A concern of Col's was that he would be exposed and vulnerable. He reported that he 'squashed' his emotions, and he held them 'deep inside'.

Col reported that if his anger and hurt could surface, his fear was that it might overwhelm him. Col also said he felt guilt and shame at things in his past that he would rather forget.

Col spoke about his grief at his father's death, three years ago. Col had not seen him for several years, and did not find out about his death until sometime afterwards. Col said he worries about losing his mother, who he is still in contact with. Col said when that happens, he will be 'all alone'.

We spoke about CAT, and he was provided with an easy read information leaflet (See Figure 9.1). Col said that he would like to feel better about himself and 'would give it a go'. My main concern was re-traumatizing Col if I did not carefully scaffold the therapy. This was discussed within my supervision group. It was agreed that I would adopt visual techniques, including drawings and objects of reference to explore Col's past and present relational patterns. My supervisor advised against using The Psychotherapy File (see Appendix 1) in the initial stages, as its potentially exposing nature may be a barrier to Col wanting to engage in the therapy process.

Figure 9.1: Easy read CAT leaflet (Dr Mark Rose)

What to expect from CAT?

- Most of the time talking therapy is helpful. It can make us feel better about ourselves and others.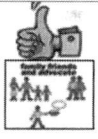

- Sometimes talking about difficult things can make us feel sad or upset. This may happen at the beginning of therapy. It is ok to feel like this.

- It is important to tell people that support you about how you feel so you can plan together to cope with these feelings. Your therapist can help you with this.

- Your therapist will write two letters to you, a "reformulation" letter and a "goodbye" letter. You will also make maps of the unhelpful patterns.

- Sometimes a therapy session will be recorded. This is to make sure the therapy is good quality.

- It is best to have therapy sessions once a week. Each session will last about 1 hour.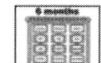

- You will have a fixed number of therapy sessions. Your therapist will arrange these with you so you know when therapy will finish.

- If you miss an appointment without letting your therapist know, your therapist will contact you to make another appointment.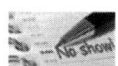

- If you miss two sessions in a row and you have not spoken with your therapist about this, your therapy sessions may stop.

Reformulation: Sessions 1-5

By applying the Procedural Sequence Objects Relations Model (PSORM) (Ryle, 1991), I sought to explore how Col's relationships with self and others had evolved and how these were expressed in his thoughts, feelings and actions. (Corbridge et al, 2018). My stance was one of compassionate curiosity. I began by working with Col to produce his genogram. The aim of this was to provide a window through which to look at how Col's early experiences had impacted throughout his life in the Reciprocal Roles (RRs) and Reciprocal Role Procedures (RRP) he had developed (Vygotsky, 1978).

Col had difficulties describing his childhood in terms of a timeline or people around him. This gave a sense of a chaotic, powerless and confusing childhood. Col's mother has a learning disability. His parents had separated before he was born and, as a young child, he had irregular contact with his father. Col had initially lived with his mother and several other adults in a two-bedroom flat. At around the age of eleven, due to child protection concerns, he was removed from his mother and placed with his father. Col said he felt punished and scared. He reported that he rarely saw his mother after this. Col did not disclose that he had been the victim of abuse. However, on several occasions, he reported feeling scared as a child. Col described his father as emotionally distant, and it appeared he had had little concern for his son's emotional well-being. Col told me that when he was away on a school trip, his father had his pet dog put down for no apparent reason. He spoke about his deep sadness at the loss of a beloved pet.

As Col talked about his life, he would often abruptly stop talking about painful and difficult memories and change the subject. Considering this in relation to the Multiple Self States Model (Ryle, 1975), I wondered if this dissociation was an enactment; a cutting off from experiences that are too painful to process. I reflected on my identifying countertransference (Ryle, 1995) in feeling apprehensive about leading Col onto topics that might be too painful for both of us.

At the end of our first session, I provided Col with a visual countdown of sixteen CAT sessions (kindly provided by Julie Lloyd). This was in the form of a pie chart that we coloured in each week to represent a completed session. This brought into the room the finite nature of therapy and allowed us from the beginning of therapy to consider its ending. It was a visual reminder each week to consider the conclusion of therapy and issues that may arise from this process. This scaffolding focused us on how finishing therapy might trigger Col's associated RRP, and the development of exits to manage what he may perceive as another loss.

Figure 9.2: Sixteen-session visual countdown

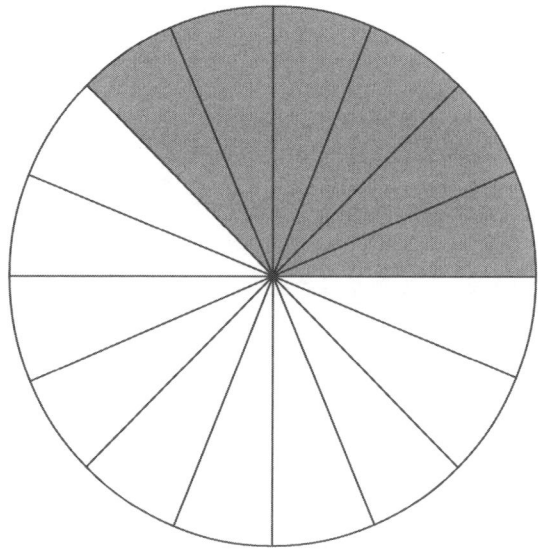

I reflected with my supervision group on Col's fear blocking us from moving forward. For this purpose, in our second session we built a wall between us using wooden bricks. This was a technique I had seen demonstrated by Lucy Morris and Phillip Clayton at the CAT, ID & Trauma Conference 2018 (Lloyd, 2019). These were taken from a Jenga block play set, which we labelled with Col's fears of therapy (Figure 9.3). This wall had a meaning that could be named and deconstructed, as described in Semiotic Object Relations Theory (SORT) (Hepple & Sutton, 2004). Using the bricks, Col was able to name his fears. We were then able to work together to start to think about how we could address these fears in our therapy sessions.

Col's core fear was that I would perceive him to be bad and that this may even result in him going back to prison. Col appeared reassured when I advised that people only go to prison if they have committed a crime. I reflected to him my understanding that he has a strong motivation to not re-offend. Col agreed with this, but said he was concerned what I would think of him. I invited Col to share with me within our sessions if he was feeling that I was judging him so that we could address this together.

Col also identified concerns about therapy reminding him of painful memories and making him feel worse about himself. We agreed to focus therapy on the present and moving forward to a life he feels better about. The use of the wooden blocks provided a playful context, offering creativity in exploring and developing Col's self-expression (Coulter & Rushbrook, 2010) which I was able to use in future sessions.

Figure 9.3: Blocks to therapy

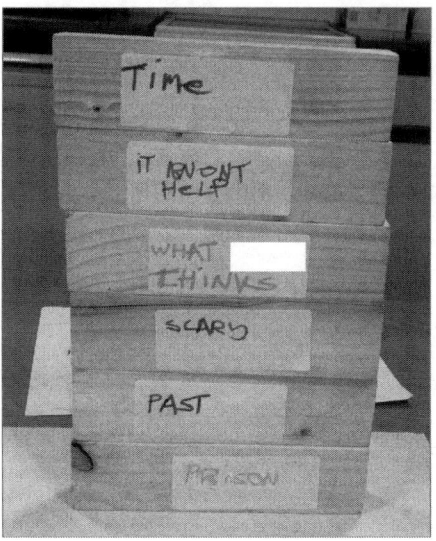

Using the theories of Boik *et al* (2000), in which sand play is used to create personal stories, in sessions three and four I introduced the medium of a sandbox. The sandbox provided the possibility, using miniature figures and the arrangement of the sand, for Col to produce an imaginary scene that represents his inner state (Kalff, 1980). Utilizing this playful and inventive approach, opportunities were provided for Col's reciprocal roles to become visible in a three-dimensional format. To begin, we used animals within the sandbox to represent family, staff and friends. Col used the donkey to represent his father, reporting it was sad, alone and frail. His mother was a rabbit, seen as sweet, harmless and powerless. In contrast, he placed staff in roles such as tigers and lions – protecting and strong. Col represented himself as a horse, a cow and a dinosaur (Figure 9.4). These appeared to represent his different self-states. Col described how the cow is 'milked' and is powerless and passive. In contrast, the dinosaur is feared and uncontrolled, like his anger, while the horse is useful, liked and admired. The RRPs of using–used and rescuing–rescued (protecting–protected) were identified.

Figure 9.4: Sand play reciprocal roles

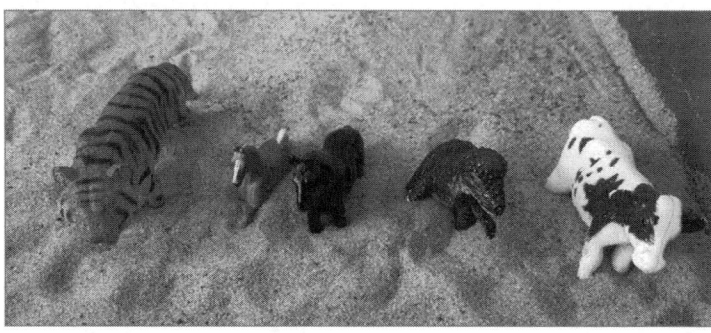

Col's limited insight into recognizing patterns in his own responses led me to consider whether it might be easier for him to express or recognize these things in a projected story (Lloyd and Clayton 2013). The Six-Part Story (Lahad, 1992; Lahad & Ayalon, 1993; Dent-Brown, 2011; see Appendix 5) is a popular tool in working with people with learning disabilities, and provides information about the person's wants, and how they perceive themselves and others (Lloyd & Clayton, 2013). We used the sand tray, and Col created a story (Figure 9.5). A key theme to come out of this work was his desire to be a powerful figure and protector of others. In the story, there were lurking, hidden dangers (thieves) and being protected by powerful others (police). This could be translated into Col's RRPs of hiding–hidden (unsafe state) and protecting–protected (safe state). The powerful protector formed the basis of compensatory fantasies of being a hero which was evident throughout the therapy. This is in contradiction to Col's lived reality of being controlled and vilified due to his offending history.

Figure 9.5: Sand play Six-Part Story

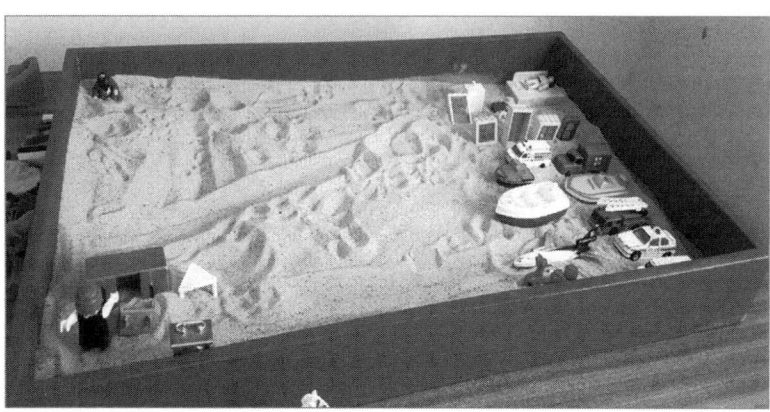

Using the identified states and RRPs, we were able to start to map out Col's current relational and emotional life. Col put being popular and liked as his desired place, with associated emotions of happiness and secure. Col identified his feared place as alone and scared, with associated emotions of anger and upset.

Col was also supported by his care coordinator to complete an easy read Psychotherapy File (Clayton, 1999). The patterns Col identified with were:

- 'Thinking I am no good' trap.
- 'Keeping my feelings to myself' trap.
- 'Trying to please' trap.
- 'Feeling I am not important' trap (this was the pattern he most strongly identified with).
- 'Upset feelings' dilemma.
- Snag: I want to feel good about myself, but my learning disability and offending history do not allow this.

We reflected on how Col had learned to hide his feelings as this protected him from exposure. However, this left him feeling alone and scared.

Guided by the information gathered during our first sessions, a reformulation letter was created of our shared understanding of how Col's experiences had led to Target Problem Procedures (TPPs), and how these continued to be sustained. The letter outlined three agreed Target Problems (TPs) to be worked on in CAT:

TP1 I don't have a voice in my own life, as I don't tell people what I want and need.

TP2 I don't like myself and don't think I deserve to be happy.

TP3 I feel scared of what other people think of me and what they might do if they don't like me.

I was concerned that in the letter, Col should recognize the story as his own, and therefore his subjective reality needed to be captured (Bakhtin, 1986). I used the support of my supervision group who made recommendations on the personalization of the reformulation letter. The letter was provided in session five.

Dear Col

Now we have had five of our sixteen sessions together, I wanted to write you a letter about what you have told me about your life, and my understanding of what you say are some of the problems you have. It is important, Col, that what is in this letter is right for you. Especially, as I know how important it is for you to please others. I want you to feel free to tell me if I have got anything wrong, without worrying that I will be upset. I promise I won't be.

My understanding of the problems you would like to work on in therapy is as follows:

1. *You told me other people make decisions about your life. You said you would like to have a voice, for others to listen to you and understand what you want in your life.*
2. *From the work we have done, it seems there are times you don't like yourself very much. You said that you want to see yourself as a good person and like yourself more.*
3. *I have some understanding of how frightened you are of what others might think of you. You would like to be less worried about this in the future.*

When you first came to therapy, I saw how scared you were. It seemed to me like you were worried that therapy might be something that would be painful for you, or that would uncover a side of yourself that you wanted to remain hidden from yourself and others. I think you have been so brave continuing to come to therapy despite your fears, and I think that, as our sessions have progressed, although still uncomfortable for you at times, you have started to take steps to talk about your feelings and problems.

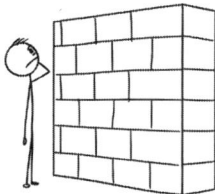

In our first session when we spoke about your childhood, it was quite difficult to make sense of it. With lots of different people, times and events all jumbled up. I wondered if this is how it felt to you as a child? You said that your mum and dad split up when you were very young,

but you don't remember when. You had half-brothers but didn't see much of them when you were growing up, and you don't have contact with them now. You said that you lived in a flat with lots of other people including your mum and her partner (who looked like a wizard) and his wife. You couldn't remember everyone else who lived in the flat, but you thought it was about fifteen people in a two-bedroom flat.

You said your childhood was happy, but you also told me about things that happened that were upsetting, confusing and frightening. You told me that your grandad once came and picked you up unexpectedly from school and took you on a road trip to Wales for a week. You said that this was fun, although you were confused about being taken out of school and you didn't know if your mum knew where you were. Another time you said the police came around to the flat you lived in with your mum and lots of other people as someone had said bad things were happening to you. You told the police you wanted to stay living with your mum, but the police took you to your dad's to live. You spoke about how angry, upset and frightened you were about this. You said you barely knew your dad when this happened. Although you loved your mum and dad very much, I really got the sense that, as a child, life was messy and wobbly, and this must have been very frightening at times, as you never knew what to expect.

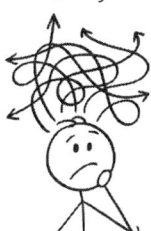

When you went to secondary school, you said you were bullied. This was really upsetting for you. It seemed like you and your family were very different from other people and this made you feel like you didn't fit in? Feeling like an outsider seems to have continued throughout your life.

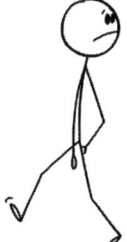 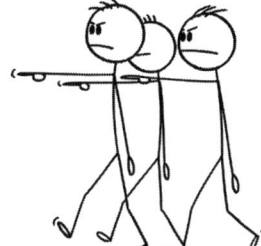

From the age of fifteen you have been shut away, first in a young offenders' unit, and still now a bit in your own flat. It seems like others have always had control over your life. This has left you feeling powerless with a bubbling anger at your life not being what you want for yourself.

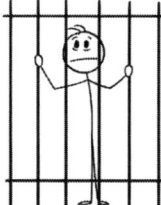

Being so much controlled by others seems to give you not only the message that you are different from other people, but also the message that others see you as too dangerous to be around people. I have noticed in our sessions that you seem scared of what people think of you and might do to you. You also seem scared that it is true, and that you are a bad person. You have described a 'scared monster'. I wonder if this is how you feel about yourself?

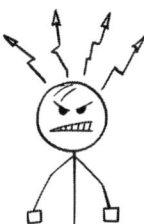

A way you have learned to manage these feelings of being a 'scared monster', is to always try to make other people happy. You do this by hiding your own feelings and not challenging what is happening to you. Sometimes your feelings leak out and you find yourself feeling so sad and frustrated that you can no longer hide it. When this happens, you start to think about wanting to end it all. You feel scared when this happens and quickly pretend that everything is fine again. You described hiding your feelings and pleasing others as being like playing a game of hangman, where you could lose at any time.

In our sessions you have talked a lot about wanting to have what you see as 'normal life' – to have friends, a wife, a job, and most of all to be respected. Basically, to be in control of your own life. While the perfect life may not be possible, I hope that in therapy I can help you to have a life you feel better about.

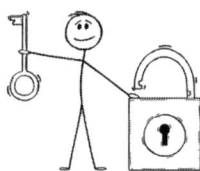

Our time working together is limited and this can be difficult, as it may be a reminder of other times you have people coming and going in your life. However, we will work together to manage the therapy ending in a way that does not leave you feeling abandoned by me.

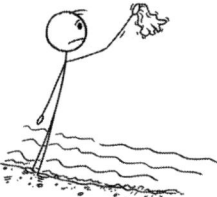

Col, I enjoy working with you. In therapy you have been kind to me even if I get things wrong, and you have lots of interesting ideas. I am looking forward to working with you over the next eleven weeks.

Best Wishes,
Sarah

Col listened intently while I read the reformulation letter. At the end of the reading, he said that it was 'brilliant' and 'just right', as if brushing off the rawness of what he had heard (hiding). Then Col began to cry, quietly and without shame. We sat with the sadness, as it felt as if something powerful had passed between us. Potter (2018) describes this as a therapeutic moment; a connection and new openness that signalled a shift in fostering an increased therapeutic alliance between us.

Recognition and revision: Sessions 6-13

In moving through therapy, it was important to keep in mind the exposing nature of therapy and Col's emotional vulnerability. We spent some time exploring how he could feel safer within the sessions. Col had shown that he finds objects and metaphors helpful, as this provides a medium to explore difficult feelings and experiences in a less personally direct manner (see Lyons, Chapter 4 & Turner, Chapter 7, this volume).

Using objects, Col selected a figure of a person curled up and weeping. He advised that this showed how he felt 'scared and sad'. Col then placed a bear holding the figure (Figure 9.6). We discussed how bears can be dangerous and unpredictable, but also strong and protective. Col stated that this bear is strong and protective as he hopes therapy will be for him. The bear became a transitional object (Winnicott, 1953) that he could use to overcome his fears about the exposing nature of therapy. We were able to use this as a grounding technique after difficult conversations and at the end of therapy sessions.

Figure 9.6: Transitional object

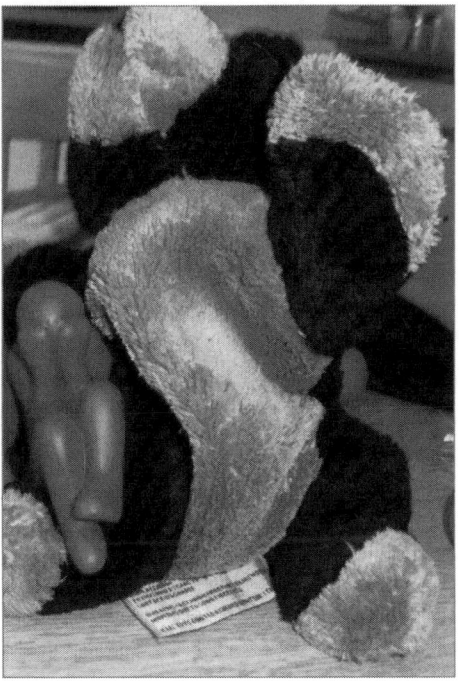

A key requirement for the therapy moving forward was to ensure that we remained within our zones of proximal development (ZPD), and for sessions to be tailored to bridge the gap between where Col was emotionally, and where he could potentially reach (Ryle & Kerr, 2020). For this purpose, and to provide a safe therapeutic space, objects were used to start to create the Sequential Diagrammatic Reformulation (SDR). The diagram was developed in the sessions through mapping together (Figure 9.7). This shared activity facilitated the shaping of Col's story into a context that was meaningful for both of us (Potter, 2010).

Figure 9.7: Initial diagram

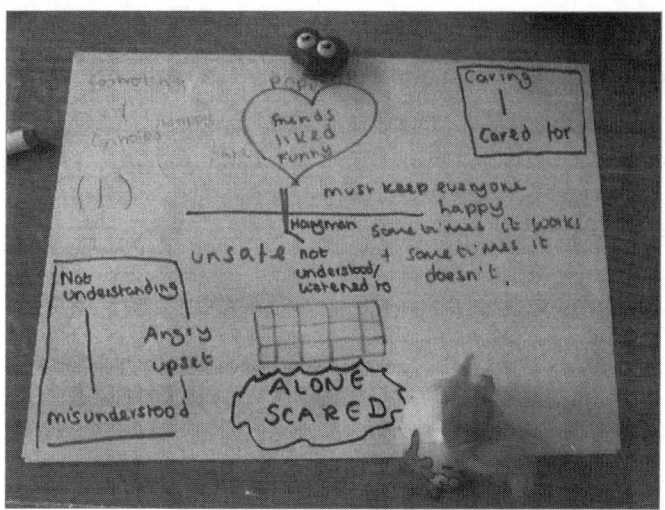

Creative and practical tools were also used within the sessions to support Col to develop skills in identifying TPPs. The reformulation letter continued to be referred to during sessions to reorient us to the core pain and helped us to formulate Col's TPPs. Figure drawings from Sunderland & Armstrong (2018) and hand drawings were used to visually capture Col's RRs (Figure 9.8) and his RRP. RRPs of hiding–hidden and controlling–controlled alongside emotional states of cutting off and blaming were described.

Figure 9.8: Reciprocal Roles

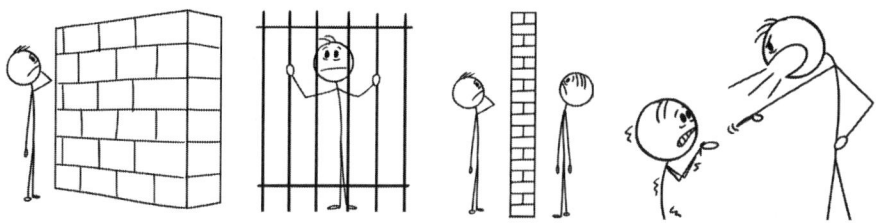

These RRs were placed on the map and extended out to show relational and behavioural TPPs. Col recognized traps, dilemmas and snags that perpetuate his cycle of TPPs. Col identified his ideal state as being a brave hero, and his feared place as being dangerous and hated – 'a monster'.

Col identified his target TPP:

'I want to be liked so I hide my feelings and allow people to tell me what to do. But I feel angry that no one understands me. I can't let people see who I am as they might punish me (reject me, put me in prison again). I feel like a "scared trapped mouse".'

Col's concern with not being exposed meant that he suppressed many of his thoughts and feelings. Using drawings, the concept of learning to hear your inner voice was introduced to Col.

Figure 9.9: Inner voice (based on Scrivener 2012).

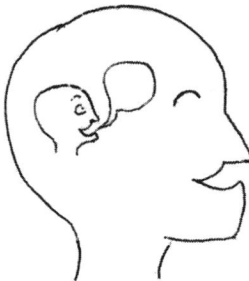

Col spoke about how his inner voice could ruin things for him, and how he mustn't listen to it. The inner voice appeared to be a 'free child' state (Berne, 1961), as opposed to the repressed adult. Col referred to it as 'my little voice'. It seemed that Col was experiencing internal battles between the adult- and child-states within him. Col identified the dilemma that either he does what people want and his voice is not heard, or he stands up for himself and gets into trouble. We explored standing up for yourself as 'having your voice heard', and how this is important in order to have a life that he is happier in. We identified that an exit for him may be to give his little person a voice, as he never had this as a child. Role-play allowed Col to reflect on what he would tell his younger self, and this provided a shift to enable him to consider how he could be compassionate to himself (Winnicott, 1971). Col identified his main aim of therapy as 'To have a voice and a life he feels better about'.

Self-reflection in between sessions was encouraged, using a TPP rating sheet (Figure 9.10).

Figure 9.10: Target Problem Procedure (TPP) rating sheet

Angry and unsafe 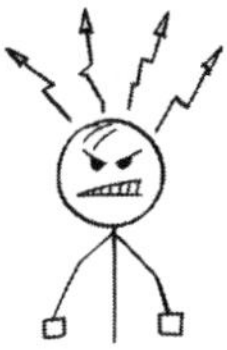	Alone and scared 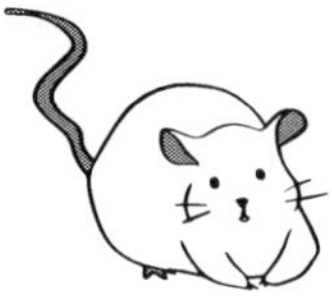
What I did:	What I did:
Did it help?	Did it help?

This also helped to recognize and address enactment, transference, and countertransference, inside and outside of the therapy. Initially, Col did not complete any of the rating scales that we had developed together. We explored this using the map RRP of 'controlling–controlled' and 'protected–protecting', linked to the emotional state of hidden. I invited Col to use his inner voice and Col reported that he wanted therapy to 'F**k off'. We explored Col's ongoing discomfort with CAT as a process. Col related that this was to do with a fear of being exposed, judged and the uncovering of painful memories. Col said that his life 'is terrible' and he didn't feel it could get any better. I gently challenged this, reminding him of tough times in his life, including being in a Young Offenders' Institution, and how life has moved on and improved since then, proving change is possible. This was a replenishing action (Clarkson, 2003), supporting Col to start thinking about exits from his TPPs.

Within the therapy, I recognized the need to model that expressing painful truths and associated feelings does not necessarily result in negative responses from others. When I observed transference taking place, such as Col's attempts to say what he thought I wanted to hear, like 'therapy is helping', I reflected upon how this felt disingenuous given the difficulties he had shared in his self-rating scale. He acknowledged this and stated that he wanted to please me. I invited him on these occasions to use creative mediums to honestly express these feelings. During session nine, when I questioned Col regarding his redirecting therapy away from a problematic pattern, Col said that sometimes his little voice 'hates you'. This allowed me to recognize the potential for countertransference in feeling punished or needing to please. I validated the challenges of therapy and reminded Col that engaging in CAT is his choice to make. Col said he wanted to continue, and we mapped out the shift that had taken place between us. Potter (2016) describes this as 'hovering and shimmering', using the map to consider different perspectives. Col's experiences of me as the therapist being listening and caring allowed him to feel heard and cared for. This was the springboard to enable future changes to be made (Ryle & Kerr, 2020).

In sessions ten to twelve, we continued to use RRPs to complete the map with possible exits. Unmanageable emotions of anger, fear and guilt were placed on the map. A toy grenade was selected by Col as a symbol of his unvoiced discontent and associated unexploded anger, which was placed on his map. Through creativity, Col's started to develop self-awareness of his TPPs using an 'observing eye' (Ryle & Kerr, 2020). This provided opportunities to consider coping strategies and exits in response to the recognition of TPPs (Corbridge et al, 2018). Col wrote on the map, 'I wish I could turn the clock back' (Figure 9.11). He said that he wished he could help his young self and began to cry. We stayed in the moment together, appreciating the vulnerability between us that this truth exposed (Stern, 1985).

Figure 9.11: Map revision

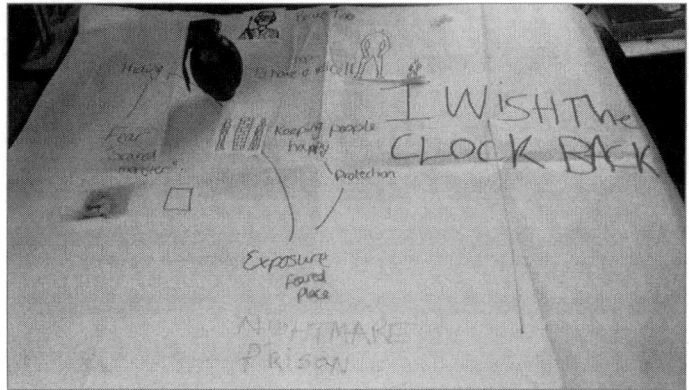

A core identified TPP was the 'fear of hurting other people's feelings' trap. Col recognized that this people-pleasing results in him hiding his thoughts and feelings. I encouraged him to think of ways in which he could start practicing having his voice heard, such as informing his support staff of choices he wants to make about his activities. Col was invited to practice ways of telling staff within the session, using role play.

Endings: Sessions 14-16

In the final three appointments of CAT, we reflected on the therapy journey. Col was able to recognize his emotional states, and how he had found the exposing nature of therapy frightening at times. We linked this to his RRPs, drawing out a TPP of his difficulties in engaging in therapy as the snag. Col recognized that he had grown in confidence and had learned about himself. We spoke about how Col had started to listen and use his inner voice to have his own needs met. We discussed that accepting the past, and that it can't be changed, is a big step forward. Col reflected on the challenges that he continued to have due to his history and resulting restrictions. We started to explore the idea that he could find a different path, to have opportunities to make decisions with the support of his staff (Lloyd & Clayton, 2013).

In session fourteen, the concept of having a healthy island was introduced, with positives that Col could use to ground and contain him during difficult times. However, Col used this exercise to develop a fantasy island where he is the protector and keeper of his own safe place. This involved him being safe and in control, as well as being protected from dangerous people by powerful others – in this instance, sharks. This fantasy appeared to reflect Col's continued desire to have control over his own world, while being kept safe and protected by his staff from potential risks. (Figure 9.12).

Figure 9.12: Healthy island

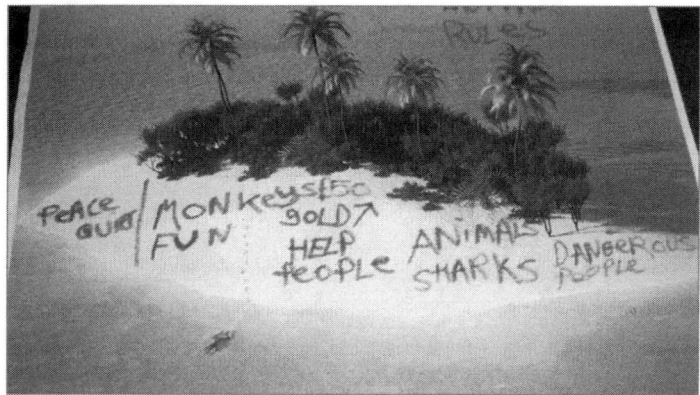

In session fifteen, I provided Col with a goodbye letter. I was supported by my supervision group to write a personal and meaningful account of Col's therapy journey. I read the letter to Col and gave him a copy. Col also wrote a goodbye letter which he gave to me. I observed in his goodbye letter the enactment of trying to please me, but also noted that he had included that therapy had been hard for him. The enactment of cutting off was interpreted as Col's strategy for coping with the ending of another relationship in his life.

Dear Col,

Now that we have come to the end of the therapy, here is the goodbye letter I promised to write you. I wanted to start by saying how brave I think you have been in coming to therapy. I remember how scared you were, 'a scared mouse' as you later described, when we first met. You have worked so hard to tell me why therapy is so frightening for you, even though this was difficult to do.

The things that make therapy painful:

- *The past.*
- *Not really trusting yourself.*
- *Worrying that people will think you are bad and might even send you back to prison.*

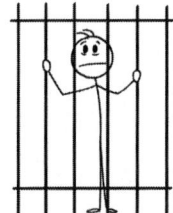

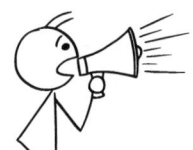

We came to understand, in therapy, that these things also cause the problems in your life that you wanted to work on in our therapy. You came to therapy saying:

1. *You want to have a voice, for others to listen to you and understand what you want in your life.*
2. *To be able to see yourself as a good person and like yourself more.*
3. *To feel less scared about making choices in your life.*

In our early sessions you kept yourself very hidden from me. You reported that everything and everyone in your life was happy and skipped over any of the bad things that had happened in your past.

By using the sandbox, the toy animals, and pictures, you started to find a way to have a voice about what you wanted from your life, which is 'to be a brave hero' and to protect others.

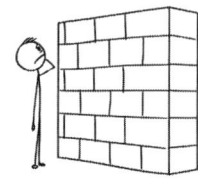

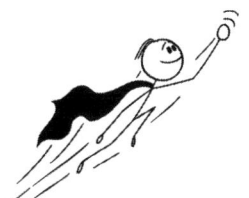

You also told me about the people who you had supported you in your life, and that you trusted, X, X, X and X. I also learned that you have an amazing imagination, and that you are a brilliant storyteller. This can be good as it allows you to escape to a different world, but I wonder if it may also cause

you difficulties at times. It may be another way of escaping from real life, or a way of distracting attention away from yourself?

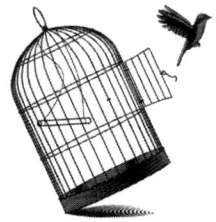

As our sessions went on, although it could be difficult and at times painful for you, you started to make steps to talk more honestly about your feelings and problems. You were able to tell me how difficult your life has been. The breakthrough came when you told me you wished 'therapy would f**k off' so that you didn't have to face the pain. You also told me that at times you 'hated therapy' for bringing out these painful feelings. This seemed a huge step, as you are always concerned about other people's feelings and making sure everyone likes you. I wondered if being able to say these things to me showed that you felt safe with me, and able to say what you really felt without worrying that you would be judged or punished. I hope that expressing your true feelings, wants and needs is something you will feel more confident to do now in your everyday life?

At times you spoke about feeling that your life is 'crap' and your sense of hopelessness that things could be better. It seems like you don't feel you deserve a good life. You often spoke about the inner you (little voice), being 'a git', 'ruining everything', and that you could not let this part of you out. However, your inner voice is part of you 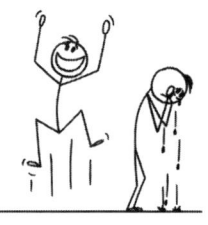 and it can be helpful. We practiced listening safely to the inner voice a lot in therapy. Maybe now you have been able to start to listen to your inner voice, without letting it get out of control?

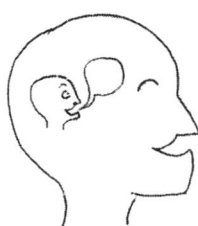

I know you feel bad about things in your past, both that have happened to you and things that you have done. You said you 'want to turn back the clock'. I felt your pain and helplessness, and I wanted so much to wipe the pain away. Sadly, this is not possible. But hopefully therapy will have helped you see that things in the future can change and be better?

I also hope that you can see what I and many other people see are the good things about you, including how much you care about people, your kindness, your fun side, and how much you never want to hurt anyone again.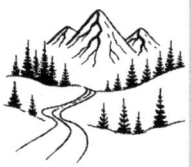

> *Towards the end of therapy, we started to look at things that may help you to have a life you feel better about. These were our ideas:*
>
>
>
> - *You would like to create a life storybook to help you remember some happy times you had in your past, because your past is part of who you are today.*
> - *You are also hoping to have a memorial to your dad, to help you say goodbye properly.*
> - *You are going to ask for regular meetings with your staff team, helped by your care coordinator, so that you can have a voice about how your support package is going and what changes you would like.*
> - *You have agreed to use your experiences to help improve the lives of other people with learning disabilities, by being part of an interview panel for staff.*
> - *Dramatherapy groups will be explored to help you use your wonderful imagination in a safe and fun way.*
>
> *Col, I really enjoyed working with you. It has not always been easy for either of us, as I tried to help you look at things you wanted to run and hide from. But with your bravery you explored, progressed and developed new ways of thinking through therapy. This is only the start Col, and I am confident that you can make the changes required to have a life that is more of your choosing.*
>
> *With very best wishes,*
> *Sarah*

In our final session, we reviewed the final map with exits (Figure 9.13).

Figure 9.13: Final map with exits

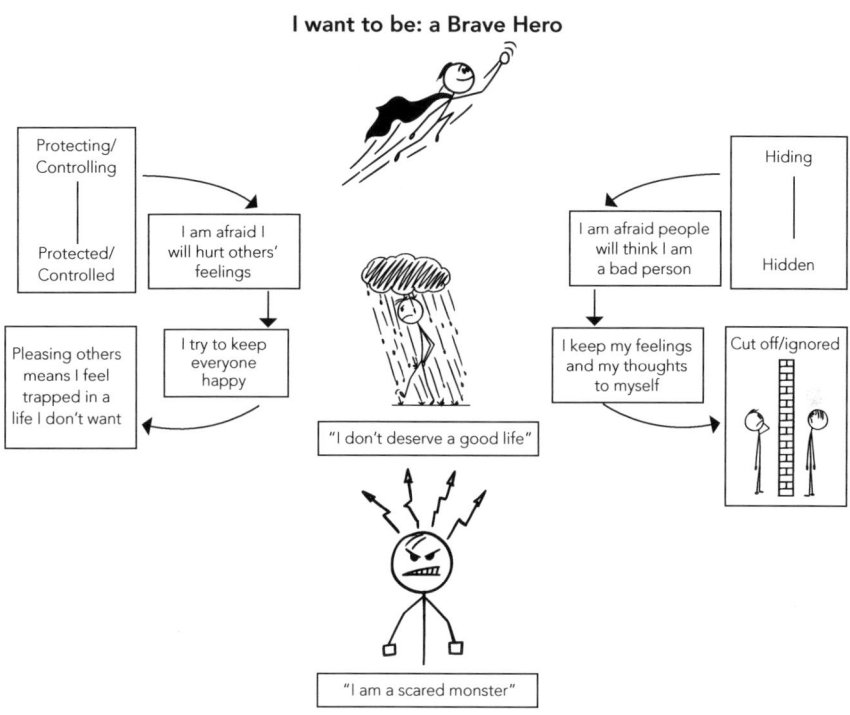

1) Having a voice	2) Liking yourself more
■ Practice in the mirror what you want to say. ■ Talk to your care coordinator. ■ Write down what you want to say. ■ Have staff meetings you run. ■ Ask your keyworker/staff to help.	■ Use your CAT tools to remember what you have achieved. ■ Get involved with groups and activities you enjoy, e.g. drama. ■ Take care of yourself, e.g. eat well, exercise.

The CAT observing eye, in self-reflection and recognition of his TPP (Akande, 2007), was considered for his future use. Col reflected that he had started to listen to his inner voice and use it to have his emotional needs met. He said that he had enjoyed the creative elements of therapy the most, especially the object and sandbox work. Col recognized that he had found talking about his past the most difficult part of the therapy process.

Col considered his ongoing difficulties in telling staff how he is feeling and what he would like. He decided that he would ask his care coordinator to support him to facilitate staff meetings.

Col wanted to feel some connection with his past and, in particular, his father. We talked about him creating a memory book. He also felt it would help him to have a memorial to his father, as he had not attended the funeral.

We then discussed Col's desire to live out his fantasy role of being a brave hero. Col was interested in joining an adult drama group to provide opportunities to safely explore being different characters.

Follow-up sessions

Two follow-up sessions were provided, one and three months after we finished CAT. In the first follow-up meeting, Col said that he now felt more confident to express his wants and needs in his everyday life. I noticed the countertransference eliciting a feeling of being pleased. I checked this with Col, and he acknowledged he wanted my praise. He said the reality is that he still worries he will upset staff, so largely keeps his own thoughts and feelings hidden. We thought about how he could feel more empowered with his staff team. We discussed that a step towards this could be his involvement in the recruitment of staff. With his care coordinator's support, it was agreed that Col is part of an interview panel for new staff and involved in their induction and training.

By the second follow-up meeting, Col had been involved in the recruitment of two new staff members. Col spoke about his initial fears, and how he had overcome them. He was also working with his keyworker to develop a training package for staff on how to support him. Col said he felt proud as he felt his views were being listened to. This new competent role appears pivotal in starting to give Col a voice in his own life and a healthy reciprocal role of 'speaking up – listened to/compassionately understood'.

Reflections

My supervision group and Suzanne Lyons as my supervisor were invaluable in supporting me in maintaining safety for both myself and Col within therapy. They also helped me to reflect on the enactments and re-enactments that took place inside and outside the therapy, and encouraged me to be brave in using versatility within the therapy.

Col's care coordinator was also an important figure in providing continuity and the link between what was happening inside therapy and Col's outside world. He not only knew Col well, but also advocated for him to be heard.

During therapy, Col never spoke about his abuse, either as a victim or a perpetrator. But it was ever present in the room as the 'scared mouse/ monster' he referred to himself as. I took the position of 'insideness' (Hepple, 2010; Hepple, Chapter 12, this volume) as I wanted to show Col that I did not see him as 'a monster'. Col came to therapy feeling unlovable, dangerous and a burden. I wanted to show Col that I heard his pain, and this enabled me to build a platform of mutual respect so that we could engage in the collaborative CAT process of effecting change. Through creative approaches I was able to move towards the position of 'outsideness' (Hepple, 2010; Hepple, Chapter 12 this volume), in which I could support Col to see that he is the catalyst to make positive changes in his own life.

Summary

The dialogic perspective of individuals evolving and responding to their relational context (Hepple, 2013) can be seen in Col, who as a victim and a perpetrator saw himself as the 'scared monster'.

'I get myself from the other: It is only the other's categories that will let me be an object of my own perception' (Holquist, 2004, p15).

By recognizing how internalized relationship interactions impact Col's sense of himself (Object Relations, Feltham & Dryden, 1993), he could then consider the development of new, healthy RRPs represented in the exits in his map (PSORM, Ryle, 1991).

CAT provides opportunities to develop and use a shared understanding of the enactments and procedures at play inside and outside the room that provide context to their personal narrative (Bakhtin, 1981). Potter (2019) talks about therapeutic moments in CAT, in which the direction, feel and relationships within the room are shaped. It is through these moments that there is a 'meeting of minds' (Stern, 2010) and the healthy reciprocal role of 'willing given to gratefully received' is modelled (Corbridge et al, 2018). Through the process of exploring the versatility of the CAT model using creative therapeutic activities, alongside contextual and developmental perspectives (Lloyd & Clayton, 2013), Col was provided with opportunities for self-reflection and to consider how to apply new skills to have greater therapeutic integration of his relational inner and outer worlds (Potter, 2019).

Chapter 10: Neurodivergence and the Multiple Self States Model

James Randall

With thanks to Petal, Jade and Leon (pseudonyms are used to maintain confidentiality).

To be neurodivergent is to see, feel and experience the self, others and the world in ways unfamiliar to most (neurotypical) people. Understanding oneself as autistic, for example, involves differences in communication and social interaction, which in certain contexts can enable or restrain an individual's socio-emotional engagement. Whether someone thrives, just about survives, or deteriorates, is very much contingent on how attuned others and environments can be to underlying neurodivergent needs in social, psychological, and relational experiences –too often overlooked.

With a guiding value of collaboration, Cognitive Analytic Therapy (CAT) promotes a curious therapy which should welcome neurodivergence. CAT offers communicative and interactive scaffolds to address relational and mental health difficulties, and the opportunity to recognize and negotiate patterns within one's life.

This chapter explores how, when facing complex and developmental trauma, CAT's Multiple Self States Model (MSSM) can be a useful framework within which to understand the impact on selves when a neurotypical world attempts to seep inside (for example, partially dissociated states of autistic meltdown, autistic shutdown, or autistic burnout). Herein lies an opportunity to empower individuals to notice and observe the relational conditions from which such emotional states emerge. Many autistic people describe themselves as having a multiplicity of self-states; describing separate and individual 'parts' of themselves, identifying themselves as 'plurals' and self-states as 'alters'. In terms of CAT and the MSSM, these self-states are often described as having varying degrees of dissociation, with some being partially integrated as opposed to dissociated.

In exploring the use of CAT and the MSSM to support autistic individuals, this chapter describes and demonstrates a handful of ways to engage creatively in such work and how practitioners can look to invite the plurality of alters into dialogue. The relevance of CAT, and the techniques and ideas developed in clinical practice are shared throughout.

Three accounts of engaging with CAT, with illustrative materials and key practitioner learning points, are shared to support readers to expand their own zone of proximal development (ZPD, Vygotsky & Cole, 1978), and most importantly, to look to better engage and support autistic individuals in CAT.

CAT can support neurodivergent people to reformulate and map out ways to develop and change for the better in a neurotypical world that does not always hold them in mind. And what this chapter can offer is a reassurance that this can be inclusive of all aspects of one's self: the dissociated and integrated states, the voiced and unvoiced states.

What is autism?

Autism is a neurodevelopmental diagnosis that is assumed to reflect genetics. However, the presentation and visibility of autism are largely shaped by interactions with one's environment and culture. Autistic traits are typically observed in children before the age of three. However, increasingly individuals are being referred for diagnostic assessment following key transitions in life, whereby increases in socio-emotional, relational and academic demands lead to a greater visibility of or reliance on autistic traits. For example, schools may recognize autistic traits in the individual when environmental changes mean that the masking of autistic traits is no longer sustainable.

The Diagnostic and Statistical Manual of Mental Disorders – Fifth Edition (DSM-5) criteria for autism includes 'deficits' in social interaction and communication (e.g., socio-emotional reciprocity, non-verbal communication, relationships), and a preference for particular or repeated regulating, balancing and/or soothing behaviours (e.g., a need for predictability, fixated interests, overwhelming or immersive sensory experiences, idiosyncratic stimming behaviours, or speech).

'Neurodiversity' is a term originating from multiple discussions amongst autistic individuals via 'the Institute for the Study of the Neurologically

Typical' and those participating in an 'Independent Living' discussion forum – but is often cited as being coined by autistic sociologist Judy Singer (Botha *et al.* 2024). 'Neurodiversity' reframes the psychiatric lens of 'deficit' or 'disorder' (which are arguably *imposed upon* autistic people within the medical/psychiatric paradigm), with an appreciation of the multiplicities of experiencing the world.

Accessing CAT as an autistic person

For a multitude of reasons, the prevalence of mental health difficulties is much greater for autistic people than it is for neurotypical individuals (Lai *et al*, 2019). Lai and colleagues (2019) note that anxiety difficulties, sleep disturbance and 'conduct disorders' are most prevalent in autistic adults, and that exposure to trauma, patterns of substance misuse, and questions of gender identity are very common.

Autistic people rarely feel well supported by psychiatric services and at times feel harmed by therapies, and so advocate that *complexity requires flexibility* (Brede *et al*, 2022). Indeed, research surveying autistic service users in Scotland (Hallett & Crompton, 2018) highlighted that:

- individuals want the opportunity to collaborate and work jointly with practitioners in addressing problems within therapy – while recognizing they may need additional supports in order to feel able to do this.
- individuals want to learn about the services being offered to them and to have a clear sense of what therapy involves.
- therapy environments need to be inclusive in terms of being sensorily and physically accessible.

What this research suggests to me, is that CAT may well be one way of addressing these needs within psychological therapy and broader systemic intervention. Service users find CAT to be a useful opportunity to gain knowledge, skills, and insight into the relational patterns most pertinent to their lives (Balmain, Melia, Dent & Smith, 2021), through time-limited, structured and collaborative means. Within CAT, neurotypical and autistic people alike, may benefit from the specific and transparent structures and transitions within the work. From the outset of therapy, there is a clear trajectory and, early on, individuals collaborate on defining the terms of the work through target problems. Specifically, this may aid in developing a more secure and safe context for the autistic person to trust in, having in my experience often experienced unexpected or poorly planned changes and a lack of clarity in aims and vision for defined endings. Table 10.1 expands on aspects of structure seemingly conducive to the engagement of autistic individuals.

Table 10.1: CAT tools when working with autistic individuals

CAT tool	How this supports autistic clients
The Psychotherapy File (see Appendix 1)	The Psychotherapy File offers: ■ Dialogical scaffolds: listing a number of example patterns and inviting individuals to identify relevance to their circumstances. ■ For example, this can be particularly helpful for autistic people who become non-verbal when faced with pressures, demands, and/or change outside of their complete control. ■ The Psychotherapy File offers a fantastic opportunity for collaboration, whereby individuals can analyse and 'correct' patterns to guide the therapist in their endeavour to build a shared understanding.
The Sequential Diagrammatic Reformulation (SDR)	The Sequential Diagrammatic Reformulation (SDR) offers: ■ A visual scaffold that is personalized, historical and situational (making it relevant and applicable). ■ It can be both complex and simple in its design. ■ It can be guided by structure in a stepped way as per the theoretical development of CAT. For example, I have used the Procedural Sequence Object Relations Model to detail 'steps' within initial mapping, such as bottom-role experiences leading to needs, to appraisal beliefs, to actions, to consequences, to top-role experiences or a novel procedure (PSORM; Ryle & Kerr, 2020)).

CAT tool	How this supports autistic clients
Recognition and revision rating sheets	Recognition and revision rating sheets offer: ■ Logical and systematic ways of identifying and tracking relational patterns. This offers a tangible and hands-on means of scaffolded recognition (which could otherwise be challenging for some to remember, rehearse and apply outside of the therapy relationship itself). ■ Either a particularly useful process for individuals interested in mathematics, social sciences and academia – complementing the need for predictability. Or an opportunity to dismantle and redesign the approach to be more personally appropriate – particularly, in my experience, where an autistic person's strengths and identity revolve around the Arts and creativity instead. ■ An opportunity for ongoing evaluation, documentation and feedback – increasing clarity about the objectives of therapy and direction.
Narrative letters	The Reformulation Letter offers: ■ An often-novel experience of witnessing one's account through the voice of another – with intentions to both validate and expand understanding in terms of the zone of proximal development (Vygotsky & Cole, 1978). I have found this to be a powerful experience – possibly due to experiences of neurotypical environments and systems, and often, previously harmful psychological therapies (that too often overlook neurodivergent needs). ■ An opportunity for patterns associated with being autistic in a neurotypical world (e.g. masking) to be explicitly named and explored together. ■ An explicit statement of intention for the therapy in naming Target Problem Procedures – increasing transparency, predictability, and empowerment.

CAT tool	How this supports autistic clients
Narrative letters	The Goodbye Letter offers: ■ A shared opportunity to identify, name and reflect on the therapy and experiences of change. ■ An invitation for clear evaluation of the tools and processes of therapy, enabling further personalization and direction – scaffolding future change.
Other tools	Within CAT, additional tools offer further opportunities, such as: ■ *The Personality Structure Questionnaire* (PSQ; Pollock *et al.* 2001) helps to explore the extent to which a sense of self is deemed 'static' or diffuse and changeable. ■ Depending on aims, the PSQ can be used to explore changes in integration and the capacity to reflect on and notice self-state meta-procedures. Used as an informal outcome measure, though not tested for reliability/validity as use as such a scale, in practice, can offer feedback on change and springboard reflections. ■ *The States Description Procedure* (Pollock, Bennett & Ryle, 2003, as cited in Bennett & Ryle, 2005) supports identification, naming and evaluation of self-states in a step-by-step manner – which in my experience scaffolds relational awareness and reflection within CAT. Namely, one is prompted to identify (a) what they experience within themselves, (b) their attitude towards others within this moment, (c) other peoples' attitudes towards them, and (d) the frequency, intensity, triggers and factors which bring about repair or closure. ■ *The Life Chart* provides individuals with a relational-focused structure to what many individuals will have experience of from engaging in other psychological therapies (e.g. timelines). Within my practice with autistic individuals, there

CAT tool	How this supports autistic clients
	has been positive feedback that focusing on how one has learned to cope or has adapted to past events, rather than 'just listing' events, creates a dynamic process of self-self reflecting and curiosity; and therefore, mitigates the potential harms of what can be felt to be 'needless repetition' or exposure to re-traumatizing life content without the rationale of underlying meaning and purpose in doing so.
	Outside of CAT, many other tools can be incorporated to further scaffold the relational approach:
	■ The Camouflaging Autistic Traits Questionnaire (CAT-Q (Hull *et al*, 2019)) is a screening measure used to identify patterns in 'masking' autistic traits (i.e. coping through efforts to hide traits or present a non-autistic persona), compensating (i.e. developing patterns that coping that mitigate the impact of autistic traits, such as copying others' communication styles), and assimilating (i.e. efforts to adapt and change oneself in social situations). These concepts clearly link with CAT procedures, and, in my experience, this tool can be used in a similar way to The Psychotherapy File.
	■ The CAT-Q also categorizes responses (along with non-clinical norms), providing some explicit feedback to clients on their patterns and procedures specific to coping with being autistic in a neurotypical world.

Little is published on CAT with autistic individuals. Victoria, a woman diagnosed with Asperger's syndrome, appears to agree that much of what CAT has to offer could help many neurodivergent people – as detailed in her published account of engaging with CAT (Victoria, 2015). Victoria detailed how she benefited from CAT structures, the focus on written communications, and importantly, how the therapist is open and transparent about their thoughts and intentions (rather than relying on service users to read and interpret non-verbal communications, for example). Similarly, I have shared my own work on the appropriateness of CAT when working with autistic individuals – particularly young people with complex and developmental trauma histories (Randall, 2023). Along similar lines, Chorlton (2023) reflected on the use of CAT in post-diagnostic support for adults newly diagnosed with autism, the usefulness of CAT in addressing the consequences of lifelong masking, the helpfulness of adapting or using CAT in more 'concrete' ways, and some of the challenges for neurotypical and neurodivergent individuals to psychologically attune to one another's relating.

From my experience working with autistic people accessing services for significant mental health difficulties, many have faced numerous adverse childhood events and trauma (e.g. childhood neglect, childhood sexual abuse, criminal exploitation).

The 'Torchlight model' (Jefferis *et al*, 2021) demonstrates how CAT requires multiple layers of synergistic scaffolding. The model describes how the beginning stages of therapy involve a CAT map which develops with the client, therapist and CAT concepts working in partnership, as the therapeutic relationship dynamically evolves. Indeed, they detail how mapping *needs* and *builds* the relationship (Jefferis *et al*, 2021). Where diversity is named as a client factor within this research, neurodiversity highlights the necessity to consider relative differences between and within the space and the dynamics which can and will emerge as a result. Indeed, something which Chorlton (2023) reflected upon in terms of negotiating differences in the need for, or seeking of, attunement within CAT.

There are, in my view, key components which either need adding to CAT to support autistic individuals, or careful, considered and purposeful adaptation, to better support the suitability of CAT for autistic people:

- An integration of embodied, sensory and neurodivergent needs early on in the work (and ongoing thereafter). Collaboration becomes a crucial tool in the process of asking, learning and nourishing these multifaceted needs within the therapeutic context. For example, this could involve dedicated space to explore what autism looks like for that specific individual, involving an explicit invitation to stim if and when needed (e.g. a preference for repeated regulating and balancing bodily movements, such as rocking back and forth or rhythmic humming) – with individuals often reporting to have restrained themselves and masked such needs in many other contexts.

- A genuine curiosity to engage with and learn from the individual's interests (sometimes described as 'specialist' or 'fixated'). These interests can inform, guide and personalize CAT tools – supporting progressive engagement in the zone of proximal development (Vygotsky & Cole, 1978). For example, Petal, an autistic young adult accessing sixteen-session CAT returned to a session having completely redesigned their CAT map with detailed sketches of teeth depicting reciprocal role procedures (e.g. others 'pulling teeth'; sensitive roots), and playfully, the observing eye was adopted as the light on the dentist's forehead; exploring, investigating, documenting and intervening (see below for further discussion on Petal's CAT). The creative possibilities are endless, but authenticity is key; meaningful integration can occur from adopting the position of genuine curiosity, interest and participation in someone's interests.

- Awareness and experience in the Multiple Self States Model (MSSM (Ryle, 1997)) of CAT appears necessary for a number of reasons, which will be explored further below. In short, autistic individuals often report a multiplicity of selves with varying degrees of integration. Dissociation is frequently reported, particularly as part of patterns in overwhelm or autistic meltdown and shutdown – which can take shape as distinct self-states. Some autistic traits, such as 'thinking and feeling in the extremes', 'all or nothing thinking', and perceived cognitive rigidity, predispose individuals to operate along similar lines to the MSSM conceptualisations of the interface of self-states (e.g. switches, partial and complete dissociation). Within neurotypical contexts, autistic individuals are also much more likely to require additional supports in terms of scaffolding 'reflective capacity', as defined by the model.

Autism and the Multiple Self States Model

The MSSM offers a framework within which to understand the structure of 'personality'. It is particularly useful in drawing attention to entrenched and chronic, 'disruptive' reciprocal role procedures that are seemingly trait-like, internalized and consolidated to the extent that they reflect one's personality and selfhood. These are proposed to emerge from adverse childhood events and environments, and so the model is often applied in contexts of complex trauma. Within the context of autism, there may be 'disruptive' reciprocal role procedures which damage and limit self-development and growth, but there is also an additional layer in which individuals may learn and internalise scripts that their procedures are 'disruptive' – when in fact they are simply attempting to be themselves in neurotypical environmental and relational contexts. Indeed, sometimes snags may come from important others in our lives or the environmental conditions in which we find ourselves. (See The Psychotherapy File, Appendix 1).

There appears to be a significant overlap between how autistic traits manifest in trauma and the psychiatric diagnosis of 'borderline personality disorder'. Traumatized autistic people often present with identity confusion and disturbance, emotional extremes, mood switches, dissociation and depersonalization, and interpersonal conflicts. Manifesting procedures frequently involve suicidal fantasies, plans and acts, repeated self-harm, substance (mis)use, complex patterns of engagement with others and with services, and targeted abuse from others, among many other experiences.

The MSSM, with its development in response to the need to conceptualise and address such concerns at the level of 'identity' (in terms of self-state composition and dynamics), appears equally relevant and applicable then, to the context of CAT with autistic individuals – whom, much like individuals diagnosed with 'personality disorder', are much more likely to have faced discrimination, exploitation, abuse and stigmatization. The MSSM provides a theoretical underpinning that can validate relational mental health in association with traits, states, temperament and, ultimately, more entrenched ways of being. It can be a helpful frame in which to understand the core structures, roles and procedures underlying these presenting problems for autistic people; poorly integrated or partially dissociated self-states, or similarly, a plurality of coherent yet fragile self-states.

Whereas within 'personality disorder' CAT, the focus may be solely on the integration of self-states, for autistic individuals this may not be warranted, wanted or even possible. Namely, the difference here is that (from a neurotypical lens) the perceived rigidity or construct inflexibility of emotional and self-states can be inherent to autism (possible reframes in an affirmative approach, could consider the 'solidness' and construct predictability of states). In this light, this perceived inflexibility of states does not necessarily need to be changed, nor can or should be – theoretically and ethically speaking. However, given the multiplicity of internalized states, some possibly more attributable to adverse events and experiences, the therapeutic process of exploration and collaboration in identifying such states and holding them for consideration within the process of change – remains important.

The MSSM involves three levels of self-state organization (Ryle, 1997). Conceptually, 'level one' of the MSSM describes how an individual's 'personality structure' may entail a narrow and restricted number of self-states. These fewer self-states are characterized by rigid and inflexible ways of relating and are often experienced as depicting an 'extreme' emotional state, distinguished in concretely 'black and white' ways – 'all or nothing' states of being.

Level two of the MSSM depicts the ways in which self-states 'interact'. Within this level, the extent of disintegration or fragmentation of self-states is suggestive of greater psychological disturbance. Whereby disturbance at level one of the MSSM depicts the rigidity, inflexibility and extremes of each self-state for the individual, level two details the extent to which these can be switched between. Disturbance at level two is depicted, then, by dissociation and partial dissociation of self-states. Namely, one may experience but be unaware of their different parts, who are by all accounts estranged from one another through dissociative processes; fragmentation that often manifests in chaotic and confusing self-state switches. Such fragmentation may not necessitate that this fragmentation results in conscious or immediate distress or problems for the individual but becomes most apparent to those in social encounters with the individual (e.g. partners, bosses).

Psychological distress associated with self-state switches tends to be contingent on an individual's ability to observe and reflect on not only the content of their self-states but also their dynamic mechanisms of change and the relating (or lack of) that takes place between themselves. 'Level three' disturbance within the MSSM depicts the lack of capacity that individuals can have in terms of reflecting on self-states and these dynamic processes of switching/changing self-states. The capacity to reflect is proposed to be chronic and inherently difficult for individuals whose personality structure is considered fractured in this way. The non-reflective stance depicted in level three disturbance is said to be established within the formative years, and to manifest through temperament and trait.

As demonstrated here, the application of the MSSM in supporting autistic people through CAT invites an openness to be challenging of the dominant conceptual assumptions held within the framework. Considering the third level of the MSSM, I suggest that a distinction between 'disturbance' and 'disruption' could be conceptually useful when using CAT with autistic people. As described, level three disturbance supposes an engrained, possibly embodied difficulty in reflecting on the nature of self-state integration, which may well be the case for autistic individuals who do not have nourishing, scaffolding and affirmative environments conducive to building reflective capacities historically or presently.

To consider the potential for 'disruption' at level three of the MSSM could help to contextualize approaches further. Namely, the ways in which society, neurotypicals, and specifically in this context, therapists, can be complicit in overlooking or neglecting foundational considerations and practices needed to support the autistic person's engagement. This may involve initial sessions thoroughly unpacking and sharing sensory needs within therapy spaces, or pre-CAT negotiations and contracting around schedules and routines, or inviting feedback on interpersonal style and needs (e.g. not all autistic people require 'closed questions'). These practices 'warm up' the relational capacity not of the individual necessarily - but of the therapeutic relationship and relational ZPD (Vygotsky & Cole, 1978). Such practices ought to nourish autistic needs, welcome expression of traits, celebrate neurodivergent identities, and, in doing so, create conducive environments for relational progress and positive change through CAT.

These practices ought not to be thought of as radical in practice, but possibly radical in principle and values. Take, for example, the notion that autistic individuals struggle to or cannot empathize – this is simply stigmatizing and discriminatory, in that it decontextualises the individual. 'Verbing the noun' is a personally useful CAT mantra, which translates this proposition to something along the lines of *empathizing-understood*. For neurotypical individuals to propose that autistic people 'lack empathy', are they themselves simply failing to empathise with the autistic person's processing, experiencing and expression of empathy? It's a reciprocal conundrum, captured by 'the double empathy problem', as described by Milton (2012), in that autistic people do not only struggle because they potentially misunderstand others and the world, but also because they are *misunderstood by* others and the world.

The relative failure of psychiatry to acknowledge the inherent relational component to 'difficulties in' empathy emphasizes the very 'top-heavy' basis to these reciprocal roles. Arguably, society and professionals specifically have disproportionately 'weighed down' on autistic people: discriminating, excluding and abusing. Figure 10.1 illustrates the multitude of factors connecting the conditions of CAT, which therapists need to consider when offering CAT to autistic clients – including a curiosity about their own relational capacity, intersectionality (which may include neurodivergence), and personality structures.

Figure 10.1: CAT therapy in a neurotypical society (Randall, 2024).

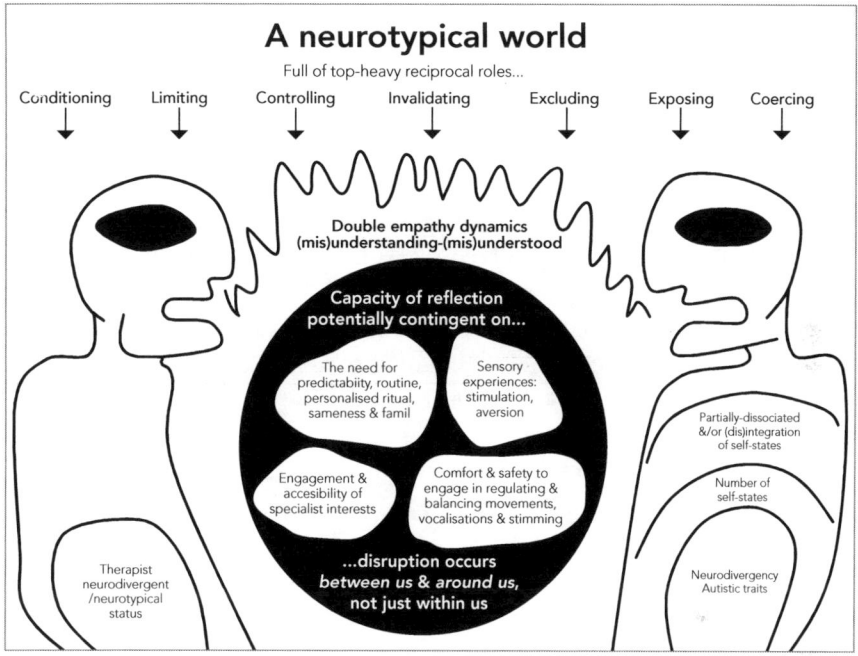

Working creatively with self-states in autism

As described, at least in the context of adverse childhood events, developmental trauma and complex relational mental health, the MSSM within CAT is a welcomed resource in conceptualizing psychological distress and associated relational patterns. Numerous clients have benefited from this approach within my practice, with reports of people feeling 'taken seriously', validated, and 'not having everything blamed on autism'. Psychometrics have continually proved to be promising, with consistent clinically reliable change, albeit not always falling into non-clinical thresholds – but indicating change in the right direction, with associated reflections on a sense of ownership and control in crafting the individual's next steps. Below, I share some of my work and experiences with clients, using various approaches to engage with self-states. I hope to draw attention to any unique aspects of applying the MSSM within CAT for autistic clients, and to highlight novel and creative means of working together.

Petal

Petal is a twenty-year-old autistic woman with a history of sexual exploitation, reported 'toxicity' and complexity in relationships, and patterns of extreme meltdown or dissociated emptiness. Petal is motivated and open to rethinking her understanding of herself and patterns of relating, having already developed a sense of some of her relational patterns, such as 'cutting off' from others. Reformulation enabled her to expand her perspective, noticing, for example, the ways in which she could 'cut off' from herself, emotionally. CAT provided a language in which she could begin to appreciate the development of reciprocal roles in early life experiences and the ways in which she internalized relational patterns. Increasingly, self-states became more relevant to her understanding, as she noted the blockages between emotional states and her inability to recall and reflect on such moments. She would feel everything all at once or feel absolutely nothing at all. At other times, she would be overwhelmed by her own sensitivities and vulnerability, becoming child-like, cradled in hurt.

Petal was tasked with recognition work early on in therapy, with a more traditional CAT map draft. She returned having struggled to use the map in practice, particularly in moments where apparent states would take over her feeling and thinking. Initially, Petal could only use the map retrospectively following these incidents, but she gradually attempted to do so within the moment, having the map available in many different places. She struggled with this and returned one week with an alternative – she revealed a partly redesigned map, based on her passion for teeth – which I encouraged her to develop further.

Eventually, Petal's CAT map was fully teeth-based, and she was then able to use sections of this to aid recognition within the moment (sections were used almost like flashcards). These images, which carried meaning for her, enabled her to begin to see the conditions which allow self-states to emerge and to develop strategies to either prevent them or ensure the contextual supports were in place to mitigate their impact (e.g. managing social contact/diaries, scheduling mindful breaks). For Petal, self-self exits enabled a management plan of her self-states, and these were only permitted by observation through our playful CAT 'dentistry'. In taking this approach, Petal was able to 'tame' her self-states in a way that meant they did not have a significant and detrimental impact on her ability to function throughout the weeks. We reduced the severity and frequency of meltdowns and cut-offs, but remained grounded in our acceptance of their roles to play – given Petal's autistic traits and sensory sensitivities.

Figure 10.2: A Reciprocal Role procedure of cutting off, getting 'at the roots' of past and present (a separate image was used to depict the internalization of this pattern)

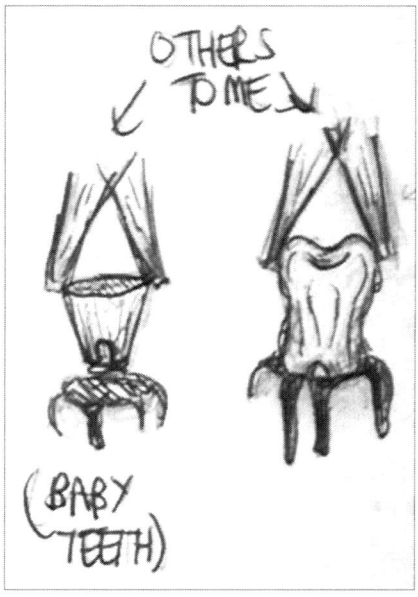

Figure 10.3. Petal's 'exposed roots' state visually depicted, with annotations aiding both recognition and revision.

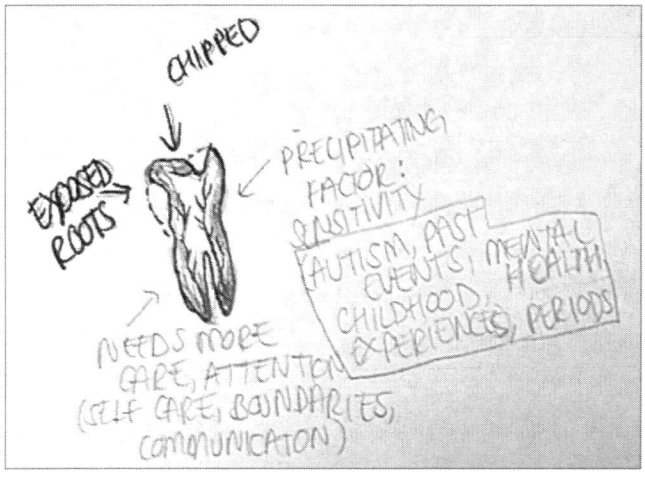

Figure 10.4. An illustration from Petal's exit map, depicting the potential of change through multiple means (within the metaphor of dentistry).

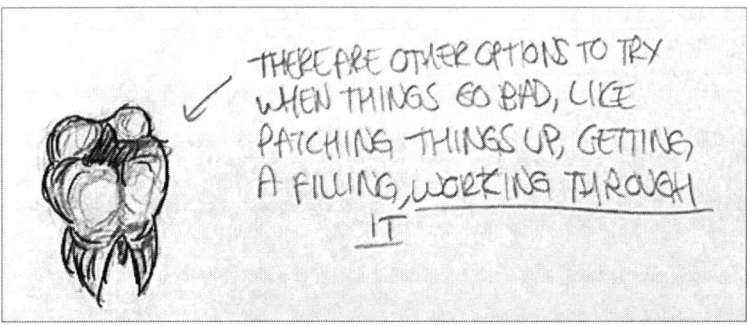

Key practice points:

- Making the task of noticing and naming self-states more tangible and practical may assist engagement throughout CAT.
- Be both person-led and passions-led; this will nourish the commitment to therapy and trust within the relationship. However, therapists should not 'chase' specialist interests – integration of these is a helpful possibility, but not a hard-line rule.
- Collaborating in the design of idiosyncratic and concrete aids will benefit the recognition phase of CAT, so therapists may wish to invite clients to redesign their maps and reassure them that 'the rules do not matter much'. When more unique or creative redesigns are brought back, the therapist and client can work together to ensure they are still working in ways which align with key CAT concepts and principles (e.g. reciprocal role procedures retained but possibly demonstrated in unique ways).
- Where the key aims of self-states-focused CAT are increased awareness and empowerment over managing (likely lifelong) cycles, a sixteen-session CAT may still be suitable (but one may wish to consider offering additional follow-ups along similar lines to twenty-four-session CAT).

Jade

Jade is a sixteen-year-old, newly diagnosed autistic girl, who reported a history of physical and emotional abuse at the hands of her father. She would experience herself to get caught up in the details when talking, losing track of where she started, but over time, learned to use her CAT map to direct and focus herself within the room. She would often notice talking *at* or *over* me at times, needing to 'finish the point', but anxious of our limited time – something she could notice, name and chuckle about, sometimes re-focusing and at other times making her choice to continue.

Jade is strong-willed, resilient, charismatic and forthright. Her CAT map (Figure 10.5) highlighted the ways in which she strived for connection, love and acceptance, but often found herself triggered into disconnection and separation – from others, but also from her values and needs in relationships. Anticipating abandonment, she would desperately 'cling on' but others would reject her, eliciting unmanageable feelings of repulsion. Jade would either unwittingly cut off from feeling and fall into her 'wise wizard' state of unemotive intellectualization, or another state switch would occur in which she would become 'psycho Jade' – enraged, dangerous and abusive. She would find herself facing a constant oscillation between 'all or nothing': from best friends to enemies, from quintessential love to disgust; from emotional overwhelm to vacant emptiness.

Jade has a passion for fiction, fantasy and history. She described how reading a book or watching a television series could help her identify how she feels and learn more about herself and her emotional states. She would connect, for example, to the afflicted villains – often rejected and ostracized by society, their emotions explode out or their actions disguise a real need for belonging and care. A key part of revision for Jade was in terms of the recognition of the relational contexts in which state shifts were triggered, and in parallel, we worked together to identify and 'thicken' alternative 'states' or personas – that could help validate, guide or respond to situations. This involved, quite naturalistically, Jade's passion for literature and the Arts.

She shared images or narratives which struck her as communicating something about her, such as Millais' Ophelia painting, which in Jade's eyes saw a dialectic of beauty and desirability, with loss and despair. This sharing evolved into an invitation, initially to guide recognition of her relational patterns – with some tentative linking of characters or art to elements of the CAT map. Over time, as this clearly scaffolded Jade's sense-making and her exploration of patterns outside of the therapy room, I invited her active engagement and reflection on the fiction she is most (or least) drawn to, and how this communicates something about the different parts of her. In reality, Jade also drew on a range of sources outside of fiction.

Figure 10.5: Illustrative re-creation of Jade's CAT map

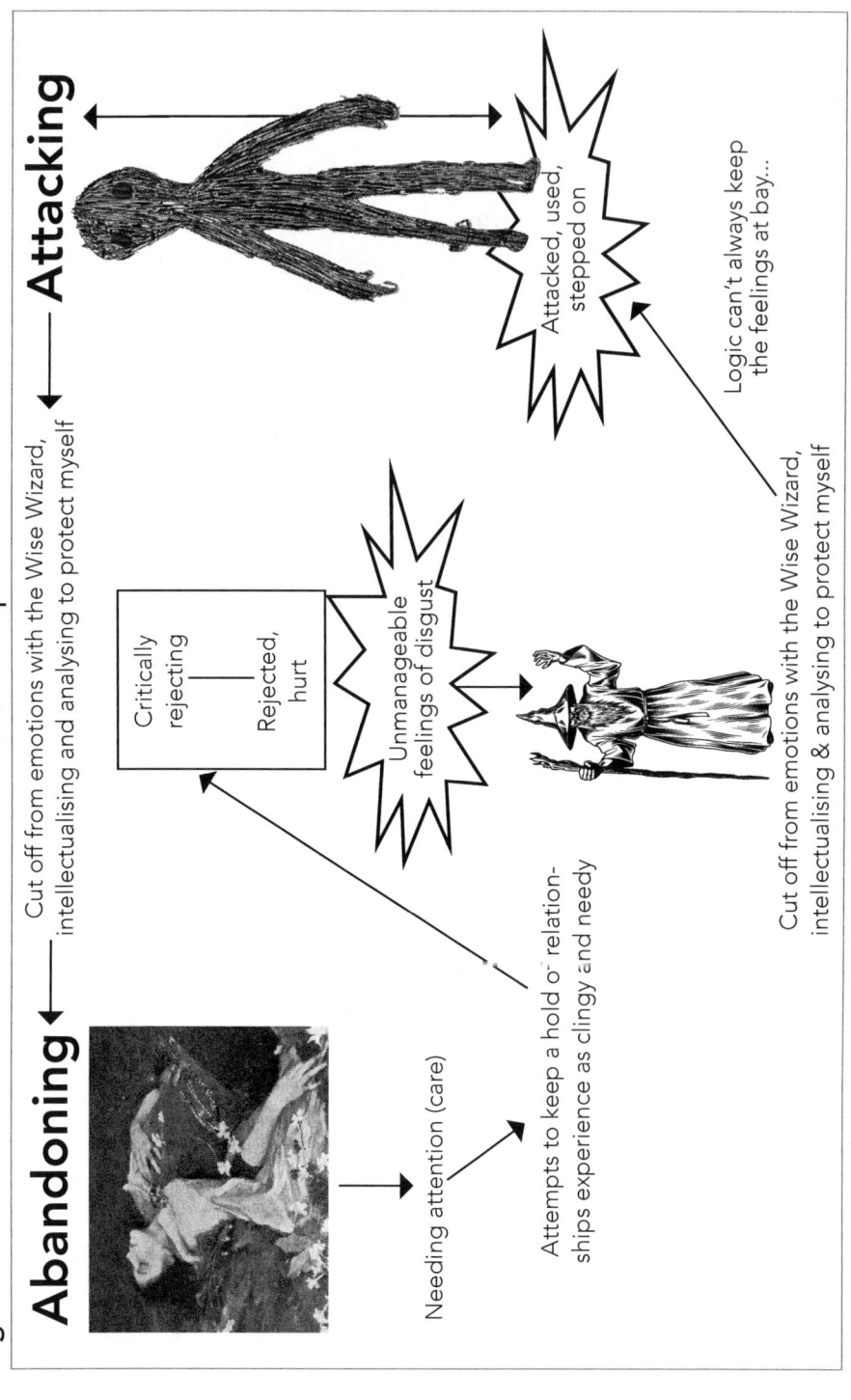

Underpinning elements of this approach was the narrative practice of the 'club of life' (White, 1997). This is a practice whereby individuals are invited to bring to mind influential others in their lives – who may be present, deceased, fictional, and more. The therapeutic notion is that these characters have in some way shaped or influenced one's life. Through joint exploration of these influencers, individuals may identify shared values, qualities or skills, such as a belief in fairness instilled by a parent, a logical mindset modelled by Star Trek's Spock, and a felt sense of feeling unconditional warmth and care from a beloved companion animal. Clients may choose to draw out what they deem meaningful, write the symbolic words or phrases, exact quotes and words of advice, use actual objects handed down by others, or many other ways of conceptualizing such influence. Therapists may then explore a range of situations with the client and explore the ways in which they can benefit from having such wide-ranging skills and support within their 'club' and work together to identify, rehearse and apply strategies that 'recruit' from this team.

For Jade, we explored her listed influential others: ranging from *The Lord of the Rings* wizard Gandalf, offering wisdom and vision; to Morticia Addams offering a celebration and confidence in beauty despite darkness around and within us; to Frida Kahlo, an artist who, for Jade, gave a permission for 'unconventional femininity', non-conformity to cultural pressures, and a confidence to be creative without care of what others say or do. There were many others whom Jade introduced into the space, and we explored their relevance, voice and influence on various situations – as guided by her map. Jade used these characters and images on paper and her phone, as if 'exit flash cards' when known triggers were anticipated, or she recognized the pull of procedures. For example, Jade could notice the temptation to desperately cling on to those she experienced as 'toxic, but present', and instead could practice confidence, belief and love in herself, and hold onto a wider perspective than her immersive 'abandonment goggles' – as supported by her team members Frida, Morticia and Gandalf.

Throughout mapping self-states and associated procedures, the naming and symbolic depiction of states became crucial aids to progress within Jade's CAT. She built the capacity to recognize and revise over time, through an active and playful adoption of vision: alternative influences to her self-states, who were well versed, rigid and often invisible to her – until we started to observe them and build a dialogue about and with them.

Key practice points:

- Invite yourself to spot opportunities for reformulation, recognition and revision activities within the passions and interests of your client. You may at first not necessarily feel they link directly to the CAT task, but remember that curiosity as a process will itself be conducive to the therapeutic relationship.

- Fiction and the arts can be important communicative symbols to anchor one's capacity for reflection and the underlying processes of self-self and self-other empathising. Fictional scaffolds can provide a shared language that mitigates the risk of the 'double empathy problem'. Using associated imagery and physically anchoring these onto the CAT map supports the recognising and naming of relational patterns.

- Integrating the 'club of life' technique (from narrative therapy; White, 1997), provides a workable framework in which more concrete, externalized and/or valued 'other'-states, can contribute to the exit work.

- The collaborative curiosity with such characters and influences creates a process in which new reciprocal roles can emerge that nourish, cater to, and join up self-states.

Leon

Leon is a twenty-three-year-old autistic trans-male who had recently started to attend a gender-identity clinic and was also working with a support worker to seek alternative accommodation to that of his birth family home. Leon talked about facing chronic emotional abuse and neglect within his family, particularly in relation to his mother - whom he described as an alcoholic and narcissist. Leon also carried a lot of anger about the ways in which society treats trans-individuals, and frequently reported feeling let down by services who misunderstood or dismissed his needs in this regard.

Leon was unsure about whether CAT was right for him at this point in time, and presented differently across the initial appointments. One week, he would seem intensely anxious, desperately trying to get all his words out, insistent on completing all points and starting from the beginning again if interrupted or asked anything – making the task of collaborative dialogue challenging at times. Another week, he would present as low, depleted and lacking initiation. Another week, he would present as agitated and enraged. Leon was struggling to recall these sessional experiences and initially, to make linkages between sessions. He seemingly had a vague sense of self-state switches, reporting that he struggled to log information or engage in reflection outside of the moment and feeling, and would be apologetic within the sessions alongside the intense presence of these states. For me, this suggested that Leon could notice state shifts retrospectively, even if just a hunch or feeling he had, and so we focused a lot on recognition work early on. We did not formally use the States Description Procedure (Pollock et al, 2003, as cited in Bennett & Ryle, 2005), but the process was akin to this – identifying and tentatively naming a state of interest, and then looking out for this throughout the weeks.

As we developed a CAT map, Leon came to recognize that he did not value the goal of integration of selves, as possibly inferred and at times explicitly questioned by me. He developed the confidence to say that what was important to him was to seek 'harmony' between his states. For him, this was about the ability to recognize and observe one another, to develop nurturing and caring relationships with one another; but ultimately, to not problematise his reality – that there are multiple, distinct parts of him. Through CAT mapping and recognition work, Leon was also able to notice the aspects of his experience or environment which would elicit a state-shift.

In developing confidence in these strategies of observation and selves-awareness, both Leon and I also witnessed an increase in confidence in himself, and he was much more able to engage in dialogue with me, possibly due to being much more readily able to be in dialogue with himselves. This process led to using an exit map that focused on the ways that this harmony could be conceptualized between states; for example, an appreciating–noticed reciprocal role enabled Leon to manage feelings of being alien or inhuman, by recognizing others' efforts to understand him and, in part, accepting some of the imperfections of others in their efforts. For Leon, it was also important for him to develop strategies that would enable his exits, such as a more meta-process of energy management in order to mitigate exhaustion and burnout.

Leon invited me to another world of his, which he was initially somewhat bashful about – having not shared his creation of characters and role-playing scenarios with professionals before. Throughout the work, Leon had had numerous issues with his computers breaking, and this was significantly overwhelming and distressing for him – he spoke of his world being lost. This was possibly meant literally also, for his laptop was his access to his selves-expressive and a soothing fictional world. Leon would create characters, plot relationships and build new worlds in his mind, through his words and through drawing. Through creating space to reflect on aspects of this world, and primarily some of the characters within, it was clear that these characters expressed elements of Leon's various states. We talked about their origins, their qualities, their values, their actions and their relationships, and how these all seemed to communicate some aspects of Leon. Leon was tentative, but also clear, that these were not 'copies' of himselves, but connections to parts of him. What was interesting was that the creation and roleplaying elements seemed to enable Leon permission to experiment with the characters, knowing they had some elements of himself in there, he could relinquish himself of needing complete control, become immersed and spontaneous within the creativity and narratives, and he spoke of sometimes 'finding himself' or highlighting for himself a dilemma or question which could guide his personal development further.

Key practice points:

- Not all autistic clients value or want 'integration' of self-states. Relational awareness and the empowerment to recognize self-states and procedures may be enough for autistic clients. Clients may conceptualize this in different ways; for Leon, he called this 'harmony'.
- The creation of characters can enable self-expression, but also observation or experimentation with selves and relationships.
- Recognition and revision experiments can be developed using character creation to guide exit-mapping (e.g. 'Can we find out what your life would be like, being this character over the next week? What beliefs would you have about yourself? What would you say to or do in response to others? Let's observe, document and review this in our next session').

Is the integration of selves always crucial?

As demonstrated through the CAT accounts above, the assumption that integration of selves is a necessity of CAT work is challenged here. There are likely to be a range of contributory factors as to why this seems to be the case here, but it does seem that autistic individuals are more likely to experience themselves as having a multiplicity of self-states and for this to not necessarily be the focus of concern or a key contributory factor to their distress.

Identity fragmentation does not necessarily equate to incoherence. If self-states are deemed multiple yet coherent – individuals may just conclude that they have multiple 'parts' to themselves, and not pathologize this. Beyond the conceptualization of such states being rigid or dissociated in some way, this idea of multiple selves and parts of selves can be observed in other theories and therapies (such as 'the community of selves' in Personal Construct Psychotherapy, (Mair, 1977). What is unique here, is the possibility that autistic traits can play a specific role in the ways in which these states are experienced, perceived and expressed. Indeed, what can also be different, in my experience, is how autistic people tend to view the necessity of shifting or changing their nature. Many autistic people come to consider themselves as 'plurals' or their different parts of themselves as 'alters', for example. Plurals identify as having a number of 'alters' (akin to self-states) and although these states often remain partially dissociated, they seemingly have greater integration and coherence in general, and there is no assumption of associated distress or impact on functioning. People describe varying degrees of control over these alters, with some having the potential to be consciously 'recruited in', and others being elicited in response to anticipations, others, or environments (which is much more in line with the MSSM in its conventional use).

Self-states, then, will have varying degrees of dissociation, with some being partially integrated as opposed to dissociated. Their relational content may well be reformulated in connection with childhood traumas, adverse experiences, and entrenched relational experiences in relation to society (e.g. discrimination of one's protected characteristics), but the dynamic processes by which they operate are likely to be unique to autistic populations, as described throughout this chapter (e.g. limits on the MSSM level three capacity to reflect due to overlooking of sensory processing/ need for stimming). The rigid distinction and demarcation of self-states, in my experience, can also elicit unusual experiences for individuals – such as voice hearing, possibly linked to partially-dissociated parts of oneself, or entrenched paranoid meta-states, whereby someone constantly feels on edge, unsure of what their self-states 'are up to'.

What I have come to learn is that curiosity is key to realizing the potential for such relational work, whereby dialogues can still be developed for parts of self that may initially be felt to be inaccessible. Many autistic clients, where these aspects of experience ring true and they have an appetite to explore themselves more fully, have noted that services too readily conclude conversations with 'dissociation' or 'voice hearing' – as if these are the end of potential meaning. The task for CAT here, for all – not just autistic clients – is to keep a hold of the curiosity. There is an opportunity for dialogical work when multiple parts of oneself are recognized and explored, and it is worth questioning where our expectations of fully integrated, static selves come from.

I wonder whether this, at least in this context, represents another neurotypical imposition – that a plurality of selves, parts and alters is deemed atypical and therefore something to be 'corrected' back into the mould of society. There will be times when integration is key, and this should be guided by the individual's wants and needs, the practitioner's clinical assessment that includes consideration of context, systems and relationships – but never based on hard-line rules that MSSM CAT work is all about integration. Many autistic clients have benefited from a different approach to this, one that invites awareness of, and harmony between, self-states – and in my practice, this doesn't seem to be a problem.

Conclusion

The MSSM offers a useful framework in which to understand the impact of dynamic shifts in moods and selves. It offers promising avenues for autistic people, who may experience themselves as having multiple parts. For autistic people, interestingly, such states are not always dissociated, and although still distinct and disconnected from one another, may still be felt to be coherent in some way. CAT can therefore look very much in-line with conventional therapy based on the MSSM where there is a request or need for integration, but there also appears to be a real need for CAT to offer a relational space of curiosity and acceptance to open up a dialogue with the plurality of selves – a divergent CAT for neurodivergent individuals, perhaps?

PART 3: Bringing our creative selves to therapy

Exploration and discovery in CAT training and supervision

Jak Smith

CAT supervision, in my experience, is uniquely placed compared to other models of psychotherapy supervision I have received in that it emphasizes co-created meaning and understanding of the therapeutic work and how this is described, explored and formulated in the supervisory relationship. One central difference is the use of mapping. Mapping offers a visually tactile, joint activity, encouraging a deepening exploration of relational patterns and procedures that may be present in the therapy and enacted in the supervisory relationship/group.

With the use of RRP and TPPs, CAT mapping in supervision offers a rich opportunity for greater understanding of phenomena such as parallel process, transference, and countertransference in an accessible language, thus enabling and promoting the use of the 'observing 'eye' – hovering, noticing, naming. I have been encouraged by supervisory relationships that foster an openness to 'explore and discover' (*together*) the many possible meanings of those relational encounters that take place in both the individual therapy and the supervisory setting. This dynamic 'openness to explore' can lead to 'shared discovery', which is central to the task alliance in many psychotherapy approaches – for *client and clinician.*

'Exploring to Discovering' may only be possible when a relationship feels safe. Supervisory relationships, marked by a contractual agreement, have contributed to my own sense of psychological safety. This agreement helps to establish boundaries, trust, purpose, and a meaningful relationship that has a shared aim and expectation, while outlining any caveats. Establishing a safe relational space (akin to a 'secure base'), in my experience, encourages exploration and reflection. It fosters an arena for the use of cognitive and analytic technique in CAT, in an integrated manner. For example, mapping 'supervisee experience to group experience', provides an opportunity to consider its relevance to the clinical work. Incorporating the tools of CAT, such as TPs, can promote effective use of the time-limited nature of CAT supervision. Joint activity fosters a sense of being alongside (*doing with*), this relational positioning, attends to the hierarchy/power(?) inherent in role difference. By using the tools of CAT, relational supervision has enhanced my learning experience, nudging me towards the edge of my ZPD, a place where we know continual growth and potential can be achieved – for all group members.

Figure 1: Relational supervision – Aim for a Shared and Central Reciprocal Role Procedure (RRP)

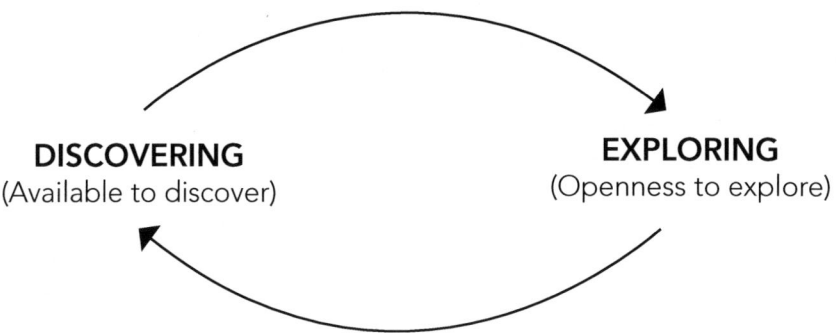

DISCOVERING
(Available to discover)

EXPLORING
(Openness to explore)

Chapter 11: Reflection as a creative process within supervision

Vicky Petratou

Introduction

I often use food and cooking metaphors in my therapy and supervision work, and talk about fresh, seasonal and frozen ingredients, recipes, and improvised meals we create as offerings for ourselves and others. Cooking, like gardening, is an activity that can symbolize our ways of relating to ourselves and the world because they are sensory and creative processes that facilitate an inter and intrapersonal space for relating. For instance, I may ask a supervisee, what are you and your client cooking here? What does it look, smell, and taste like?' Or I might ask 'If your relationship was a garden, how are you both attending to it?' In this chapter, I will provide some reflections on using metaphor and creative action in clinical supervision. I will share some creative experiences that were co-cooked/co-gardened in supervision sessions and will share supervisees' feedback on how they 'tasted' and 'what fruits they produced'.

One of the essential aims of clinical supervision is to provide a welcoming and fertile space for reflection, integration and dialogue between different states of being to emerge and flourish. CAT is a therapy that emphasizes the development of this self-reflective capacity. In this chapter, I will advocate that reflective practice and reflexivity requires creativity, and that reflection is an act of creativity (Williams, 1995, Hilton, 2006; Patterson, 2020).
As Elaine Patterson defined it, creativity is a way of being and doing that reshapes the old and/or brings the new into existence; it 'helps us to break old ways of thinking, relating and seeing while spewing fresh approaches to life' (2020, p9). In CAT, we promote 'the reshaping of the old' by collaboratively reformulating with our clients their presenting problems and usefully reflecting on their target problem procedures. We also aim to 'bring the new into existence' by the process of revising the problematic patterns and developing exits that can expand Reciprocal Role repertoires

towards more creative and caring ways of relating with the self and others. Furthermore, the CAT approach views such recurrent coping patterns (conceptualized as traps, dilemmas and snags) as limiting people's freedom to choose and to reflect and engage with life creatively.

Developing a playful, imaginative space can act as an enabling experiential bridge that can help us to explore conflictual and/or restrictive relational patterns in our CAT supervision and therapy practice. Supervisees often bring to supervision various moments of crisis and challenge in their clients' personal, social, physical and spiritual worlds, and we need to provide a process of learning how to rise again and regain our capacity to respond, reflect, revitalize and re-invent ourselves and our worlds in fresh and integrated ways (Van Deurzen, 2021). Creativity and improvisation can help with this process (Shohet & Shohet, 2020).

In supervision, when we don't pay attention to the body and instead rely on our verbal reflections, we may neglect important bodily experiences that are stored as body/sensory memories (Panhofer *et al*, 2011). Based on the notion that reflection in CAT supervision is essentially a creative process, I will argue that the presence of embodied, imaginative and playful approaches can enrich the practice of CAT supervision. For this to happen, a safe-enough playful space needs to be created where collaborative exploration of different perspectives can take place 'in the immediacy of the moment', without which such a 'dialogical process can be inhibited' (Seikkula & Trimble, 2006, p:466).

I will discuss some key creative elements that can enable connectivity, openness and reflection. Facilitating a playful, containing and energized atmosphere in supervision, can reduce anxiety in new therapists and encourage self-disclosure in a 'non-spotlighting' way (Blatner & Glass Collins, 2008, p143). I will demonstrate that this can assist CAT therapists in supervision to be more aware of the impact of non-verbal communication and to reflect in ways that help them to access their own potential for openness and creative responsiveness.

Creative supervision can expand supervisees' perceptual and relational capacity and reduce a sense of feeling stuck and entrapped (Gilbert & Evans, 2000; Tselikas-Portman, 1999). In this way, the supervision process becomes a creative bridge that can contain, address, express and reduce our supervisees' anxieties, in order to help them gain courage and widen their perspective.

Later in the chapter, I will provide examples of how the House of Self States (HOSS, Petratou, 2019) technique can be used in clinical supervision as a creative means of externalizing intrapersonal and interpersonal relational patterns and in exploring countertransference issues. I will also include some examples of how improvisation, storytelling, song lyrics and poetry, creative work with sensory play and symbolic representation (using art, clay and objects), role play, and movement work can inspire and promote creativity in CAT supervision.

Feedback from supervisees on creativity in supervision

In preparing for this chapter, I invited several supervisees to provide written feedback on how creative experiences in supervision, including engaging with their own 'Houses of Self States', have affected their clinical practice. This feedback was gathered by sending a questionnaire to fifteen of my current supervisees (from the NHS and private practice), who attend both group and individual supervision sessions, and are both trainees (eight) and qualified/experienced therapists (seven). The questionnaire invited them to provide feedback on their experiences of using the House of Self States technique and other creative supervision activities, anything specific they have found helpful or unhelpful with regard to creative supervision, and any amendments they would like to recommend along with a list of potential positive effects.

The responses are summarized in Table 11.1. The answers of the supervisees suggest that many of them find creative activities particularly helpful in developing their empathy, expanding their reflective capacity, helping with feeling stuck and developing their capacity to work creatively with their clients.

Table 11.1: Areas where creative work in supervision has contributed positively to respondents' CAT practice

Clinical domain	Percentage of respondents who felt creative methods were helpful in facilitating this
Dealing with moments of feeling stuck	86%
Gaining more perspective on your client's presenting difficulties	86%
Feeling more empathic towards your client	78%
Working with the client in more creative ways	78%
Helping the client engage with the therapy process in a more embodied way	64%
Tolerating and working with distressing moments in the therapy	57%
Developing therapeutic scaffolding skills	50%
Facilitating the client's capacity to mentalize	50%
Encouraging the development of exits	36%
Repairing a rupture	28%

For the remainder of this chapter, more detailed comments shared by the respondents have been used to illustrate the core themes that emerged in this process. Their comments are coded R1-R15 (Respondent 1-15).

Creative CAT supervision – a way to scaffold reflective playfulness

Creative supervision can be defined as a playful, welcoming process that encourages supervisees to feel safe enough to express, share and explore difficult relational dynamics in therapy, using metaphors, images, stories, and embodied enactments (Lahad, 2000; Jones & Dokter, 2008, Petratou, 2007, Chesner & Zografou 2014). Establishing a space in supervision where supervisees are encouraged to be imaginative and to have a spirit of playfulness and improvisation can enable CAT therapists to engage with their creative potential in therapy work. To make clinical supervision beneficial, supervisees need to be able to trust the process. An enabling and caring/whole-person approach from the supervisor is essential in promoting this, facilitated by a variety of creative activities. Keeping creativity alive is not always easy and requires perseverance and flexibility. As Bravesmith (2008) argues, being open to the unknown, developing trust, and playing with various ideas and possibilities 'allows supervisees to use their imaginations in order to explore relationships creatively in the service of learning about the self and about others' (cited in Edwards, 2010, p251). Creativity in supervision also requires supervisees to feel secure enough in the space to be vulnerable when sharing their uncertainty, fears and challenges in supervision. This can feel risky, so suitable support and containment becomes even more important (Edwards, 2010).

Creative explorations in supervision can provide helpful scaffolding when needed to enhance therapists' relational repertoire and reflective capacity. There are a number of key areas that I keep in mind when using creative approaches in supervision:

- Using metaphor, storytelling and projective techniques as containers to help therapists develop their empathy and their reflective skills.
- Creative checking-in and checking-out to help contain the supervision process.
- Expanding empathizing and reflecting ability via creative activities that fit supervisees' zones of proximal development.
- Creative use of the observing eye when reflecting on maps/diagrams of relational patterns.
- Bringing in embodiment, role and movement to the work.
- Facilitating creative experimentation when feeling stuck.

The use of metaphor

In CAT theory and practice, metaphor has proved useful in containing, understanding and recalling core relational patterns, tools and experiences (see Chapter 7 in this volume). In the CAT literature, metaphors have often been used to refer to some core CAT tools, such as the 'observing eye' (ability to engage actively with a mindful meta-perspective of relational patterns) the 'broken egg' (a diagrammatic depiction of polarized states of being), 'the map' (which refers to a diagrammatic reformulation of problematic procedures), the helper's 'dance' (a list of relational stances/ positions therapists can take) (Ryle & Kerr, 2020; Potter, 2010; Potter 2013). More recently, the metaphor of the 'House of Self States' has been developed as an accessible way of initiating the process of mapping that contains four key relational areas of states of being: the desired, the dreaded, the interpersonal and the intrapersonal) (Petratou, 2019).

Using objects for symbolic representation and images can help with concretizing painful relational experiences and feelings and giving them space (Chesner, 2008; Chesner & Zografou, 2014).

Box 11.1 summarizes some supervisees' responses to how metaphor can be helpful in their therapeutic work.

Box 11.1: Using metaphor in CAT supervision

R3: I really like the use of metaphors – for me this helps to observe the topic from a distance, which feels easier to think about things and also aids understanding. It also for me brings to life the subject.

R15: Sometimes I may get stuck or find the process less enlivening… but even then, this is telling me something about the dynamic and the therapeutic process that feels helpful.

R1: Metaphors have been helpful in illustrating repetitive non-helpful behaviours and relationship dynamics in a non-shaming way.

R3: For me, there is something about using images and pictures when I describe how I respond, which helps me to make sense of the experience. My particular roles are highlighted, and this helps me maintain awareness of what I may be invited into and be reminded of my own tendencies, and observe them carefully, but also playfully.

Using group activities that embrace helpful metaphors in group supervision has been particularly useful during challenging moments in therapy. For example, sometimes I encourage group members to provide each other with the *gift* of a specific image that might be helpful to them when engaging with a relational difficulty that has arisen:

> **R3:** '[I found] The sharing of "gifts" [in group supervision] helpful – something metaphorical we could offer each other as supervisees if we found a situation difficult. I think this is such a lovely idea, it helps move away from things that feel overwhelming and also provides an exit to feelings of being overwhelmed or stuck-ness. I also find it so interesting what each member of the supervision group might envisage or come up with – how fascinating this process can be and what interesting images people can share with each other. It really is a gift!'

Checking-in and checking-out

Checking-in and checking-out rituals are very helpful in supervision. Over the years, I have used this with all my supervisees, both in groups and individually. As a process, it helps them to pause and notice what emotional state they have entered the session with. By acknowledging this state and 'putting it to one side' until the session is over, the supervisees are encouraged to create a more available and fresh perspective and to notice what might get in the way of being fully engaged in the process of supervision. Such rituals can help supervisees to de-role from the state/activity they were in immediately before the supervision started, and en-role (become more available and open to engage fully) into the supervision process. This ritual provides an opportunity for creativity.

For instance, a creative check-in that I have used online and in person has been to pay attention to what the supervisee is feeling in the moment at the beginning of the session. Then they name their feeling and/or come up with an image that describes the emotional experience they have. During the COVID pandemic, in online group supervision sessions, I sometimes encouraged the participants to replace their on-screen names/surnames with a feeling/image of how they were at the time i.e.: 'Maria Cloudy', 'Katerina I Need Some Fresh Air'. Other times, in group supervision (both in person and online), I use a simple warm-up drama game called 'name and action' in which each person in the group states their name and does a short movement and/or sound that connects with their present emotional state; the rest of the group members then copy this name and the action. This ritual helps individuals to embrace physically and emotionally an 'acknowledging to acknowledged' Reciprocal Role ('self-to-self' and 'others-to-self') while at the same time activating the 'connecting to feeling-connected' Reciprocal Role ('self-to-other' and 'other-to-self').

Another purpose of the check-in is to help supervisees engage more fully with the reflective task of supervision, to notice and to release any restricting and/or emotionally charged states they currently have, helping them to be more in the present. Supervision should provide an environment that promotes honesty and courage, welcomes vulnerability, and strengthens creativity and reflexivity. Check-ins contribute significantly to setting the tone for creating such enabling environments. The check-out ritual helps with completing the ending phase of a supervision session. For example, each participant names what they want to take with them from the session (it could be a verbal reflection, or an image, verbally or physically expressed). Sometimes doing a spontaneous short drawing or drafting a quick poem can be helpful too.

In Box 11.2, three supervisees describe how they found check-ins helpful.

Box 11.2: Check-ins

R3: Using an image, a movement, or an object to describe how we feel when we join the supervision space is really helpful. It helps us to name and identify our current state and identifying it in such a way does help me to observe it helpfully and try to put it aside as we start the supervision process.

R2: I like the style of introduction at the beginning, and using imagery, body work and metaphors to support understanding of where I am at emotionally and relationally, and as a nice example of exercises I can do with patients.

R1: I have found drawing/creating images at check-ins is a nice metaphor to carry on throughout the supervision – e.g. an image of being a 'cracked egg', feeling overwhelmed like my yolk was spilling out helped me understand how to manage a tricky client.

For a supervision process to be a useful and facilitative space, it needs to provide experiences and structures that can be used to contain, express and reflect upon painful and problematic relational patterns that might be challenging for the therapists. We should not assume that because these groups are not therapy, they shouldn't be caring and supportive. Supervision is a learning, reflecting and enabling process and we need to pay attention to its dynamics and to care for the well-being of all involved – the clients, the supervisees and the relational systems they operate in. Many supervision groups in the NHS only allow time for therapists to briefly summarize their clinical material and reflect, receive and discuss feedback as there is often no time for check-ins and check-outs. In my experience, supervising therapists holistically, *human to human*, rather than just as professional *providers* of therapy, makes therapists feel more acknowledged, able to be open, and more willing to learn from any difficult experiences they may have had with their clients. When facilitating clinical supervision sessions, I have found it helpful to offer five or ten minutes for supervisees to check in and check out, whether we are meeting individually or in a group format.

Expanding supervisees' playful zone of proximal development

It is important to remember that using a creative activity doesn't guarantee creativity. The supervisor needs to be familiar with creative and embodied processes before they introduce them in supervision. In CAT, we often strive for clarity; we attempt to make sense of chaotic or rigid relational states of being in our narrative and diagrammatic reformulations. We try to help therapists and clients not to collude with habitual problematic patterns, but in doing this perhaps we can miss opportunities for deeper engagement when we are too focused on reflexivity (naming and noticing). We need to be able 'to be' (actively present, taking on roles in flexible and engaging ways within an uncertain and at times confusing process – less distant) *and* 'not to be' (stepping back to reflect/witness and gain perspective over our ways of relating to internal and external worlds – more distant). This flexible interplay between active engagement and reflective mindfulness is necessary for establishing a well-attuned therapeutic space in terms of distance, that values creativity and playfulness both in therapy and in supervision.

It is useful in supervision to consider the emotional availability and/or distance of all parties involved. A few questions we may ask are: What is the emotional distance of the therapist? How do they interact with that of their client? If both client and therapist are over-distanced or under-distanced, emotionally, how does the supervisor help the CAT therapist to decrease/increase their emotional distance to be able to work effectively with the client? Introducing playful activities in supervision can help therapists to become more flexible and emotionally attuned to their clients. Therapists who find it difficult to connect, understand and empathize with their clients' emotional states might benefit from under-distancing, such as embodying, role-playing activities and songs/lyrics. There may be times when therapists are too immersed in their client's emotional states. In these situations, they might benefit more from stepping back, distancing and reflecting activities like mapping, spectrograms, genograms etc. Supervisees who need space to engage and explore their experiences of the 'therapist-client relationship' could benefit from using creative media, such as objects in sand trays, creating relational constellations with clay or Play-Doh, furniture, or sculpts made by other participants in the group, writing poems and no-send letters to their clients. Identifying and working with a supervisee's zone of proximal development and thinking about emotional distance are two ways of helping to develop an environment that is safe enough to try experimenting with new and creative ways of doing things which can often lead to positive and sometimes surprising results.

Box 11.3 illustrates some creative activities that the respondents particularly connected with.

> **Box 11.3: Creative experiences in supervision that the respondents found particularly helpful**
>
> **Role play and embodiment**
>
> **R15:** Role play is very powerful.
>
> **R8:** I liked to watch role play. As a witness, it seemed to help grasp the situation and the relationship between client and psychotherapist more accurately. I felt I could share easily emotions triggered by what I saw in a more efficient and impactful way with the therapist who was role-playing.
>
> **R6:** I have found using role play, working with spectograms, metaphors and image work all very useful.
>
> **R1:** Role play has been helpful in re-enacting and understanding a difficult dynamic between a patient and their father.
>
> **R1:** It has been very helpful to do chair work in supervision to embody clients and the process.

Lyrics and songs

R1: Lyrics from songs have been helpful in understanding unhelpful relationship patterns in a non-shaming and playful way.

R10: I found examples of lyrics in songs to be really helpful as a way of understanding a patient's perspective as a clinician- – I think it was, 'Maybe This Time' from Cabaret which was quoted as a way of understanding the need for a relationship and the need for fulfilment in someone with emotionally unstable personality disorder. The sense of longing in the song, to be fulfilled in a very intense and painful way and not be alone, really encapsulated the sense I had from my patient and allowed me to think about this with them.

Poetry

R1: What I have found most helpful is how you identified creative ways of processing which came naturally to me e.g. poetry and drawing. I loved that you noticed how these were ways I enjoyed expressing myself. This helped me to feel empowered in my processing.

P11: I really like the co-creation of poems – using words that we have all come up with has felt so lovely and a way of bonding us together as a group and sharing our experiences and imaginations with each other.

Storytelling and story making

P4: I did enjoy using the six-part story, where we each created a character and told the story to each other – I have a client currently who enjoys writing short stories so would benefit talking through this in session – this activity helped me to understand how to introduce this into a session and the step-by-step process to take.

P12: I have always particularly appreciated my supervisor's use of metaphor and storytelling – something I have incorporated into my own practice. Story telling seems to help me to see things from a different perspective, gain insight, see another aspect of a situation, or help me to relax and put it into perspective.

Projective object work

R10: I also found object work interesting as a way of allowing states and emotions to be articulated, it might take more confidence to actually get me to use it!

Drawing and images

R11: I've found pausing to draw or write very helpful; again it taps into a different mode. I've done this with clients too, having tried it first in supervision. It helps to bring some variety to how I am with clients. Particularly with clients with whom I might get stuck in wordy mode and not be able to easily access more feeling modes.

R8: I particularly enjoyed working with images as I found that sometimes it is difficult to provide all the layers and subtleties of the client / psychotherapist relationship. As a mirror I also started to use more image works with clients when they are stuck with words.

R12: Drawing myself and a client as an animal was helpful.

How do we help CAT therapists experiment with being more creative?

Box 11.4 illustrates some of the methods used in supervision that have helped them experiment with trying sometimes new and unfamiliar creative approaches in their therapeutic work.

Box 11.4: Creative methods in supervision
Modelling of how to use the House of Self States in supervision

R9: The House of Self States would often be drawn out in group supervision and my supervisor would often use stories or metaphors to make links between the levels.

How metaphor helps group supervision:

R3: 'Walking on hot coals' – This example really stuck with me and helped me really recognize how incredibly difficult and frightening it might feel for any of us, particularly some of the vulnerable people we meet, to make changes – it can feel very scary. This really helped me to develop empathy and compassion for him and what it was we were trying to ask him to do in challenging himself in life.

A clearer window on personal processes:

R1: [Using creative reflective methods] helped me to relax and become more present with my client after, rather than to feel reactive. It took the charge out of my conditioned responses.

Keep innovating/don't get complacent:

R1: I liked that [the supervisor] didn't stick with these creative activities but used others too. This kept sessions vibrant and interesting. It left me curious. e.g. Play-Doh, cope/OH/Blob cards, postcards, small body cut outs, movement and pebble trays.

Unlocking new perspectives:

R2: I particularly liked working in 3D with Play-Doh and pebble trays, because it bought my senses alive and allowed movement and fluidity. This allowed me to drop into my experience in an embodied way, which added a depth to my processing I really appreciated.

Breaking out of over-thinking/intellectualizing:

R7: I also find story, music and drawing useful to connect to emotional processes, especially if I have become stuck in a cognitive cycle of thinking and need to reconnect my mind and body.

Doing together/creating together:

R2: An important part of the process was that you [my supervisor] would use these tools at the same time as me, so that we each reflected on our experience of the client, which was very beautiful.

It's important to be able to recognize, listen and respond to a supervisee who might not be feeling positively connected to a specific activity. The following respondent comments on this, emphasizing how working within her zone of proximal development has been important for her in this regard:

R3: I guess I am finding the edges of what I feel comfortable with, what is within my ZPD, and I wouldn't be able to use all methods with all clients all the time, there's some need to find what will work for me with each different client to help us without pushing beyond what works. So that would be a good area to explore.

It is important to have regular reviews with supervisees to get some feedback on what works and what might need some consideration/alteration or extra training (i.e. sometimes it is important to slow down and take helpful steps in teaching/introducing/altering activities in ways that meet the needs and interests of the supervisees). When using creative methods in supervision, the supervisor needs to have significant experience in using creative experiential methods in supervision before they introduce such activities.

The observing eye: creating different perspectives

How do we train/develop our observing eye's capacity? Under what circumstances do we lose our ability to observe/notice/be with our relational worlds in a non-intervening, non-blaming, and non-shaming way? In CAT literature, this observing eye is often depicted as 'hovering' above the maps that we make with our clients, as if it has a privileged perspective on the clients' problematic procedures/patterns, and therefore has a 'better' reflective capacity than if it was 'lower down'. However, the need for it to always be depicted hovering above in order to take a 'meta-perspective' can be limiting at times.

When working creatively in CAT, one realizes that, when it only hovers from above, the observing eye can be too remote and fixed, allowing for only one *over-distanced* point of view that shows how the problematic procedures are maintained. However, is the most useful perspective always from above (like a drone which can never land) or might it at times be more useful to be like a helicopter (Hawkins & McMahon, 2020) or even a bird or bumblebee, which can shift perspective, moving between higher and lower vantage points and all levels in between? Additionally, the remote, all-seeing observing eye as a metaphor at times can be problematic for some people. This is because this perspective can be associated with a god-like and potentially persecutory metaphorical meaning. So, using different observational metaphors can be important, particularly when working with clients from different cultural backgrounds.

Sometimes, creating 3D constellations/depictions of our maps and diagrams (using big objects in the room, or small figures/objects in a sand tray for example) can be helpful in expanding possibilities for noticing other viewpoints/intentions and the impact of Reciprocal Roles and their corresponding procedures/self-states from different points of view. Our cooperative observing ability is enriched when we are able to look at maps of relational patterns not just from above but also from below and many other points of view, in three dimensions, all around the constellation. Looking from each character's/state's/role's point of view allows one to notice and understand different experiences and also what is illuminated or obscured/hidden from specific viewpoints.

When supervisees and clients are feeling emotionally dysregulated, it is very difficult for them to engage with their reflective capacity. Using our calm 'observing eye' in these circumstances requires us to step out of identifying with harsh, rigid and limited role procedures and strong feelings. Naming self-states and procedures can be useful, but how do we help ourselves as therapists and our clients to notice our relational identifications and enactments? Under what kind of circumstances do we lose our capacity to notice our patterns in non-judgmental ways? Usually, when there is too much fear, anxiety, anger or shame, it is very difficult to engage with our reflective observing eye capacity. How do we recover from unsettling, unregulated states of being?

When therapists are emotionally dysregulated, creative and embodied grounding/calming activities can be generated in supervision to help this process before attempting further reflection. Such activities can help us to regain our capacity to step away from our habitual identifications and relational perspectives. In this way, creative CAT supervision can stimulate a space where, in Edwards' words: 'the attention of the supervisor and supervisee can move playfully up and down, backwards and forwards, in and out of the material under consideration… when the supervisee is helped to do this playfully, they will be better able to refine and renew their practice in ways that are truly creative and truly therapeutic' (Edwards, 2010, p257).

Embodiment

> *'Human imitative behaviour is what both relationships and theatre are originated from.'* (Barrault, 1962)

In CAT supervision, the focus is often on reformulating, naming, noticing and revising problematic relational procedures and self-states. As supervisors, our key contribution is to help the therapists maintain a therapeutic alliance with their clients and to assist them with their verbal narrative and diagrammatic reformulations and revisions. But one question that remains is how the therapist engages with the client in a creative and embodied way. This might be neglected in CAT supervision if we don't pay attention to how the body expresses/reacts/responds. How can the therapist develop their empathy on a non-verbal, relational level?

Creative embodiment activities can help therapists to relate to their clients' roles non-verbally. For example, in one exercise, the supervisor can facilitate the supervisee to take on the role of the patient for a few minutes 'as if they are in a silent movie' playing a scene from the therapy or a scene from a story they have discussed, using no words, and miming how they move physically. This embodied experience can provide another layer of relating with the patient that might usually be hidden, or not acknowledged in the verbal domain of communication. Taking it further, in group supervision the therapist can pause and watch other supervisees miming the same roles non-verbally. The experience of the therapist taking on the physicality of the client and then seeing it again in the playback enactment of the other supervisees (or the supervisor herself if working individually) can provide fertile opportunities for forming a deeper connection with the client's relational processes. Following such enactments, the supervision group can comment on their experiences with enriching reflections.

Noticing how your client walks, where they put the weight of their body, with which part of the body they lead, how they breathe, how they sit, how they use eye contact, where they carry tension, what happens to the face, the chest, the waist, the pelvis, the feet, the pace and rhythm of how they move – all of these dimensions can be valuable in gaining an appreciation of how they relate to their body and to others interpersonally. Often in CAT supervision, the therapist and/or the supervisor will notice some of these physical expressions in themselves or in the patient. This is good, but the use of a creatively embodying process where physically embracing your client's non-verbal presence offers the therapist embodied empathy and expands their appreciation and understanding of their client's lived experience. It can also help the supervisee notice something that they would not have noticed otherwise. For example, one supervisee, when asked in supervision to role play the way their client walked, noticed that they moved with such purpose and vigilance that they lost their capacity to be curious about other people in the space or use their peripheral vision to engage fully in their environment. This provided them with an opportunity to empathise with their client's unique perspective on the relational world.

A creative embodied activity like this can help supervisees and their clients to engage with the concept of Reciprocal Roles through the witnessing of a simple and communicative moving sequence of mimes. CAT therapists benefit from also attending to how non-verbal elements, expressions and contributions in therapy influence/impact the relational 'play' between client and therapist. In supervision, providing therapists with experiences that help them develop more flexibility and attunement in their practice can be invaluable, as demonstrated by the following respondents' comment in Box 11.5.

> **Box 11.5: The use of role play and embodiment**
>
> **R15:** Embodying/playing the client and allowing someone else to be therapist especially often brings real insight into how it may be for this client navigating the world. New thoughts, feelings, insights, empathy and understanding are reached through direct embodiment, using their catchphrases, posture etc as 'ways in'.
>
> **R14:** I found role play and embodying my clients particularly valuable because it helped me have a have a better sense of how they experience being in the world and see our relationship from their viewpoint.
>
> **R7:** Yes. I find role play challenging, but it helps me to experience the perspective of the patient and always facilitates a deeper understanding of their position and needs.
>
> **R3:** Physical work on Zoom! That was initially quite unexpected, different, a bit awkward, and I felt self-conscious to begin with. But it quickly tapped into a rich source of information, helped my creativity and sense of openness, flexibility, disrupting the usual routine of static words, but also complementing the words.

The House of Self States – a therapeutic tool that can be used as a self-reflective exercise in supervision

The House of Self States (HOSS) (see Appendix 4) is a creative mapping technique that can be used both in therapy and supervision. The supervisee draws a simple house with four areas that accommodate some core relational states of being (attic: desired states, basement: dreaded states, ground floor: interpersonal/performative/public states and first floor: intrapersonal/private/unseen states).

Sometimes, before the therapist introduces and co-constructs the HOSS with their client, it can be helpful to encourage supervisees to create two House of Self States in supervision: one that identifies/portrays/accommodates the self-states of the client (as viewed by the therapist) and one that identifies/portrays the relational states of the therapist toward the clients. Putting these two depictions next to each other can help with identifying unmanageable painful states, unattainable expectations, and potential countertransference issues and problematic relational recruitments. This can be useful in helping the therapist to have a clearer perspective on the different roles she adopts in her relationship with a patient.

The HOSS can be a useful creative reflective mapping experience for trainees in supervision, even before they start seeing clients to help them reflect on their own aspirations/desires, fears/dreads, interpersonal/performative/habitual tendencies and intrapersonal relational patterns and states with regards to their role of CAT therapist and the task of therapy. The supervisor can facilitate this process by using some questions, such as:

- What kind of therapist do I want to be and what do I hope my clients will achieve through therapy (attic)?
- What am I dreading/don't want to happen (basement)?
- What kind of therapist am I in the room (ground floor – interpersonal styles of relating, e.g. an empath, a pleaser, a teacher, a guide, a clever thinker)?
- How am I with myself when I think about my role/task as a therapist (first floor – my internal/private ways of being with/relating to myself when I think about this work, 'self-to-self' reciprocal relating)? For example, do I catastrophize and/or ruminate on anxious thoughts, do I distract myself/procrastinate with writing letters or do take care of/support myself to engage with the task?

One example of this work is demonstrated by a supervisee's comments below. It provides a clear description of how this creative therapeutic technique can be used as a reflective exercise in supervision:

> **R14:** I created a HOSS for myself to explore my countertransference with regards to a client who repeatedly missed sessions. I explored how my client's willingness to seek therapy in her ground floor, prompted my own ground-floor state of caring and connecting with her.

> However, her anxiety and inability to attend her sessions elicited my first-floor anxiety, rumination, and a wish to withdraw from the relationship. In my attic I wished to be useful and save her but, in my basement, I feared to be inadequate and a failure. Opening these different states in supervision helped me find ways to tolerate my anxiety, assert my own feelings, and find helpful ways to remain open to the needs and difficulties of my client. This allowed me to keep on trying to remain collaborative and relational with my client, avail of the support from my supervisor and fellow supervisees and maintain a caring and professional stance.

The HOSS can also be a useful creative reflective activity in the training of CAT as well as at the beginning of supervision in helping therapists to become more aware of their aspirations, fears and habitual intra and inter-relational tendencies, as demonstrated below by two respondents:

> **R4:** I've created a HOSS for myself but not in relation to my client as of yet – it has helped me to think through what I am 'striving' for as a therapist and whether the client's aim for therapy is in line with my own.

> **R5:** I did [a HOSS] in supervision and was able to look more deeply at my feelings towards my client and the reasons behind my own actions and motivations in therapy. It also highlighted my concerns for the client and what my role was to them.

Putting the therapist and the patient's Houses of Self States next to each other has helped supervisees expand their perspective on the various relational stances acted out in therapy. As two supervisees reported:

> **R13:** I have found doing my own HOSS in comparison to our clients invaluable for understanding transference and countertransference processes.

> **R3:** Clients have really liked it because it seems to allow them to acknowledge the less comfortable and accepted parts of themselves, as well as to articulate who they want to be, and to value and show what qualities are important in themselves.

Reflecting upon the various self-states located in these houses and their interactions can be of value in the process of recognizing and working with both helpful and problematic relational dynamics (Petratou, 2019). Here are some reported examples of how using the HOSS in supervision helped my supervisees deepen their reflection and their awareness of their countertransference, summarized in Box 11.6:

> ### Box 11.6: Supervisees experience of completing their own House of Self States exercise
>
> **R15:** [In my HOSS] one of my basement characters feels helpless and deflated. If I feel this in countertransference without mentalizing or noticing, I may act from my own attic and 'strive' to 'fix' or 'rescue', hooking into an 'idealized mother' or 'caregiver' archetype which is unhelpful.
>
> **R9:** Using the HOSS, we spelled out how the high standards that I set for myself was driven by a clear picture in my mind of what a bad therapist would look like. By putting my HOSS alongside my client's, it was helpful to notice the behaviours that I was modelling to the client, both during our sessions and in preparation. Ultimately, I found it a bit easier to let go of trying to write the 'perfect' reformulation letter by acknowledging that I was not the therapist that I had constructed in my basement and that I didn't have to be the therapist in my attic either.
>
> **R1:** [Drawing a HOSS with clients] helped me to unpick the complexities of states in a simple yet profound way. It allowed me to clearly see transference and countertransference.
>
> **R11:** It has helped me to understand how I am different with different clients, and as above, helped me to understand particularly the harder to acknowledge basement feelings, as well as the attic hopes and intentions. I like the imagery and sort of concrete form, that helps me to use what can sometimes feel quite an abstract and hard to use concept.
>
> **R11:** I also mapped my own HOSS in supervision and was able to look more deeply at my feelings towards my client and reasons behind my own actions and motivations in the therapy. It also highlighted my concerns for the client and what my role was to them.
>
> **R7:** Creating a HOSS to explore my countertransference helped me to recognize the parts of myself that responded to a patient in sessions; by exploring these defensive and 'not-good-enough' parts in supervision, I was able to notice them more readily as mine which resulted in a more open and allowing dynamic in the therapy room, contributing to a shift forward in the patient's process.

> **R8:** It helps to understand the dynamics between me and a client with narcissistic traits. They were looking for perfection in everything they were doing and receiving, and I wanted to be the perfect psychotherapist. I understood that I needed to put the right distance and that my feelings of being a failure with this specific client who was disappointed by not being saved, was part of the work. Instead of staying on my shameful feelings, it helps me to address it and discuss the limitation of psychotherapy with my client if they stayed passive during the treatment. It was a shift in the relationship, and she started to make progress.
>
> **R7:** I have been facilitating a therapy group within a prison setting, and the HOSS has supported me to recognize and explore my expectations, fears, hopes, fantasies and emotional responses to the work. This tool in particular has helped me to understand and subsequently implement boundaries that are useful for the group members, the staff and for myself. I have also been able to recognize my own needs within the setting and to create rituals to connect with my internal resources, helping me to feel grounded at the beginning of each session.

For the last five years, I have been using the HOSS with many supervisees and clients. It became apparent to me that the use of images instead of words to name the states presented was at times more valuable in emotionally engaging with them and keeping them in the memory of the supervisees and their clients. One supervisee describes this process vividly:

> **R3:** [The HOSS] allows the possibility of objects to describe self-states which can feel very descriptive and accurate e.g. drawing a clam to imagine someone's clammed-up state in relation to others. It really helped me to identify with this patient who would become so emotionally wound up and felt restricted when having to interact with work colleagues – we both found that the image of a clam in the public/living room space really summed up his experience of interacting with others. It helped me to understand how uncomfortable this felt for him, and I think this helped him feel understood.

My supervisees who have used the HOSS to portray their relational repertoire in their role as a therapist with particular clients have found it useful in acknowledging hidden, fearful and desired self-states and in recognizing intra and interpersonal states that are activated and that often portray previously unnoticed problematic patterns. Also, when feeling stuck, it can help them to regenerate their compassion towards patients and their ability to contain challenging relational dynamics that they were having difficulties with. Below, some supervisees illustrate how this activity helped them in their work:

> **R12:** I have [used the HOSS] in supervision. It helped me see how some of my own material was playing out in the patient-therapist relationship. My patients need to be rescued or taken care of was combining with my own anxious perfectionism and desire to 'fix' or be a perfect therapist. My own fears mirrored some of the patients' fears.
>
> **R1:** The HOSS was helpful to match/compare my basement to my client's and think through how that might present in the therapy. For example, my fear of being dropped and abandoned or hurting/abusing a client stopped me from challenging them at times when it was needed.
>
> **R15:** It helps to guide and inform interventions and step outside dynamics I feel stuck with, to find new and playful ways into understanding where the client is and what they might need in our being together relationally.

In the survey, some supervisees provided examples of how they had used the House of Self States in flexible ways and adapted the activity when needed. Box 11.7 summarizes some examples.

Box 11.7: Adapting the House of Self States (HOSS)

R15: I find that the client and I will often remember and refer back to rooms in the house in later sessions – i.e., if they are describing an experience, I might say 'is this the attic-self speaking, do you think?' or 'it's a bit like how you described you feel in the bathroom, getting ready to face the world'.

R6: I have often spoken about ideas of changing the wallpaper, moving furniture, redecorating and these are nice metaphors for change.

R8: Once they completed a first version of it, I like to ask how to build stairs between the different levels.

R6: Yes, I have done this on a few occasions. I find it helpful to ask patients how they find it if I or somebody else moves between the

> different rooms. Which rooms are they more comfortable with people seeing, which rooms are they less comfortable? I also sometimes ask if there are any 'other rooms' not here, and this can be an interesting way to explore other parts. On a few occasions the house image has not sat well with some patients. For instance, one patient who was abused as a child in her loft bedroom found the metaphor difficult, and another who watched a lot of horror movies found it difficult not to picture bad things happening in a home (particularly basement or loft).

With regards to the last comment, the important element to keep in mind is the four core relational spaces (desired, dreaded, intra and interpersonal states of being) within an accommodating structure that works for the client and the supervisee. Most of the time, the metaphor of the 'house' is accepted as helpful, but at times when this is not appropriate, it may need to be replaced by another type of accommodation (such as a boat, castle, train, guest house, apartment or bedsit). This allows the concept to be used when working with a wide diversity of people who have a variety of domestic living situations.

Conclusion

Creative practice in supervision can promote opportunities for playful polyphonic dialogue, insight, empathy and flexibility, and can be useful in developing CAT therapists' zone of proximal playful development.

Such processes can also aid in expanding therapists' relational repertoire (their ability to move more fluently between acting roles and stepping back to reflect) and in listening and responding more intentionally and collaboratively. Embracing embodied and imaginative activities can wake the senses and one's ability to be more effective in improvising and engaging in attuned ways. It can illuminate the therapy dynamics and relational patterns in ways that help therapists to use their imagination and improvisation abilities.

Using projective work with objects and stories as well as embodiment and role-play experiences encourages CAT therapists to embrace the body and imagination in supervision and therapy. The survey completed by fifteen supervisees who had access to creative CAT supervision offered overall positive feedback and gave clear examples of how the exercises and activities were helpful in working with therapeutic relational processes and in enriching their experience of supervision. Creative metaphor, embodiment and understanding of different role reciprocations and patterns can be accessed through a variety of creative activities. These can provide useful ways to familiarize, communicate and validate all kinds of experiences, including those associated with feeling stuck, confusion, fear and anger.

In creative supervision, it is important to be able to move between 'being' (actively involved and identifying with something) *and* 'not being' (stepping out, reflecting, dis-identifying from what you do and who you think you are). Playing with metaphor through meaningful verbal and non-verbal activities can provide scaffolding for therapists to become more creative. In that way, through playful activity in supervision, therapists can engage their spontaneity, imagination and improvisation skills and develop their ability to connect more fluidly with their clients.

Chapter 12: Human development and Shakespeare's 'Seven Ages of Man'

Jason Hepple

Introduction

I have long had an interest in Shakespeare, and I have directed several Shakespeare plays for amateur groups over the years, including an outdoor production of *As You Like It* for the Amateur Players of Sherborne. I also started out my career in psychiatry with a strong interest in later life and in looking at psychological development across the whole lifespan. This led to my editing the *CAT in Later Life* book with Laura Sutton (Hepple & Sutton, 2004).

When asked to write about creativity in CAT, it seemed a natural choice to combine these two interests by putting a CAT lens to Shakespeare's famous 'Seven Ages of Man' speech. Shakespeare's insight into human nature is striking, especially considering this was all written a long time before Freud and Jung! I hope that by laying out the Reciprocal Roles embedded in each of the stages and using insights from more recent psychotherapy theory and dialogism, I can suggest creative and healthy exits to the challenges of existing within 'this mortal coil' (*Hamlet*, III, 1, 1760).

First, the speech itself:

> **Jaques:** *All the world's a stage,*
> *And all the men and women merely players;*
> *They have their exits and their entrances;*
> *And one man in his time plays many parts,*
> *His acts being seven ages. At first the infant,*
> *Mewling and puking in the nurse's arms;*
> *Then the whining school-boy, with his satchel*

> *And shining morning face, creeping like snail*
> *Unwillingly to school. And then the lover,*
> *Sighing like furnace, with a woeful ballad*
> *Made to his mistress' eyebrow. Then a soldier,*
> *Full of strange oaths, and bearded like the pard,*
> *Jealous in honour, sudden and quick in quarrel,*
> *Seeking the bubble reputation*
> *Even in the cannon's mouth. And then the justice,*
> *In fair round belly with good capon lin'd,*
> *With eyes severe and beard of formal cut,*
> *Full of wise saws and modern instances;*
> *And so he plays his part. The sixth age shifts*
> *Into the lean and slipper'd pantaloon,*
> *With spectacles on nose and pouch on side,*
> *His youthful hose, well sav'd, a world too wide*
> *For his shrunk shank; and his big manly voice,*
> *Turning again toward childish treble, pipes*
> *And whistles in his sound. Last scene of all,*
> *That ends this strange eventful history,*
> *Is second childishness and mere oblivion;*
> *Sans teeth, sans eyes, sans taste, sans everything.*

(As You Like It, II, 7, 1037)

In this famous speech from *As You Like It*, Shakespeare, through the words of the character Jaques, condenses the lifespan into seven ages 'played' by seven characters. The characters are all men (except perhaps for the baby and nurse) and are presented as a series of foolish and superficial performers trying to deny the inevitable and linear journey towards bodily decay and death. It is a brutal analysis.

Is there wisdom in this or just contempt for the frailty of human existence? What does a CAT lens make of this progression, and are there any exits?

The first and most important thing to note is that these are the words of a character and are utterances spoken by Jaques and addressed to the banished duke, among others, in the play and, of course, to the audience/reader.

Mikael Bakhtin's concept of 'utterance' is part of the dialogic underpinnings of CAT theory. An utterance is complete in that it is ready to be put out into dialogue and receive a response. Bakhtin's '…word, which always wants to be heard, always seeks responsive understanding, and does not stop at immediate understanding but presses on further and further (indefinitely)'. (Bakhtin, 1986, p127). It is addressed to one or more addressees, with sometimes a 'sideways glace' (Bakhtin, 1984a) to hidden or imaginary addressees.

To put this simply, everything that is put out to receive a response (words, gestures, a poem, a novel, a piece of music) is crafted and designed for the real or imaginary others that are its addressees. If the addressees had been different, then the utterance would have been crafted differently.

So, to analyse what Shakespeare is saying about the lifespan in this speech (the utterance), it first needs to be contextualized by understanding the character who is speaking and those to whom it is addressed.

Jaques

Jaques is a former nobleman of the banished Duke Senior who lives without seeming care for his physical comforts in the forest of Arden. He does nothing to advance the plot itself but is a melancholy observer/philosopher who entertains banished courtiers and country people with his wit and cynicism and claims comfort in this role and in his isolated, Diogenes-like lifestyle.

> **Jaques:** *I thank it. More, I prithee, more. I can suck melancholy out of a song, as a weasel sucks eggs. More, I prithee, more.* (II, 5, 830)
>
> **Jaques:** *I thank you for your company; but, good faith, I had as lief have been myself alone.* (III, 2, 1353)

There is an isolated grandiosity going on here for those used to a CAT lens, with an idealized self-state of admired (for seeming renunciation of mortal pleasures) to admiring (as if a voiceless disciple) and a second self-state of contemptuous (of human frailty viewed in others) to contemptible (mocked/shamed).

This has been described as: 'Conspicuous non-consumption… a situation where consumers abstain from or reduce their consumption of material goods or immaterial services and at the same time advertise their non-consumption and related motivations to others. This can be done in many more and less subtle ways. As with conspicuous consumption, conspicuous non-consumption will not work without observers and admirers.' (Sørensen & Hjalager, 2020).

In Jaques' case, this stance could be seen as an escape from acute awareness of human mortality as applied to oneself: '…an illusion of self-love and self-sufficiency that actually depends on the desire of the other to sustain it. Metaphysical desire, in which the self is experienced as insufficient or inadequate in relation to the other, is humiliating and painful: a way of avoiding this is by imposing it on others.' (Pollard, 2008)

The banished duke begins to see through this when he connects Jaques' contempt for others to a projection of Jaques' own shame from his previous life as a 'libertine':

> **Duke:** *Fie on thee! I can tell what thou wouldst do.*
>
> **Jaques:** *What, for a counter, would I do but good?*
>
> **Duke:** *Most mischievous foul sin, in chiding sin;*
> *For thou thyself hast been a libertine,*
> *As sensual as the brutish sting itself;*
> *And all th' embossed sores and headed evils*
> *That thou with license of free foot hast caught*
> *Wouldst thou disgorge into the general world.*
>
> (II, 7, 957)

Jaques' 'map' can be summarized in Figure 12.1.

Figure 12.1: Jaques' 'map'

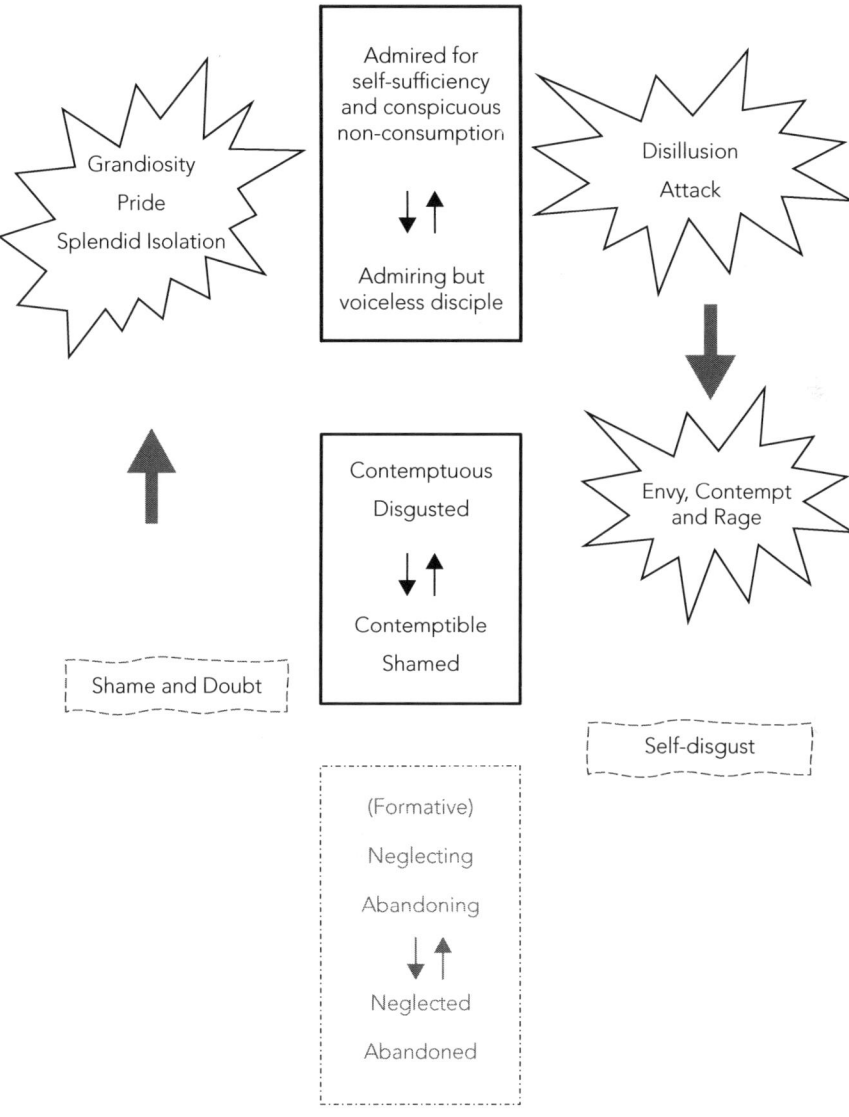

So, with this understanding, the 'Seven Ages of Man' speech could be seen as a contemptuous attack on humankind in general, broken down into seven ages, each with its own cause for scorn and mockery. Jaques claims to have transcended this mortal procession towards oblivion and we can understand this distancing as his own defence against the shame and vulnerability of his own human condition.

But should we be invited into a dismissive response to this seemingly nihilistic analysis, or is it possible to see through the attitude of the *character* Jaques to a deeper wisdom that Shakespeare is alluding to? There is no doubt that the journey is recognizable as part of our human lifespan, but it is so harsh! It is perhaps one of the fundamental qualities of a joke that someone or something is brought down to earth, and as this tirade is about all human beings, we are all the victims (including Jaques). This may be part of the speech's fascinating draw. In some ways, this speech pulls us together and points out our similarities rather than our differences. This has been called, in dialogistic parlance, 'insideness' (Pollard, 2008).

'Insideness' presumes that there is such a thing as common humanity, that there is an essential similarity between any two human beings, regardless of how great the differences between them might be ... we can potentially know other people from our 'interior' knowledge of ourselves. Pollard coins 'insideness' as a counterpoint to Bakhtin's 'outsideness' or 'surplus of vision'. 'This ever-present excess of my seeing, knowing, and possessing in relation to any other human being is founded in the uniqueness and irreplaceability of my place in the world' (Bakhtin, 1990, p23).

'Outsideness' offers objectivity and detachment. 'Insideness' offers empathic connection and ultimately human affection. Bakhtin acknowledges that this 'outsideness' or 'surplus of vision' must be offered to the other with care: 'The most important aspect of this surplus is love… This surplus is never used as an ambush, as a chance to sneak up and attack from behind. This is an open and honest surplus, dialogically revealed to the other person…' (Bakhtin, 1984a, p299). This, in a nutshell, is the task of the therapist – to offer reformulation and perspective in a way that is beneficial and digestible. The Reciprocal Role freely giving to gratefully receiving (Hepple, 2010; 2022).

Finally, Jaques' speech well illustrates Bakhtin's concept of 'carnival', where the commonality of the body and bodily functions are mocked and made grotesque in order to provide relief from oppressive control (death) by allowing rebellious irreverence and temporary escape through the medium of the carnival (Bakhtin, 1984b). It is perhaps through this shared subversiveness in the face of our human frailty that we may find connection, fraternity and, ultimately, love. Maybe this is what Shakespeare had in mind after all…

I would now like to go through the seven ages of the speech offering an antidote to Jaques' mocking narrative and trying to find the positive, reparative, therapeutic alternatives. The first self-state represents Jaques' attack on the seven characters (self-to-other but also himself-to-himself). The second, a reparative therapist-to-client then client self-to-self relationship.

The seven ages
The first age: The infant

'At first the infant,
Mewling and puking in the nurse's arms;'

The verb 'mewling' encapsulates vulnerability and helpless animal distress. The 'puking' provokes disgust. The infant is unloved and reviled and left to the care of the nurse. This is in contrast to a loving start in life – the baby as special and cherished. As Kohut famously said: 'The most significant relevant basic interactions between mother and child usually lie in the visual area: the child's bodily display is responded to by the gleam in the mother's eye' (Kohut, 1971, p117).

The infant and its unmanageable bodily functions may be speaking to Jaques' own vulnerability as he ages and resonates with the 'second childishness' of his seventh age yet to come. The task of the psychotherapist is to offer acceptance and respect that can be internalized in time through a self-to-self relationship (Figure 12.2).

Figure 12.2: The infant

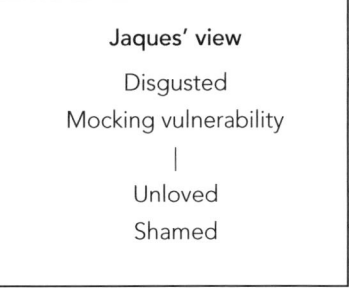
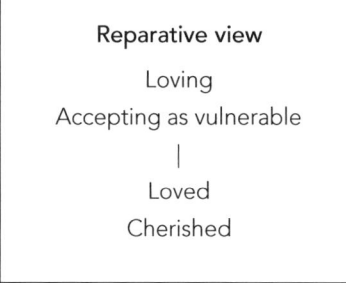

The second age: The schoolboy

> 'Then the whining school-boy, with his satchel
> And shining morning face, creeping like snail
> Unwillingly to school.'

This is a complex portrayal. His 'shining morning face' seems to allude to new hope and a new generation beginning the journey of self-development, but there is no enthusiasm here, as if the boy is already tired and cynical about the drudgery of his life ahead. I see this as Jaques' own cynicism, possibly looking back on his own early aspirations that have been disillusioned as his life progressed.

A reformulation of the character would see a child who has been discouraged or intimidated by his first experiences of school and that children who are positively encouraged and supported can develop resilience and curiosity to engage in creative play. This, for Donald Winnicott, is the primary task of helping a child develop and a fundamental part of a healing psychotherapy encounter: 'It is in playing and only in playing that the individual child or adult is able to be creative and to use the whole personality, and it is only in being creative that the individual discovers the self' (Winnicott, 1971, p54).

Figure 12.3: The schoolboy

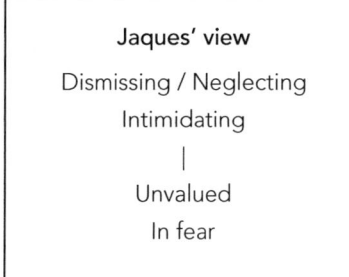
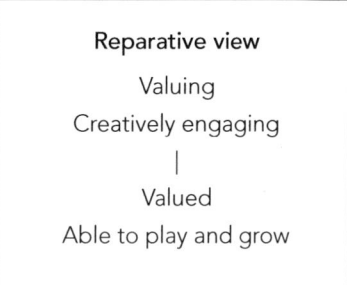

The third age: The lover

> 'And then the lover,
> Sighing like furnace, with a woeful ballad
> Made to his mistress' eyebrow.'

Here Jaques pokes fun at a young lover full of passion and emotion in a way that suggests it will soon be shown to be a brief mirage of an infatuation and, ultimately, a source of shame and disillusionment. This does not credit to the role with enthusiasm and hope that may mark the start of a new relationship (including a therapy relationship). 'Instillation of hope' is one of Yalom's key therapeutic factors in group psychotherapy (Yalom & Leszcz, 2005).

It is common in psychotherapy for there to be an initial 'honeymoon' period in the relationship between client and therapist that later faces challenge when conflict or disagreement evolve as Reciprocal Roles are re-enacted in the relationship. It is the task of therapy to weather this potential therapeutic rupture and work towards repair and an acceptance of the 'good-enough' nature of the work (Winnicott, 1953; Daly *et al*, 2010). This may, of course, be true of many relationships we negotiate throughout life.

Figure 12.4: The lover

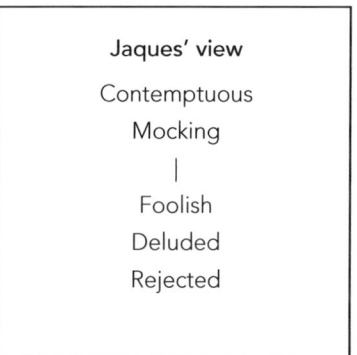
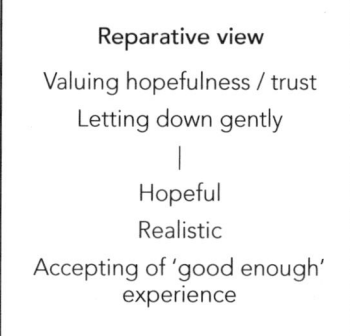

The fourth age: The soldier

> '*Then a soldier,*
> *Full of strange oaths, and bearded like the pard,*
> *Jealous in honour, sudden and quick in quarrel,*
> *Seeking the bubble reputation*
> *Even in the cannon's mouth.*'

The soldier seems to have found a way to conform and do what is expected of him at this stage of adulthood. He has joined his 'tribe' and has assumed the appearance and behaviour of the group in order to fit in. The bravado may be seen as a defence against the fear of annihilation and loss when involved in combat.

Jaques mocks the soldier as lacking any individual self-identity. 'Bearded like the pard' may refer to a leopard which would only have a soft downy beard not 'a full set'. The soldier is ridiculous as his sham bravery and willingness to die for his cause are all for nothing as reputation is only an empty bubble without lasting legacy.

Many people have experienced in their lives the need to conform to a norm to avoid rejection and alienation. People try their best to fit in and be successful in terms of the group they have joined, but there can be a disillusion and a later feeling of not fitting in after all, and needing to unravel what may have been a lengthy lifespan commitment.

In CAT, we sometimes think of this as a 'false self' – a placatory self - created to please critical and neglecting voices from earlier in life. Elliot Jaques description of a 'mid-life crisis' (Jaques, 1975) is about the questioning of these false self-states and the need to engage in creative play and dialogue to re-invent the dialogic self into later life.

Figure 12.5: The soldier

Jaques' view	Reparative view
Ridiculing of status	Respecting of sacrifices
Dismissing for conformity	Giving permission for re-invention
|	|
Foolish, a sham	Valued for service
Pointless sacrifice	Free to create and play

The fifth age: The justice

> 'And then the justice,
> In fair round belly with good capon lin'd,
> With eyes severe and beard of formal cut,
> Full of wise saws and modern instances;
> And so he plays his part.'

The justice seems to get off quite lightly, with just some envious attack on his apparent success and well-fed status, with some acknowledgement that he is at the top of his game (for now). The attack comes through Jaques' foresight of the sixth and seventh ages to come – how the justice will 'slip' into the next age after he has 'played his part'. This reminds me of a speech made by Macbeth:

> *'Life's but a walking shadow, a poor player*
> *That struts and frets his hour upon the stage*
> *And then is heard no more: it is a tale*
> *Told by an idiot, full of sound and fury,*
> *Signifying nothing.'*

(Macbeth V, 5, 2381)

The justice may be full of 'sound and fury', but this all amounts to nothing in the end. The justice may represent a different sort of mid-life crisis. In contrast to the soldier, whose task may be to re-invent his self and values, the justice may feel justifiably proud of his career and the achievements he has worked hard for through his life. But how to accept the end of this stage and to 'slip' into later life without feeling that all ultimately signifies 'nothing'?

William James wrote about the extension of the self and self-esteem after one's own death as part of one's 'legacy': 'The greatest use of life is to spend it on something that will outlast it.' (in Perry, 1935, p289). The role of the therapist in helping someone make this transition into later life can be both to validate the legacy that has been set in motion (be it children, family, occupation, creative works, people helped and supported over the years...) and to ease the transition into retirement and a creative 'third age'.

Figure 12.6: The justice

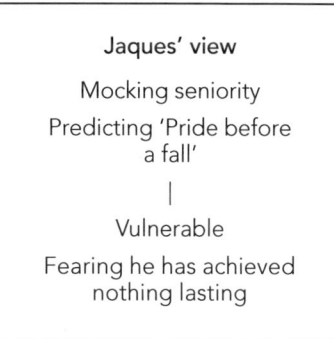

Jaques' view	Reparative view
Mocking seniority	Valuing achievements/legacy
Predicting 'Pride before a fall'	Encouraging a creative transition
|	|
Vulnerable	Proud of legacy
Fearing he has achieved nothing lasting	'Still more to do'

The sixth age: The pantaloon

> *'The sixth age shifts*
> *Into the lean and slipper'd pantaloon,*
> *With spectacles on nose and pouch on side,*
> *His youthful hose, well sav'd, a world too wide*
> *For his shrunk shank; and his big manly voice,*
> *Turning again toward childish treble, pipes*
> *And whistles in his sound.'*

This is Jaques' longest and most cutting commentary. It may be the character he most despises as it is the one he most resembles. It picks up on a foolish elderly male character in the Italian commedia dell'arte who wears baggy trousers. The justice has transitioned into a rapidly ageing and laughable shadow of his former self. This is an ageist defence that projects ageing into other people to protect the self. As ageing is universal, ageism is, paradoxically, a prejudice that is often most difficult to challenge in both client and therapist:

> *'It is difficult working psychotherapeutically with older people. Ageism is deeply ingrained in modern Western society and is inevitably represented in both therapist and client as a series of negative stereotypes, unchallenged assumptions and unconscious reactions which exert a profound influence on therapeutic work. So difficult has it been to see the wood for the trees in this area, the theoretical models underpinning modern psychotherapies themselves providing some of the most glaring examples of ageism around. To top even this obstacle is a medical and psychological model of ageing where increasing age and decline in function are synonymous and inevitable and where there can seem no alternative but to chart deficits and monitor deterioration rather than measure strengths and encourage adaptation and development.'* (Hepple, 2004, p46)

Working therapeutically into later life requires a balance of respect and acceptance of changes, losses and transitions that are an inevitable part of ageing, avoidance of 'you are only as old as you feel' defences as well as hope for contentment, re-invention and gracious transition into elderhood where wisdom and perspective are valued and nurtured.

Figure 12.7: Pantaloon

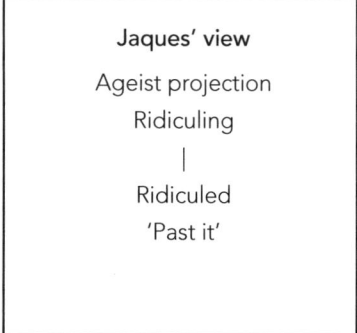
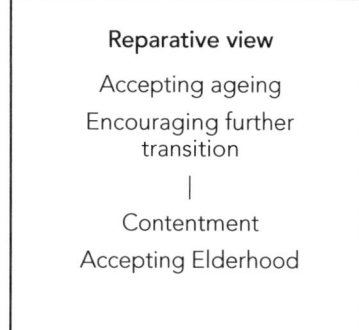

The seventh age: The last scene of all

'Last scene of all,
That ends this strange eventful history,
Is second childishness and mere oblivion;
Sans teeth, sans eyes, sans taste, sans everything.'

This is again a brutal reduction of a life to the dying body and its disabilities, limitations and humiliations. This seventh age is a seeming justification for the contemptuous attack on all the stages that have gone before. Just the brief 'hour upon the stage' before being 'heard no more'.

There is no therapeutic antidote to this reality of human death other than acceptance and compassion, and an awareness of the shared 'insideness' of our commonality and transient embodiment. For the reparative roles here, I can only return to where we began.

Figure 12.8: The last scene of all

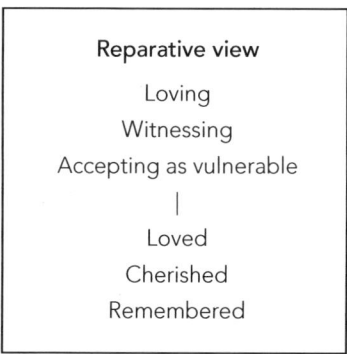

Concluding thoughts

I hope that, through this CAT analysis of one of Shakespeare's most famous speeches, we can see through the layers of characterization and parody to an acceptance of the wondrousness and challenges of being mortal and the brilliance of the four-hundred-year-old legacy of Shakespeare himself.

I invite the reader to look at other Shakespeare plays for similar insight and inspiration: *King Lear* as an account of 'narcissistic collapse' in later life, *Macbeth* for a study of power and how its acquisition can corrupt and embroil, and perhaps *Titus Andronicus* to find out where revenge can lead!

Chapter 13:
The roots and heart of Cognitive Analytic Music Therapy (CAMT)

Stella Compton Dickinson

> *'Creativity is the act of conceiving something new, while innovation is the act of putting something into practice.'* (Stone, 2022)
>
> *'Violence is immoral because it thrives on hatred rather than love. It destroys community and makes brotherhood impossible. It leaves society in monologue rather than dialogue.'*
>
> (Martin Luther King Jnr., Nobel Lecture, University of Oslo, 1964)

Introduction

Martin Luther King's words provide a source of reflection when applied to the therapeutic treatment of people who have a serious mental illness (SMI), such as schizophrenia, who have committed violent offences. Rather than being sent to prison, they may be sentenced through the criminal justice system to secure hospital treatment on the grounds of diminished responsibility for an indefinite period, until they are deemed to no longer pose a threat to others. On admittance, they become patients with very limited access to the public. They receive multi-disciplinary treatment to help them develop an understanding of their offence and the reasons as to why they committed it. Almost without exception, in my clinical experience, they have been victims of childhood abuse, bullying, neglect and domestic violence.

In this chapter, I consider the roots of mental ill health through a cognitive analytic lens, in the relationships of childhood. Winnicott (2005) in *Playing and Reality*, addresses the origins of creativity and how we develop it as infants; playing in an adult sense becomes possible in jointly created dialogical musical improvisation. This form of dialogical creative self-expression is at the heart of Cognitive Analytic Music Therapy (CAMT). I will describe specific creative therapeutic techniques that are used, more of which continue to emerge within CAMT.

The development of this model took place in the UK during twenty years of clinically based research in the National Health Service (NHS) high and medium security forensic mental health services. These patients have very limited choices because they are living within a 'closed environment': movement is restricted, the doors are locked and there is limited access to the general public. The National Institute of Care Excellence (NICE) guidance (2010) therefore stated that treatment options must be evidence-based for these patients who are incarcerated. Hence, by following the NICE guidance, the method, techniques, aims and objectives of CAMT were systematically developed, researched and ethically approved.

The challenge in forensic music therapy research and clinical practice is to explore how psychopathic traits may or may not be mediated through musical, vibrational effects in jointly created musical improvisation, because anti-social traits impact wider social functioning. The potential for disingenuous or dissociative responses creates a massive challenge in developing a genuinely relational therapy in which empathy and connection may emerge (Taylor *et al*, 2022). Non-verbal, unexpressed feelings frequently precede words, yet as neurological changes occur during jointly created musical improvisation, emotional recognition may awaken, thereby contributing to the development of 'affective' (subjectively felt) empathy which may follow from cognitive (understood) empathy (Compton Dickinson & Jolliffe, 2021).

In the clinical setting, I have observed and witnessed this process when mental integration develops with patients who were known previously to 'talk the talk' of recovery and integration yet without feeling it. They may understand cognitively what they think that they are supposed to say, yet without emotionally recognized empathy to their situation.

The CAMT model enables patients firstly to feel the vibrations from a choice of instruments, then they can choose an instrument with which they identify and resonate vibrationally as their individual 'sound print' (Compton Dickinson & Hakvoert, 2017, p139-140). From this, they may then create a relationship with their sound print instrument, safely recognizing their own feelings and responses. Following this experience of relating to an object of self-expression, they may go on to develop a shared interpersonal relationship with the music therapist, from which a new relational understanding may occur.

Development of music therapy in forensic settings

The challenge in the twenty-first century for clinicians working in high secure mental health settings is to understand and explore the treatability of people with co-morbid diagnoses. Yet, for people who may not wish to accept diagnostic criteria, for example, of schizophrenia and/or personality disorder, CAMT provides a creative therapeutic means by which to understand themselves better (Compton Dickinson, 2021). Some patients have been incarcerated and institutionalized for decades.

For those with lifetime criminal persistency, there are treatment challenges regarding whether internal relational and empathic change may be possible. In forensic mental health settings, emotional recognition and regulation within the process of musical self-expression in CAMT is central to risk assessment to ensure that over-arousal is not encouraged.

Overview of music therapy and CAMT

There are many ways of using music in therapeutic settings. These range from active listening, songwriting and lyric analysis to clinically based improvisational music making. The latter is favoured in the UK as a means by which the therapeutic relationship and creative self-expression can develop within musical interactions that reflect the internal and relational states of the individual.

In secure hospitals, listening to pre-recorded music is used in many contexts by patients, in relaxation and educational groups. A community choir may be led by the music therapist (Maguire, 2020). This way of being together – literally using the vocal cords to sing, by which these vocalized vibrations resonate between people being together – can frequently provide a harmonious introduction to music making. This experience may lead to more intensive engagement in structured 'evidence-based' forms of individual or group music therapy.

Evidence-based models of music therapy are based on, and sometimes integrated into, existing psychological principles such as psychoanalysis, Cognitive Behavioural Therapy and, as described here, Cognitive Analytic Therapy (Ryle & Kerr, 2020). Music therapy models that have been clinically tested in research trials usually begin in a specific clinical context due to the need to maintain research conditions during a research trial. (Campbell *et al*, 2007) Cognitive Analytic Music Therapy (CAMT) is one such model.

In 2018, the World Federation of Music Therapy commissioned a review of models, approaches and methods of music therapy (McFerran *et al*, 2023). Given the diverse settings in which music therapy has developed over the past fifty years, the above authors aimed to update the literature to ensure that novel and rigorously tested models, as well as approaches and methods of music therapy, are both defined and categorized. The purpose being to ensure that music therapy is fit for purpose for the diverse cultural, ethnic and social needs of twenty-first century societies across the globe. Within this process, CAMT was recognized as an 'integrated relational model' of music therapy.

Over time, some models of music therapy have been extended for use with other populations. For example, the Nordoff Robbins approach (Nordoff & Robbins, 1985) was first used for children with special needs and then much later evolved to embrace a community music therapy approach (Pavlicek & Andsell, 2004).

The Cambridge Institute of Music Therapy Research (CIMTR) approach was originally based on psychoanalytic principles (Odell-Miller, 2014). This centre is now conducting international studies across five countries for music therapy for people with dementia who are living in their own homes, as well as mapping neurological changes in brain studies for those receiving music therapy.

CAMT is now being used with looked-after children in care as an early intervention. These children have been fostered and are sometimes separated from their siblings. They frequently have avoidant and ambivalent attachment patterns having suffered separation, neglect and feelings of abandonment as infants. They discover in CAMT how to develop a trusting therapeutic relationship with a developing ability to be creative, discovering how to play, have fun and to experience joy with another person.

CAMT: Research and development as an integrated intervention

CAMT was developed specifically to fit in with the over-arching treatment models and the structured treatment pathways of multi-disciplinary forensic mental health treatment. (Lawday & Compton Dickinson, 2013). My relief was palpable when I first presented positive clinical changes and outcomes in a ward round through using this integrated music therapy approach. Team members responded positively to the common language of CAT by which we could understand each other when thinking about a man who had anti-social traits, and who had not responded to any other form of therapy (Compton Dickinson, 2006).

The CAMT model was initially tested within the sixteen-session CAT model, with a gradual layering of greater complexity of musical resources and harmonic structures.

From Compton Dickinson, (2015) the primary hypothesis of the feasibility randomized controlled trial that my team and I conducted was:

> 'Musical improvisation delivered to men who have committed violent offences and who are receiving secure hospital treatment in groups, through manualised Group-Cognitive Analytic Music Therapy will improve their relating to others compared with the control group who receive standard multi-disciplinary treatment as usual, as measured by The Persons Relating to Others Questionnaire (PROQ2) (Birtchnell & Evans, 2004) and The Manual for the Chart of Interpersonal Reactions in Closed Living Environments (CIRCLE) (Blackburn & Glasgow, 2006).'

The music therapists who delivered the trial initially completed an introductory two-day course in CAT. Since the validating paper was published by Kellet *et al* (2018), several music therapists have trained in and gained CAT accreditation, with permission granted to complete one of their qualifying case studies in CAMT. Others simply benefit from CAT supervision. The British Association of Music Therapy provides introductory study days in music therapy which may be of interest to CAT therapists.

At the time of writing, the CAMT model is delivered in several UK NHS forensic services by music therapists registered with the Health Care Professions Council (HCPC). It is used in Finland in a secure mental health setting as well as being used in music therapy charities for prison inmates, and it is proving to be effective in early intervention for looked-after children in care homes.

Myself and my colleague Laurien Hakvoort together published the *Clinicians Guide to Forensic Music Therapy* (2017), which provides information for music therapists and for serious mentally ill patients on our two individually developed and tested models. The two treatment manuals are included for future use should a multi-centre trial ever be funded.

The four structured stages of CAMT

The pilot project through which CAMT was developed and tested as clinically effective was implemented in an enhanced medium secure unit for women. The over-arching multi-disciplinary approach was that of dialectical behavioural therapy, hence CAMT was developed within the accepted interdisciplinary language, which was understood by both patients and nurses. Readers are invited to refer to the published chapter on how this worked (in Lawday & Compton Dickinson, 2013, p184-285).

The stages of time-limited CAMT are:

1. Musical mindfulness.
2. Emotional recognition.
3. Distress tolerance and conflict resolution.
4. Interpersonal effectiveness.

These stages employ specific CAT tools to support the development of self-reflection and self-awareness. Musical mindfulness involves observing and describing through each of the senses in turn, gradually moving towards emotional recognition within musical self-expression, then progressing to distress tolerance which is often represented by dissonance and resolutions facilitated by the music therapist within musical improvisations, finally aiming for new exits in the form of relational changes that amount to interpersonal effectiveness. As a result of this scaffolded CAT approach, the music therapist can employ musical techniques that become increasingly subtle and complex.

The musical components of CAMT

Jointly created musical improvisation is a shared dialogical activity. The CAMT model offers structure and scaffolding within a time limit that is designed to be compatible with modern interdisciplinary treatment pathways. When a musical improvisation is created in dialogue, it can be a remarkably intimate form of engagement. As a collaborative process, similar to verbal interactions, it is about far more than imitation. When the music therapist tunes in by using their embodied sense as felt from the client, a musically empathic response is created. This can be heard and perceived by the client, as if being understood, who may then feel a relational connection.

Clinical example

The following example from a CAMT session demonstrates how this process may however create a rupture in the therapeutic alliance. A woman who had experienced abuse subsequently enacted an abusive offence. She was in a dilemma of *either* fearing intimacy and of being intruded upon, *or* in a reciprocal enactment of the abuse in which she would get close and intrude upon others.

In the session, having initiated a musical motif, the patient suddenly stopped when I picked this up in a musical response. She exclaimed 'Oh! You stole that from me!' I felt shocked and on reflection I realized that I had got too close. By so doing, I had triggered a fearful feeling that restricted her own creativity. On hearing her life story, she explained that when she was a child, learning the piano in her own space, absorbed in a reverie, her abuser would interrupt her musical practice by taking her by surprise, and then smacking her for no apparent reason.

In a CAMT group session, the opportunity for movement around the room from instrument to instrument facilitates embodied responses in the therapist and patients. The music therapist can create appropriate distance, as well as opportunities for dialogical sharing and the development of attachment bonds in proximity. Schore (2003) explains how these therapeutic connections result in neurochemical changes in the prefrontal cortex where feelings are regulated both consciously and unconsciously. The effect of attuned musical vibration on the corpus callosum connects the two hemispheres of the brain, which in music therapy may promote mental and emotional integration.

Recognizing Reciprocal Role (RR) enactments in CAMT such as the RR 'intrusive to intruded on' described above, can help the music therapist in supervision to understand the transference relationship of what or who they may represent at any one time in relation to patients with whom they are working. This enables awareness of potential enactments of the dilemma of *either* becoming the abuser in collusion with an offence-related response, *or* of rejection *creating* a rupture and the risk of disengagement.

Participants in a music therapy group may choose to leave their seats, observe others, and explore various selected instruments. Instruments are accessible for anyone to play without having learned or practiced formally. For example, an ocean drum can conjure up the imagination of a journey or the memory of a scene, yet this could elicit a range of emotions, such as fears linked to negative memories, feelings of loss, or of wistfulness or over-arousal that could lead to a violent enactment. The role of the music therapist is to notice, contain and work with whatever may arise.

In our study (2015) we noted how frequently the various instruments were chosen. The most popular were the tuned percussion bass instruments and the sounding bowl[3].

Figures 13.1 & 13.2: The rear of this bowl has a different texture and a hole in it. This 'flaw' was part of the original ash tree from which the bowl was crafted, but this does not affect the tuning, instead providing ample metaphors.

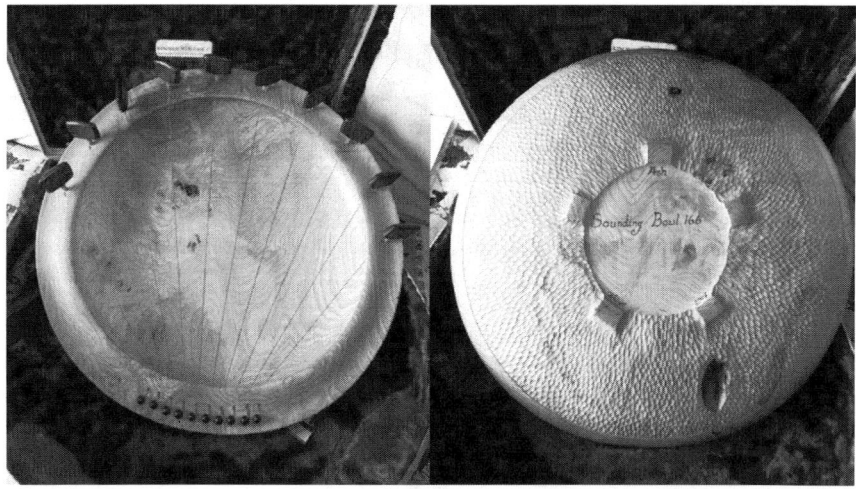

---

3   https://soundingbowls.com.

Sounding bowls are different to Tibetan singing bowls; they are made in the UK by Tobias Kaye in Devon from different tree species that have various inherent healing qualities. Their unique design and sound facilitate safe exploration without preconceived ideas such as those associated with the guitar and its uses. Exploration takes place through sight, touch of the varied textures, smell as well as sound. Tobias tunes these instruments to different modes and scales as can the music therapist.

Initially, and uniquely to the CAMT model, the music therapist will support group members' ability to find their musical 'sound print' (Compton Dickinson, 2015, ibid); to empower them to experience the vibrational qualities that most resonate with them in the moment, at the time of each session. For example, one person who came to music therapy who frequently expressed feeling untouchable, on seeing the sounding bowl, explored the different textures considering both 'the rough and the smooth' as a metaphor for his life. Only then did he explore the sounds that could be produced.

The music therapist explores each of the senses in turn, building up mindful self-awareness in a scaffolded manner, by which relational and self-reflective skills develop. These techniques are all explained in depth in the *Clinicians Guide to Forensic Music Therapy* (Compton Dickinson & Hakvoort, 2017, p138-141). By following these stages as a guide, music therapists can feel grounded and confident in their musical therapeutic techniques and underlying theoretical concepts by which to understand clinical presentations, and possibilities for intrapsychic as well as interpersonal change.

In CAMT, as in CAT, the patient may learn non-didactically both actively and responsively with the fluidity of jointly – creating a musical improvisation. For example, if the music therapist first plays the ocean drum or the sounding bowl to set the scene based on the feel in the room, the group member may observe and sense a calming and containing form of self-expression towards promoting a safe environment, or alternatively the music therapist may pick up an indication of unrest, such as agitated behaviour, which it may be helpful to reflect through subtle musical mirroring techniques.

Sound, atmosphere and silence

Music incorporating silence is a powerful therapeutic medium that may be used both positively (for example in palliative care by Dr Colin Lee (2016) and negatively (for example to manipulate crowds). With mental health patients in music therapy, it is not uncommon for a patient who has suffered traumatic abuse and who has a severe mental illness to do a final crash on his instrument after everyone else has finished. Thus, destroying the silence. Given the different qualities of silence, such as the pregnant, expectant pause at the end of a meaningful piece of musical improvisation, the music therapist may contain and support the ability of others to safely 'feel' the qualities of silence and carefully address what that final crash might mean.

The philosophical concepts that underpin CAMT and my personal healing journey are from the works of Hazrat Inayat Khan. He was an Eastern philosopher and great musician, who brought to the Western world an ancient message through meditative practices of love, harmony and beauty. In *The Music of Life* (1988) he begins by explaining that the ancient Sufis believed that the whole of life in the universe began with a single vibration in the silence of the void. He explains that from the silent life, a vibration is a creator of vibrations, motion causes motion, as with the plucking of a violin string. In this way, the silent life becomes active, which may disturb peace. It is the grade of activity of these vibrations that accounts for the various planes of existence. Hence, with the varied vibrational frequencies, altered states of consciousness may be accessed through playing or hearing music that is attuned to the situation and circumstances.

Silence has the potential to elicit a whole range of feelings: e.g. fearful, calming, peaceful or persecutory. Silences may be experienced as peaceful and restful or agonizing within a highly emotive hospital environment. They may range from signalling distress to creating a calming atmosphere if the therapist can hold the space. The 'silencing to silenced' Reciprocal Role is a frequently unrecognized then painful response for people who have suffered domestic abuse and trauma. With these patients feeling the quality of the silences can be crucial in supporting therapeutic engagement. Our own need for silence may or may not match that of others.

CAMT musical improvisation, polyvagal mapping and the Multiple Self States Model

Polyvagal theory

Usually, a session of CAMT starts with musical mindfulness. This first stage includes breathing exercises that encourage reflective thought. Diaphragmatic breathing is significant in promoting internal feelings of safety and self-reflection because the auditory nerve, according to John Stuart Reid (2023) receives 'clear crosstalk from the auricular branch of the vagus nerve'. This suggests that of our five senses, that which we hear, can trigger a trauma effect in a particularly profound way. Reid (2023) clarifies that only the vagus nerve can send a slowing down signal through the exhalation of breath as the heart beats slightly faster on the inspiration of breath than on the aspiration of breath. (These terms are used intentionally by me, as it is through 'inspiration' that we gain insight as oxygen activates the brain and the body through the lungs and heart. It is through 'aspiration' rather than expiration, that we seek to aspire to our goals, rather than to give up and 'expire'.)

The autonomic vagus nerve according to Reid (2023) requires distinction between the neurophysiological aspects of the autonomic system's two sub-branches. The sympathetic (acceleration) and the parasympathetic (brake) functions. Thus, providing a two-directional neural connection between our organs and our brainstem. In clinical practice this is born out empirically in Matthew Green's (2015) book *Aftershock: The Untold Story of Surviving Peace* in which he concludes that body-based approaches to therapy can ensure that ex-military personnel suffering from PTSD are not labelled as 'treatment resistant'. He states that by demonstrating the power of working with the parts of the brain that words cannot reach a profound gift is offered to trauma survivors. The diagram below (Pseudonym 'Dom') maps out how this poly vagal understanding was applied and integrated within CAT for a client suffering debilitating physical symptoms of performance anxiety.

Fig. 13.3. The diagram of a performing artist: 'An embodied approach to a bodily problem

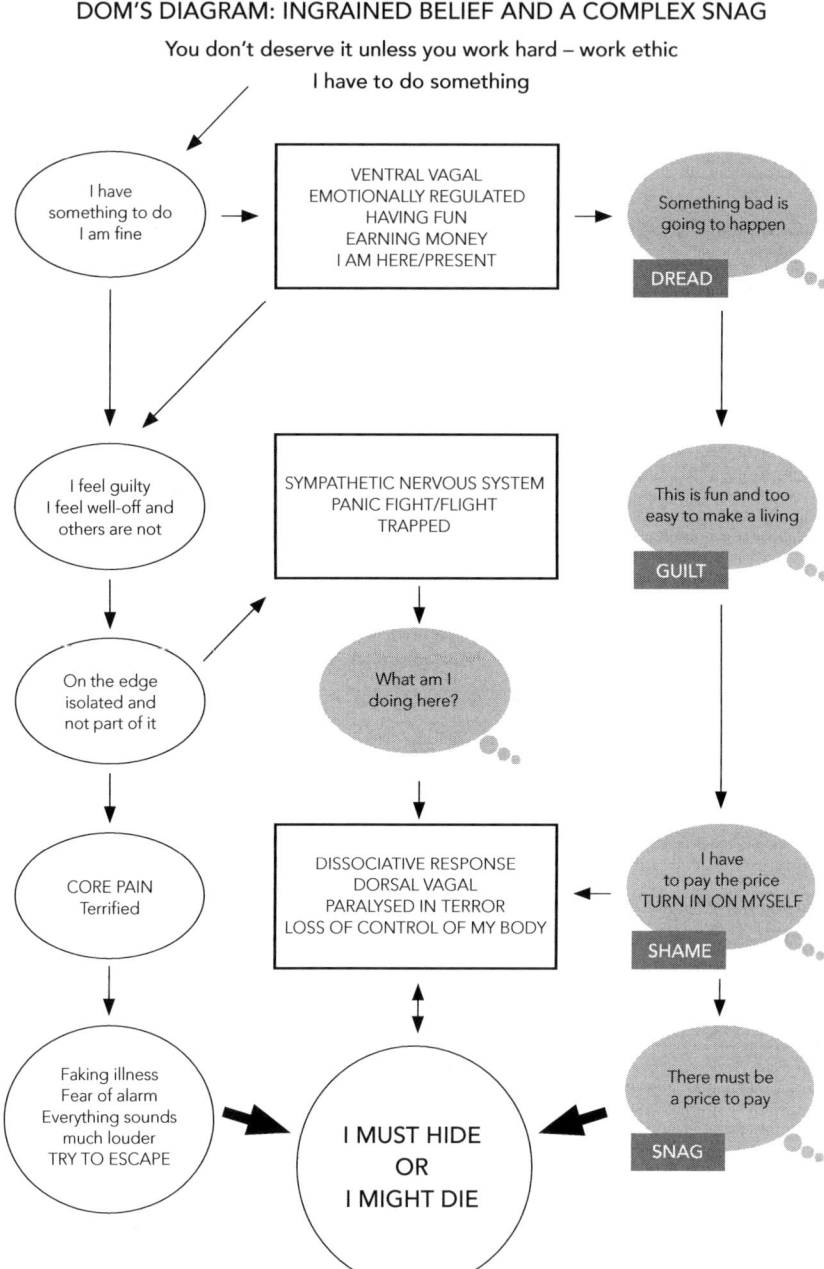

A personal example of the trauma effect that was controlled through that slow exhalation of breath as explained by Reid (2023) occurred some months after my being thrown violently from a rearing horse: when then watching at close quarters some racehorses in flight jumping a high fence altogether, I was taken by surprise when my brain registered the rise of the horses '*as if*' they were rearing. At this point, my eyes involuntarily filled with tears. In fact, the horses were jumping as in a herd. I was not in danger of being thrown anywhere. Yet I experienced for a moment the same disabling fear and shock of the initial incident through the optic nerve of the eye. This is the trauma response to which Mathew Green (2015) refers. At that point for me, it was quickly followed by my frontal cortex comprehension and recognition of the false similarity. I breathed deeply and recovered.

This personal example demonstrated how the brain in effect plays tricks with our hyper-sensitivity to threat stimuli. The trigger may in fact have very little to do with the actual traumatic event. Hence, within the personal narratives of this client group, which may be reformulated through the CAT Multiple Self States Model and within the dialogical therapeutic process of CAMT, trauma effects may be better recognized and understood and treated nonverbally in CAMT.

Dissociative trauma responses are horrible to experience, and people who have been violent to others frequently also have a traumatized child state. Given that the area of the brain that is activated is deeply unconscious, with an interaction between the hippocampus and the amygdala, the above personal example demonstrated to me that the therapeutic task is that of helping the patient to recognize that trauma triggers may not be the same as the original traumatic event. The task is to develop sufficient cognitive resilience by learning how to breathe into and pause, rather than to react to the impulsive effects that occur in complex post-traumatic stress syndrome. Hence the development of CAMT stage one of musical mindfulness. Reassurance occurs in understanding the plasticity of the brain and the capacity of the hippocampus to grow and regain its former resilience when it is no longer overwhelmed by emotional stimuli.

The music therapist will work non-verbally in effect by tuning into the overall *feel* received from the patient. This can be viscerally felt as explained in polyvagal theory by Porges (2001), in which additional to the sympathetic nervous system which activates the flight/flight mechanism, the parasympathetic nervous system can support health.

Growth, rest and digestion have an embodied sense, which is called the ventral vagal state, in which a person is emotionally regulated. This is why musical mindfulness is followed by emotional recognition and regulation in the CAMT model. Porges (2001) considered that in the ventral vagal state, social engagement, therefore relating to others, is connected to the nervous system, in effect all is well, whereas in the dorsal vagal state, which is a defensive dissociative state a shutdown occurs with the freeze/flop mechanism.

This concept fits well with the Multiple Self States Model (MSSM) model as described by Ryle in The Psychotherapy File (see Appendix 1) and expanded on in the self-states' descriptions tool. Ventral vagal emotionally regulated states can be mapped out, and stimuli can then be recognized and tracked as the patient recognizes their triggers, which may lead to the dorsal vagal 'flop freeze' states via the sympathetic nervous system fight/flight responses.

In other words, by tuning in musically, which in my experience involves *an embodied countertransference*, and then reflecting this quality in sound, as described by Daniel Stern (1985) and Trevarthen (2011), a non-verbal connection is made with the mentally ill patient that may bring them into a relational state.

CAMT as a group

> 'I had to write a requiem for all those who died, who had suffered. (...) But how could I do it? I was constantly under suspicion then, and critics counted what percentage of my symphonies were in a major key and what percentage in a minor key. That oppressed me, it deprived me of the will to compose.'

> 'I've read about Toscanini's conducting style and his manner of conducting a rehearsal. He screams and curses the musicians and makes scenes in the most shameless manner... Conductors are too often rude and conceited tyrants.... And in my youth, I often had to fight fierce battles with them, battles for my music and my dignity.'

> (Shostakovich, 1979)

Shostakovich describes oppression while aiming to be creative and courageous under Stalin's terrifying regime. He also describes the tyrannical behaviour that a powerful albeit great conductor could impose on his terrified musicians. Toscanini's ferocity remains legend to this day. It is within this power imbalance that internal validation may be lacking and eroded for all concerned, particularly in Shostakovich's situation where external validation was controlled by the state, until his 'Testimony' was smuggled to the Western world. His courage when confronted by compromise and oppression demonstrates how creativity can overcome adversity with the ability to innovate. This led me to think about the common human fears and sense of restriction in self-expression that occurs for people who were initially oppressed and who may later be restricted through incarceration in secure hospitals.

The example from Shostakovich's book 'Testimony' highlights the difference between performance under a dominating leader and the shared and cohesive experience in a structured music therapy group, which is facilitated according to group therapeutic principles. Making music in both forms can create bonds that last through a lifetime of friendship and memories. This process has implications in the clinical setting for the potential to internalise positive feelings rather than fear through the jointly created process. This method supports the need for a collaborative approach regardless of social or hospital hierarchies, and with respect for varied levels of musical skill.

There are numerous demands on the skills of the cognitive analytic music therapist. Group members are supported to feel ownership of their own part in the musically creative process of the group in which multiple musical dialogues are woven together. By using the groupwork principles of Foulkes (1983), social feeling develops so that patients can share their experiences within the group and their thoughts and feelings may be therapeutically ameliorated. The temptation or need to perform could otherwise too easily overwhelm others who may never in their life have played an instrument before.

CAT recognition in improvisation

CAMT, as a relational model, enables the recognition of feelings from the underlying emotions that are reflected through the emotionally attuned qualities of jointly created improvisation.

Jointly created musical improvisation is a dialogical activity that occurs in the same way that Vygotsky's (1978) activity theory works in that *'what the child does with the more experienced other today, she may do on their own tomorrow'*. This concept was novel in music therapy when I started to develop CAMT. The feeling of collaboration and connectedness that develops can support mutual trust and a safe form of intimacy with the patient, who in the forensic treatment setting, it must be remembered, has in the past hurt others. Attachment patterns may then be reworked over time if the therapeutic boundaries are held safely, hence relational patterns are reformulated and revised.

Impulsive actions rooted in childhood emotional, physical and/or sexual abuses, relational trauma, neglect, and high expressed emotion are predisposing factors that can lead to violent offence-related enactments later in life. Patients can reflect, without words, on the musically expressed feelings which may represent aspects of past unspeakable acts. These can be expressed through musical consonance and dissonance. When improvisations accurately reflect verbally expressed issues, the improvisation may then reflect life circumstances from past or present interactions, which may then be revised or ameliorated. The reformulation of offence-related behaviours therefore occurs through being visibly witnessed and audibly heard.

Vignette: George

'George' (not his real name) shared his life experiences through improvisations that were named after places and people. Initially he recognized that he felt 'supported' in his improvisations and these had a child-like but chaotic quality, as if he, as a boy, was chattering to me on a small, tuned percussion instrument. Given that this was a long-term therapy, George's interactions developed through a dependent and timid child-like state to an adolescent hormonal teenage state. His improvisations were objectively evaluated by my supervisor, thereby helping me to stay safe from over-involvement and seduction (Odell-Miller, 2013). To stay safe meant consideration of the Analytic in CAT; represented here in the Reciprocal Roles of mothering to mothered and then the seducing to seduced. The musical representation at this point and on reflection, felt both cloying and smothering. This mirrored the close relationship that George described as having had with his mother.

Individuation then became possible as we worked towards saying farewell. This is a high-risk time for the music therapist and any patient who has killed, for fear of an offence re-enactment. George was initially anxious and then able to mourn the impending separation and closure of therapy, eventually able to go his own way in musical expression without me. After several years of individual music therapy, George was able to listen to others and to integrate into a CAMT group. All members had completed some individual music therapy prior to joining this group. They were carefully assessed as having sufficient self-awareness to benefit from being with others. The group process enabled these men to safely resolve everyday differences with each other and to receive shared comfort in and understanding of their losses and challenges.

Recognition and the index offence

The multi-disciplinary collaborative approach is essential for the safety of all when working in a secure hospital. Central to the overall approach are the combined efforts of the team to understand why the patient has committed his serious offence, thereby recognizing the impact of their mental illness on their thinking and responses to others.

The Psychotherapy File (see Appendix 1), when used sensitively with the patient, can help in the initial recognition of the most prevalent trap, dilemma or self-state that may have contributed to offence-related behaviour.

These patterns can become visible in group interactions, without direct verbal reference to the nature of any offences committed by group members[4]. For example, a patient who finds it difficult to choose an instrument for a group improvisation may defer to the most dominant member of the group, and if this perpetuates the music therapist may explore and name the 'trying to please others trap' or the 'fear of hurting other traps' as this is recognized in the group interactions and reflected on by the group so that they can discover how to consider others.

In musical improvisation, qualities of musical timbre, mood, varied dynamics and percussive attack emerge which may reflect the conflict or distress that erupted earlier in the patient's life. When recognized in the moment, also when reflected on in a recording of the improvisation, then recognition of the original feelings of rejection, abandonment, exclusion and subsequent uncontrollable rage which preceded an offence may be re-avowed safely. Ultimately, the retributive aspects of shame and punishment within the criminal justice system may shift to those of restoration and remorse as the patient's story unfolds.

---

4   It is part of this secure hospital culture and guidelines that patients do not talk openly about their offences other than in specific offence -related treatment programmes- because there is a hierarchy of offences within these communities.

A case example from Compton Dickinson (2021a)

'George' came to understand that he was triggered into rage at the time he committed his offence by a derisory comment which he perceived as directed at him about the person whom he loved most. He was confused about whether this came from a real person or from his hallucinatory voices at the time of the offence. He reported psychotic experiences and fearful thoughts about being attacked by men. On mistakenly hearing words that George attributed to an innocent victim, this man had tragically represented to George in his confused and grieving state his original abuser. When in treatment, George recognized that he had been tricked by his psychotic experience and that he had made the most horrendous of mistakes. He was full of remorse and wanted to write a musical Elegy for the victim.

It is not always that, over the course of time during forensic multi-disciplinary treatment, a person who has committed a serious crime may genuinely come to understand what on earth went wrong in their life. To feel remorse and a desire to make amends following a multi-disciplinary treatment approach having developed victim empathy is the ideal.

CAMT and reformulation

Many aspects that are reformulated that contribute to the MDT's overall understanding are seen visually in the relational responses that occur in CAMT as Reciprocal Roles emerge. Hence 'naming' a Reciprocal Role at a timely moment can be helpful. These responses are far more than simply 'behavioural' – they are relational. As such, over time, within the therapeutic musical relationship, challenging responses can be contained and ameliorated when the music therapist can work alongside the patient in the emotional sense.

Case example

'Jacob' (Compton Dickinson, 2013, p89-104) is an eighteen-year-old man in an active psychotic state. Together, by matching Jacob's pacing across the room, I was literally alongside him, and then by tuning in to contain his terror which he described as 'nuclear', we played the congas:

Each of us having one conga drum, whilst facing each other, Jacob was musically invited to express himself, to stand up and move about actively. This felt valuable, yet without undue eye contact that he often perceived as threatening.

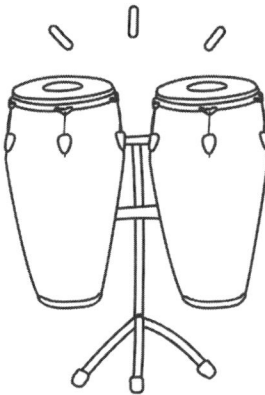

In a call-and-response interaction, we thrashed out the sounds until the feelings of fear and a need to fight off an attack were worked through and recognized. The music therapist is always observing and understanding how to contain the rhythm and pace, gradually allowing it to disperse. All the time supporting and enabling the musical expression to be that of the patient's internal world and how this related to what he may have referred to verbally as an issue. The non-verbal musical interaction was held and ameliorated eventually within what may be understood as a containing parenting to parented Reciprocal Role that was expressed with vigour in the musical enactment. This form of expression symbolically told us something relational about a past and an existing problematic relationship, thereby indicating a new relational exit as well as contributing to the reformulation process.

Enactments of anti-social Reciprocal Roles in CAMT

During the CAMT research trial we witnessed the emergence of potentially harmful anti-social relational roles in some patients that included narcissistic and intentionally cruel personality traits and responses that could not be ignored. These behaviours were visibly enacted in the group work, thereby throwing light on them as representations of offence-related responses.

Clinical example: A patient who at birth had been abandoned, and in adult life had committed murder, battered the djembe drums in an overwhelming frenzy. I stopped interacting with him. He then stopped in surprise. I said that I felt as if I was being attacked. Until that moment, he had no idea of his effect on other people. He was in effect metaphorically enacting the murderous offence, and on realizing his impact on me he was mortified.

A clinical explanation: In polyvagal theory it is possible to diagrammatically track the state shifts and procedures. If traumatically triggered, the 'ventral-vagal' emotionally regulated self-state may shift to the dorsal vagal dissociated state of over-arousal. When, as above, this occurs, an archaic embodied trauma trigger response might lead to a violent enactment (see figure 13.3).

The 'Different States' section of The Psychotherapy File (see Appendix 1) identifies the 'fight–flight' mechanisms of the sympathetic nervous system and how these states may shift and disintegrate further into the 'freeze, flop' dissociated self-state. There may be no recall in some patients of how they have shifted from one state to another; the patient may feel *'like a zombie. Cut off from feelings, cut off from others, disconnected.'* This offers an explanation as to how patients who are referred to high secure treatment may have genuinely 'forgotten' key events that led up to their index offence, through a complete dissociation between self-states.

This neurological response manifests in the dissociated states that Kellet (2005) describes in his CAT understanding of dissociative identity disorder. The 'freeze, flop' response occurs with the immediate threat to life, such as being close to annihilation and death as an abandoned infant as in the above example, from which the mentally ill patient who committed an offence may reciprocate with an annihilating violent offence.

These extreme states bypass what Ryle (2004) called the 'good enough ordinary world'. So, by qualitatively describing and understanding the re-activation of self-states in music therapy, new exits, new ways of doing things, may be explored within the collaborative therapeutic relationship.

Therapeutic endings

Preparation for endings and changes for patients in the forensic treatment setting constitute a time of heightened risk of an offence re-enactment. In CAMT, various non-verbal emotional responses and behavioural challenges arise when approaching the end of a time-limited therapy. Observation by the music therapist of such enactments can be reflected on by the group, explored and at best ameliorated thereby providing an opportunity for safe self- expression and a new sense of relational harmony. Within musical improvisation, the many ways that the music comes to an end can represent a crucial symbolic act. If the music ends suddenly, others in a group may feel quashed and surprised.

This is where the music therapist may question what has just happened. Whereas when an improvisation closes harmoniously after cathartic release and with group cohesiveness, there is a sense of acceptance and connectedness with an ability to separate safely.

Reflection by the group within the group of a representation of a potentially destructive act mitigates a re-occurrence of an impulsive unconscious behaviour so it is given reflective supportive space without judgement.

One such example was of a man who decided that his target problem was 'to control his anger'. He chose to play the loudest instrument. He had firstly to 'hear' his anger, and to feel that it was heard by others. The music therapist and group members were long-suffering in this cathartic process, so the music therapist limited these deafening improvisations to 'two minutes duration'. While the patient is always supported to feel ownership of their musical input, within a groupwork setting, they may discover how to then consider and to listen differently to others. This process involves careful reflection in supervision as described below.

CAMT supervision

During the research study, the music therapists who delivered the CAMT treatment adhered to the CAT model. Enactments of multiple self-states could be experienced through the embodied countertransference of the music therapist and recognized in the reciprocal musical interactions. Self-states identified in supervision could then be named and mapped out in the CAMT group sessions. Some highly dangerous self-states were heard and witnessed in these responses and mapped out as Reciprocal Roles, for example, predatory or negative behaviours, such as 'stalking to stalked'. The music therapist and patients could then recognize and track the processes and triggers that led to sudden, often dangerous self-state switches.

Clinical example: The group together engaged in CAT mapping with the music therapist while sitting together around a table after having improvised together. The group together described self-states including 'the dark pit of hell'. One patient, who had committed a murderous stalking offence, prowled round the perimeter of the group, thereby creating a 'threatening to threatened' enactment within the group. He was unable to sit down or to integrate as a member of the group, thus his RR repertoire, due possibly to early neglect and abuse, had shown how he could be excluding of others because he had previously felt like an excluded outcast. This offence re-enactment was sinister, yet he was able to recognize that the group dynamic and cohesion were stronger than he was, thereby enabling him to start to communicate with group members.

Within group cohesiveness, with a collaborative and at times challenging interaction, a mirroring occurred of the patient's early developmental patterns. During supervision, having reflected on the meaning and interpersonal responses of each patient within the therapy sessions, dysfunctional relational patterns could be mapped out as Reciprocal Role procedures in a groupwork map. The 'sharing to shared' reciprocity in this creative process enabled commonalities to be discussed with acceptance of dreadful experiences which were safely thought about in a compassionate and safe therapeutic environment.

Conclusion

Kellet *et al* (2018), in their secondary analysis of the feasibility randomized controlled study to which I refer in this chapter, concluded that that:

> 'This study has particularly developed the evidence base for Music Therapy by adding in an evaluation of relationality and evaluating an avowedly relational Music Therapy model. Group-CAMT appears to offer a grounding theory, therapeutic relationship, tools and techniques that make it possible to consider and change relational dynamics rooted in and mirroring early developmental traumas (Ryle & Kerr, 2020), within a structured and containing short-term group environment.'

The relational changes were measured on the Persons Relating to Others Questionnaire (PROQ2 (Birtchnell & Evans, 2004)) for which a free-to-access online scoring tool is available for quick and easy evaluation. (Birtchnell, 2020)

CAMT is recognized as effective, not only in older treatment-resistant men who may have been incarcerated for much of their lives, but also in community-based treatment and most recently in early interventions with looked-after children as young as six years old. Play with creativity remains a central aspect for innovation in both adult and early life: this aspect is too often missed in the lives of people who are oppressed, stigmatized, neglected, othered or abused.

Acknowledgements

To 'George' and to 'Jacob' for their informed and anonymised consent. (as referenced here with no direct quotation from earlier publication). To all supervisors, advisers, collaborators, colleagues, funders, my family, my cats who kept me company when writing up, and to music therapists Victoria Sleight and Claire Newman who delivered the research treatment groups and who subsequently qualified as CAT practitioners. Particular thanks to Dr Gill McGauley who advised on research methodology and implementation and to Dr Anthony Ryle for his encouragement and endorsements along this tortuous journey.

N.B. All vignettes are composites from my clinical practice with some details changed to ensure confidentiality is protected.

Chapter 14: Training films for psychotherapeutic education

Kathryn Pemberton

This chapter will explore the making and use of training films for psychotherapeutic purposes, specifically CAT. Working as a production manager, director and writer on two series of training films to date (totalling almost twenty individual films) has provided me with a unique overview of the processes involved in producing training films for this particular audience. The idea of making training films for a CAT audience was conceptualized by Catalyse, a non-profit organization which promotes CAT through training and other forms of professional development. My role was only made possible through working closely with the team of consultants at Catalyse who shared their considerable experience in CAT, ensuring the films would be high-quality products.

Before qualifying as a clinical psychologist and later on as a CAT practitioner and supervisor, I worked as an actor and director. Early on in my career, I acted in many training videos (of variable quality) and later in my career, enjoyed working in film and using other multimedia in my role as a director. So, I was familiar with the production process involved in making training films and some of the technicalities involved in making films, although certainly not an expert. However, what I couldn't appreciate at the beginning of this journey was the extent to which CAT would not only be central to the content of the films but also the extent to which a CAT 'lens' would inform and guide some of the key decisions made during the production process.

Planning

The first series of films all started as an idea reflecting a need. A series of high-quality, affordable and accessible training films on CAT. Working with a team of CAT consultants at Catalyse, we started with a blank slate and lots of questions. What did we want the films to show? What was their function? Should we use actors or 'real' people or a mixture of both? Improvised or scripted? Should we show examples of 'good' therapy and then 'bad' therapy? What were the aims of the work? What were we hoping to achieve and how could we do this given the boundaries of time, resources and budget? As in therapy, the introduction of boundaries means being realistic about what you are able to achieve with the resources you have, and this demands innovative thinking and creativity. Intrinsic to this process, for me, is imagination and play.

At this point in the process, we had more questions than answers, so we focused on what we *did* know. We knew that we wanted the films to be multi-functional; a training tool for different courses and services and they needed to be useful for individuals training in, or already trained in, CAT. We also knew we wanted to demonstrate skills using both content and process. Finally, the way the information was communicated needed to be in line with the ethos of CAT. It needed to be collaborative, scaffolding and encouraging the viewer to be an active agent in their learning.

As this was the first set of films to be produced by Catalyse, it felt fitting to start with the fundamentals, and we came to an agreement that for the first series of films we would aim to demonstrate core CAT skills on film. The next consideration was the target audience. The CAT community is diverse, with a whole spectrum of experience from seasoned practitioners who have been a part of the developmental history of CAT to current trainees just embarking on their journey. So, our potential target audience spanned therapists interested in CAT to trainee CAT practitioners in the first year of training, to more experienced practitioners wanting to refresh their understanding of the key components of CAT. We needed to consider how to provide a product that could be mindful of and flexible to each viewer's zone of proximal development (ZPD), providing the scaffolding required to enable engagement and usability of the product. We used this thinking to help inform the actual content and structure of the films.

In preparation for the filming, I watched as many therapy-training films as I could find. Some were produced with a slickness which felt intimidating, whereas others looked cheap, clunky and badly staged. I noted that the demonstration of different skills through multiple client/therapist dyads was the most common format, particularly when the learning structure, or therapeutic approach is diagnostically informed.

Reflecting on our aims for the films, and the centrality of the therapeutic relationship in CAT, demonstrating disjointed fragments of a CAT therapy, particularly for these first set of 'core skills' films felt like we were missing something. In the same way that a function of a reformulation letter is to help clients develop their observing eye through the consolidation of multiple, sometimes fragmentary experiences, the importance of showing the whole journey of a sixteen-session CAT, and the development of the therapeutic relationship, took shape. To this end, we planned to show the most salient parts of a sixteen-session CAT therapy over the course of twelve films. Using the same therapist/client dyad, we wanted to cover the fundamental skills such as determining a target problem and collaborating on the development of target problem procedures, diagrams and letters, providing a structure which captured task and process-based learning objectives on micro and macro levels.

So, to a great extent, the aims of the work and the target audience dictated the structure and content of the first series of films. In comparison, a further set of films produced with Catalyse had a different aim and target audience. Following on from the 'core skills' series, a further series of five films focused on *working with challenging situations in CAT. The aim here was to show a range of difficulties that can arise during therapy with the aim of stimulating reflection and debate about possible therapeutic responses.* These films had a different structure and content to the earlier films and were mostly relevant to those with more experience in CAT or second-year CAT practitioner trainees. This second set of films was topic or scenario-led (for example, exploring countertransference, difficult endings and working with self-states) and the whole process was markedly different to the earlier series.

Pre-production

Once a clear aim, learning objectives, target audience and an idea of the structure of a film or films has been established, the next stage is pre-production. This involves the planning, processing and execution of every task required in order for the project to be realized. From the sourcing of a film production team, recceing of potential locations and finalizing budget details to organizing where vehicles will be parked on the filming days and what people are going to eat for lunch – all these aspects need to be considered, agreed, and actioned.

Particularly salient in training films for psychotherapy purposes is the question of and decision making around whether to use 'real' therapists or actors, and, relatedly, whether films should be scripted or improvised, or somewhere in between. When it comes to the decision as to whether to use actors or therapists, the choice may not be quite so stark. I found several CAT therapists who either had some drama or acting experience, or were comfortable in front of a camera, and there will of course be actors who are also experts by experience. In the 'core skills' series for example, the therapist was played by a CAT trainee with experience of acting and film work, and the client was played by an actor who was knowledgeable about CAT.

The dilemma of whether to script or not to script is an interesting one, with both options having pros and cons attached and each possibility determined by multiple considerations. The 'core skills' series used scripts, whereas the 'challenging situations' series all featured improvised roleplays. I learned that both options require very different creative processes.

Scripting the scenarios so that the actors learn the script verbatim enables full control over the whole process from the start, keeping the aims of a film tightly matched to the post-production and editing processes. If using actors who have little or no knowledge of or experience of CAT or psychotherapy, then clearly it makes more sense to use scripted material written by someone knowledgeable about the subject matter. I learned from the first set of films that the combination of having rigid learning objectives for each film (i.e. core CAT skills) meant that, although the actor playing the therapist did have some experience of CAT, in order to meet the aims and ZPD of the target audience, their words would need to be scripted.

When you are part of the writing process and working with scripted material, all of the decision making, planning and overview of the project is required to be in place, meaning that the bulk of the work takes place before a single shot is filmed. Decisions made at this stage will be of significance in the post-production stage of the work, for example the voice-over script (if this is to be used), on-screen text or any animation incorporated, and will need to be included in the directions on the script alongside the actors' words.

The first stage in writing a script is the development of the characters, in this case the client and the therapist. In the 'core skills' series, it was important that both the client and therapist had a back story and that these were shared in the films, enabling a deeper understanding of enactments, countertransference and difference. There will clearly be a relationship between the viewer and the therapist too, particularly in terms of perceived power, dictated in part by the positioning of the competency of the therapist. Holding this in mind, we knew that we wanted the therapy to be realistic, and therefore imperfect, but 'good enough'. In doing so, we wanted to encourage debate and to encourage the viewer to be active and reflect on their own practice rather than try to simulate the actions of the therapist on screen. Lisa, the therapist in the film, is flawed, but she provides 'good-enough', competent CAT. The reasons for this were twofold: to aid a position of empowerment and relatability as well as to invite a response, and to provoke the engagement and voice of the viewer.

The next stage of writing a script for me is similar to watching a film, or even reading a book; the mental images are revealed as the words unfold, and the characters you are writing for take a role in guiding what is written. What you know about the characters begins to inform, almost with a separate agency, what happens and how it happens. The mental images generated are useful to note for the subsequent task of creating a storyboard; a series of sketches not unlike a cartoon strip clearly depicting and composing an image for each shot, building on salient plot points as well as enabling a visual suggestion and sense of 'flow' of the overall finished film.

Knowledge of the different camera angles available is useful in the storyboarding process, together with an understanding of what relational message each angle is likely to communicate. The next time you watch a film, notice the camera angles used by the director, and particularly the power differentials between the viewpoint of the camera and the characters depicted. An example is the 'eye level' shot, which reflects how we usually see others and suggests an intimacy and closeness between the actor and audience. A 'two shot' on the other hand (an over-the-shoulder shot or from the front for example), encapsulating the whole of the dyad provides different information, such as unspoken signals and signs through body language and clothes, the use of a clipboard and so on.

So, with scripted films, there is full creative control during filming. When scenes are improvised or semi-scripted, I found that the creative control comes through the editing process; this is the creative scripting of the scenes and is a very different process than when the content is known from the start.

In the second series of films, rather than using a pre-written script, members of the consulting team each wrote a detailed, imaginary scenario featuring individual client and therapist backgrounds, with 'plot points' highlighted to guide and provide a semi-structure to the scenes. This decision was again informed by the aim of the films and topic areas, the target audience, and the 'cast'. Rather than following a course of therapy from start to finish, the second series of films depicted challenging situations ranging from working with states and self-states, using countertransference, working online with strong emotions to difficult endings, and working through a rupture in therapy where the rupture is based on values and the therapist and client hold different beliefs.

Each of the five films featured different therapist/client dyads, a decision made in considering two important differences from the first series: the cast and the target audience. In the second series, all apart from one of the cast of ten were qualified and experienced CAT practitioners who were familiar with the scenarios depicted. The exception was an actor who was an expert by experience in CAT. As highlighted earlier, the target audience for the second series was also different to the first, geared towards practitioners who already had a knowledge of the core skills. Given these two differences, the use of scenarios being improvised worked well, with several of the films requiring only one or two takes.

It could be argued that there are more moments of authentic therapy captured in improvised films, particularly when experienced therapists are used, for example, micro-moments of surprise or confusion caught in real-time. The camera magnifies these moments, providing an insight into the inner world of the characters on screen. In the countertransference film, for example, the inner thoughts of the therapist are made explicit through the use of voice-over, but for all the films, this authenticity allowed for and encouraged discussion as highlighted in the supporting materials which were provided alongside both series of films.

Production

Filming days are an intensive experience. After months of preparation in pre-production, it can all come down to a couple of days of frenetic activity. There is still much to organize, but also a sense of calm and freedom in that everything that can be planned for has been done, and anything that goes wrong will simply need to be dealt with in the moment. The process of directing for me has parallels to therapy. You can prepare for a session with a client, but you don't really know what is going to happen until you are in the room. For me, directing a scene is not about being didactic or telling actors what to do, rather it is about 'doing with'; listening and exploring together and being respectful of what they are bringing to the work. The director is perhaps able to hold a slightly different stance or wider 'helicopter view' than the actors at times, and the sharing of this, the wider context of what is happening in a particular moment or scene, is part of the role. The result is a genuine collaboration and a product that is greater than the sum of its parts, elevated beyond what would have been possible without being able to 'play' and explore things together.

Post-production

In therapy, there is an ongoing consideration of the client's ZPD and the importance of 'pushing where it moves' and providing scaffolding to ensure the accessibility of the work. This ongoing assessment, consideration and attuned responding of a learners ZPD is obviously not a possibility when the 'other' is a film. However, as in any other relationship, the act of watching a training film establishes a relationship, and a multitude of Reciprocal Roles between the viewer and what/who is being viewed, bespoke to the individual.

In consideration of this, alongside the voices of the client and therapist, it was important to have a third voice, present throughout (either in the form of the narrator or on screen prompts) and after the films (in the form of the supporting materials), commenting, summarizing and supporting the viewer to reflect on what they think throughout the learning process.

In this way, the viewer is being scaffolded and, through actively engaging with the process, supported in working within and expanding their ZPD.

In post-production, the voice-over script was finalized and recorded, accompanied by salient learning points emphasized through on-screen text. Any animation was also included and particularly for the second series of films, a detailed process of editing and honing the final product which required working closely with the film production team.

The writing of the supporting materials for the films also took place in the post-production stage. Two sets of materials were developed for the first series of films, one for individual learning and the second for group learning or from a trainer's perspective.

The 'core skills' series depicted a 'good-enough' therapy, and in order to provide an objective assessment of what would constitute a good-enough CAT therapy, the supporting materials explicitly highlighted the areas of CAT competence depicted in the films using The Competence in CAT (CCAT) measure (Bennett & Parry, 2004).

The first set of supporting materials provided the running time of the films, an overview of the content of each film as well as the relevant CCAT domains demonstrated in the films. Exercises for both individual and group study are offered together with further resources including all the CAT tools which would have been used in the therapy.

The supporting materials for the second set of films assume a deeper and more sophisticated understanding of CAT and this is reflected in the content. In addition to individual reflection and the application of the films to therapeutic situations for example, the reader is invited to think about the wider application of CAT skills, for example in consultancy and supervisory roles. This was again in consideration of the target audience already confident with the basic knowledge and training and CAT skills.

Feedback and reflections

The first set of films has now been viewed far and wide, including on CAT practitioner training courses. The feedback received was very positive and the value of the films as a training resource has been widely endorsed.

Several themes were apparent in the feedback received, which suggested our aim of providing high-quality and accessible products had been realized. The feedback came from trainee CAT therapists who had viewed the films as part of their CAT practitioner training, as well as trainee Clinical Psychologists who had seen them during their doctorate training. There were also qualified CAT therapists who had purchased the films for their own individual access. In the feedback received, people spoke about how the films had helped to make CAT language and concepts more manageable and accessible; that the films had slowed down and explained the process of CAT therapy. The usefulness of viewing the films over time and at different stages of training in conjunction with the expansion of an individual's ZPD was also highlighted.

Interestingly, the feedback received from some of the trainees on the CAT practitioner training courses reflected that the therapists' portrayal of a 'good-enough' CAT practitioner and good-enough therapy was not always welcome. Several trainees wanted perhaps an expert position and a 'perfect' therapy. This perhaps reflects parallels with therapy, where it is understandable that someone may wish to be told simply what to do in order to 'get better', but learning, as we know, requires reflection, being active in the process, and seeing the value in the less than perfect.

In all the films I have been involved in producing, the main aim has been to enable the viewer to engage in the process of observing examples of CAT practice and to stimulate discussion and debate. Through being an active part of the process (rather than a passive observer), it is hoped the films provide a bespoke package for each viewer, enabling the assimilation of new skills and a deepening of their understanding and, ultimately, practice in CAT.

Acknowledgements

Many thanks to Rhona Brown, Dawn Bennett, Glenys Parry, Mark Evans, Frank Margison and all the CAT therapists involved who worked so hard to support the creation of the CAT training films.

Chapter 15:
Bringing our stories to life through animation

Rhona Brown

Introduction

In this account of animation as relevant to CAT practice, my perspective shifts between different positions, from curious observer to active learner, playful experimenter, depleted consumer, self-directed creator, hopeful communicator, novice facilitator, enthusiastic collaborator, despairing proto-editor, and, through the opportunity writing this chapter offers, reflective commentator. I hope that these movements and transitions are tolerable for the reader and help to tell a story that engages interest. My intention is not specifically to educate about the rationale and technicalities of animation, as there are others much better qualified to do so. I have referred to two of the pioneers of this approach in therapeutic work, occupational therapist Helen Mason and art therapist Tony Gammidge, both of whom have scaffolded my own exploration of animation. Interested readers may wish to follow up their publications and other channels documenting their work in this developing area.

Visualizing CAT

Soon after commencing as a year-one CAT practitioner trainee, I was released from day-to-day NHS pressures through maternity leave following the birth of my second child in late 2006. Both the richness of the CAT training and a second foray into parenting stimulated my imagination. In response to an open invitation by National Endowment for Science, Technology and the Arts (NESTA), an idea emerged about 'visualizing CAT'. At that time, data visualization technologies were beginning to develop, offering new ways to present, move and manipulate data using electronic means. The techniques being taught to me for mapping sequential diagrammatic reformulations in CAT relied largely on pen and paper, whether handwritten or reproduced in a digitally produced print format.

Despite a wish to learn and practice this powerfully succinct CAT tool, I felt limited by the boundaried edges and flatness of paper and pen. Given the dynamic and fluid character of experience in the world, perception, emotion, thought and action, I was frustrated by attempts to render such complexities to a single, two-dimensional diagram. As a more experienced practitioner, I now better understand how a CAT map can and should be amended in simple ways as a therapy progresses and understanding unfolds, that it is offered in a tentative form and that there are many different ways to use mapping techniques flexibly and creatively in CAT.

My CAT North (now Catalyse) trainers at that time were generous as consultees in this process and my more technical partner and I felt supported to submit a proposal to NESTA. In brief, this outlined ways in which emerging technologies at that time could enable a CAT map to be a more dynamic, editable and flexible entity, to which therapist and client could return in order to co-develop over the course of the therapy, and potentially beyond.

Ultimately, our proposal was not supported by NESTA. Fast-forwarding seventeen years, advances in digital engagement, accelerated by the COVID pandemic, mean that everyday technologies such as whiteboards and shared collaboration spaces are now commonly available and used as part of CAT practice. So, what my partner and I imagined back in 2007 no longer warrants particular attention.

Helen Mason's animation in therapy – the seed of a practice

Engagement with the NESTA bid process, however, opened another door to my imagination and eventually to action. News of our unsuccessful bid was quickly followed by a feature about the winning application. Occupational therapist Helen Mason had been funded to support collaborations and pilot projects bringing together artists and therapists to reflect on the use of stop-frame animation in therapy, and to pilot related tools within a range of clinical settings. Mason went on to set up an interactive website showcasing examples of this work, providing further materials to aid learning about animation in therapy, and additionally offering a number of levels of training on the approach. More information on the development of Mason's work is outlined in Ashworth and Mason (2010).

What Mason described in examples included on her website extended my own much more embryonic thoughts on bringing diagrams to life in a more animated fashion. One notable animation, 'Richard's Story 2', told the story of a young boy who had developed obsessional compulsive difficulties in the context of difficult early relationships and events (Animation Therapy HM, 2013). The viewer was presented with an account of the development of this boy's difficulties, but with an emotional engagement and a visual impact which, for me, went far beyond the story itself.

In the first person, the narrator explains how, through therapy, he externalizes demanding and intrusive thoughts through conceptualizing these as a character called Ball. Ball joins what has been a two-dimensional, hand-drawn animation as the first three-dimensional character, a small ball of red paper scrunched up inside the protagonist's head. A human hand picks this out of the drawing and places it outside of Richard's head. From that point the paper takes on a life of its own, unrolling into a more personified character with a face.

Ball is juxtaposed with Jet, a smaller, yellow paper character who Richard describes as his strength. Together with the narration, the action illustrates how Ball morphs into a much larger presence, showering Jet with a deluge of hostility and fear-provoking thoughts. A shielding umbrella suggests how Richard and Jet learn ways to combat Ball. The shape, size and colour of these characters change, and the human hand returns to push and mould Ball downwards, effectively shrinking him to a more manageable size. The narrator describes how, with the help of his family and therapist, he learns to keep Ball as a small scrunched-up presence that merely 'buzzes around'. The story ends with the affirmative statement 'It's good to know I'm back in control again'.

What I felt I was hearing in this animation was the conclusion of a therapy, like parts of a goodbye letter but addressed to the world 'out there' in an attempt to communicate the sense he himself had made of his distress and symptoms. Mason refers to the piece in her early 'Daring to Dream' paper, describing how this collaborative animation work, involving the whole family, provided a means by which parents could support their child with his mental health difficulties. She notes their report that 'being able to create figures to support him was also helpful in enabling them to enhance communication as a family and feel like they had found a new way of being there for him in the film' (Mason, 2009, p113).

The placement of this animation on a public website (with permission from the family) seemed to make it a very open and declarative utterance, sharing both problem and solution in a way that could invite and encourage others struggling to find ways to manage anxious thoughts and neutralizing rituals. Its naïve but striking hand-drawn visual style brought an emotional immediacy which drew me in powerfully to the narrative as a viewer.

Moving towards animation in my own world

When I discovered Mason's work, I was not in a position to fund or justify undertaking the Level 1 Animation Therapy training. I knew this type of work would not be supported in the NHS primary care/adult mental health setting in which I delivered psychological assessments and talking therapies. The tipping point for determining to make this happen was meeting fellow CAT Ella Knight at ACAT's 2012 annual conference in Manchester. Learning about Ella's shared interest in animation and the use of objects in therapy spurred me on to enquire about the next Animation in Therapy Level 1 training. I completed the practical taught part of this later in 2012.

The Level 1 course involved two days of practical introduction to animation which was largely experiential in a small group setting. Literally within minutes of the course commencing, we as participants found ourselves creating short stop-frame productions together. This was facilitated initially as a whole group, using the technique of pixilation. We made small changes to pose around the room, which was captured in brief frames, and then run together to demonstrate how movement could be simulated, and effects created to embellish what is possible in real life. In smaller groups, we moved on to sharing tasks such as positioning a webcam, choosing and moving objects, and operating the animation software in order to create other effects which could be achieved simply. The facilitators suggested a range of easily manageable scenarios and helped with direction and any technical complications that arose. Additionally, while we could re-run and view our animations within the software as they developed, the facilitators and technical staff polished these into more complete standalone pieces shared as show reels shortly after the training.

By the end of day two, each of us in the group had moved on to more ambitious storytelling. The enthusiasm of Mason and her co-facilitators cut through any reticence, and the two days became a soundly playful and creative space in which we moved from uncertain novices to excited collaborators taking our first steps in improvising brief films. Facilitators held the zone of proximal development (ZPD) for all participants clearly in mind throughout, and tasks progressed in a way that meant we could each contribute, stretch ourselves and learn without becoming overwhelmed.

The learning I took away from the two days enthused me to invest in an affordable suite of stop-motion animation software and a decent webcam so that I could experiment at home. Before long, I had produced a number of short pieces alone, then subsequently with my two children. Then aged five and eleven, they had grown up consuming animations of one sort or another through television, video and DVD. Besides ample studio-produced digital style cartoons, as a family we had regularly watched more 'retro' materials using stop-frame such as Oliver Postgate's 'The Clangers' in addition to the popular Aardman Studio productions such as 'Wallace and Gromit'. They grasped animation concepts and techniques with ease and did not seem disappointed by the rather clunky nature of our homemade productions. Engaging in animation provided them with many opportunities to think creatively, imagine and develop stories, and create action. Some actions possible to depict through animation are otherwise difficult to create in the real world, such as an explosion, or even a travelling' bogey' emanating from the nose and traversing a bemused sibling's face before taking residence in the opposite nostril.

Furthermore, providing them with the means and support to animate gave them, as Mason and colleagues had provided me, the opportunity to build on initial inspiration, spontaneous ideas and creativity through using more executive skills such as ordering, planning, sequencing and waiting. Through these, the movement of objects and interaction with hardware and software helped to capture and transpose ideas, or pictures in our minds, into repeatable visual stories, sometimes accompanied by sound effects (foley). Eventually, we would revel in what was co-created, and each completed piece seemed to spark another idea for a new project or story. Not only was animation an entertaining form of play but it also became a regularly requested medium through which to complete homework assignments.

A few months later I marked my forty-eighth birthday with a facilitated half-day event for a small group of invited friends and family, including both adults and children. In small, self-selected groups and pairs, we produced brief animations, plus one pixilation in which all partygoers took turns to appear and disappear under the shared prop of an oversized hat and coat.

Life happens; death happens

At that point, in late 2012, my own life and the direction it was taking was cast into question when I received a diagnosis of Grade 3 breast cancer. This forced a pause in many directions while receiving life-protecting treatments over the following six months and coping with their substantial impacts. Diagnosis of a potentially terminal illness brings many challenges. However, one of its gifts is a pressing existential awareness not only that life is short, but that one's own life may be shorter than most. As part of a recovery process from the cognitive and energy-limiting assault of treatments, resulting in extreme fatigue and 'chemo-brain', animation again played a role. This was both as a component of my emotional journey in surviving breast cancer, and as a self-directed practical preparation for resuming a work role.

The road back to working was not an easy one; there were few opportunities for workplace rehabilitation or supportive steps towards becoming fully fit to resume clinical duties. Interestingly, neither my own psychological knowledge nor the more and less compassionate approaches of friends and colleagues steeped in psychotherapeutic approaches seemed to offer the 'key' for progressing beyond profound exhaustion, slowed and interrupted thinking and limited working memory. The invisibility of cognitive struggles and the difficulty in articulating changes in one's day-to-day functioning, especially in as complex a skill as psychotherapy, seemed to lead to a dilemma. Extreme poles could be described as others either struggling to see and comprehend what had changed, minimizing, denying or questioning attempts to describe it, or else reported changes being viewed as global, irreparable and permanent. Thankfully they were not. Over time, and with the right support and opportunities to practice and adapt, recovery was possible. But at times I experienced despair that, despite holding on to life, or at least slowing its departure, cancer and its treatments may have taken away or spoiled fundamental aspects of my 'self', my identity, and perhaps my livelihood.

It was in fact an occupational therapy perspective, first accessed through a well-being drop-in setting at my local oncology unit, that set me on a more activity-focused road to recovery. No queries were made about motivation, secondary gain, nor eyebrows raised while questioning the evidence base for chemo-brain. Instead, the therapeutic enquiry centred on what I liked to do, what gave me pleasure, what was the smallest amount of it that I could do before it felt unmanageable or later caused a debilitating crash. Three sessions of constructive and compassionate enquiry in this vein helped set me on a path back to myself using self-directed walking, engaging with the life-death-life cycle of nature, and a range of very unambitious creative activities. Some I could do alone, and some were welcomed also by my then-six-year-old, who enjoyed nothing better than a post-school 'makey' session.

When the opportunity to attend Mason's Level 2 'Re-animation' training, more focused on therapeutic applications of animation, arose in early 2014, this initially seemed out of reach. Satisfactory completion of Level 1 Animation in Therapy training to allow progression to this level required submission of a written assignment reflecting on how the initial learning integrated with practice, and this was outstanding. At first, finding the energy and breaking through the brain fog in order to undertake a writing project seemed impossible, as did the prospect of organizing and surviving a journey and staying in Exeter for what would be an intense couple of days. I drafted an email to Mason outlining the obstacles and declining the opportunity with regret. However, somehow, in the space of a few hours, I found another exit to the 'it's impossible' trap that I'd co-created with ill-health. My memory (as for many things over that period) is sketchy, but the email that made it out of my drafts and secured my place on the training told a different story of determination to get myself there and push on through the mental fog to produce the required written work on how CAT and animation might interweave. Looking back, those few hours in early 2014 were quite pivotal in a process of recovery towards re-animating myself, enabled by listening to and acting on the 'life is short' narrative.

As part of more local, regular, self-directed CPD as preparation for return to work, I'd also recently attended a day on the Six-Part Story Method with Kim Dent-Brown, (see Appendix 5) organized by Catalyse. This approach invites the story-maker to contemplate both obstacles and resources in relation to the task of a story's protagonist. Looking back, these ideas probably also helped me become mobilized into action rather than resignation. Joining with that group of fellow cognitive analytic therapists for a powerful and replenishing day, after a long year of isolation and uncertainty about whether or not I still belonged in a therapist world, was another nourishing resource. A co-attendee on that CPD day was Regine Blattner, with whom I'd previously completed my practitioner training. Since qualifying, we had maintained periodic contact for the purpose of informal peer CPD. This proved to be another sustaining factor through my subsequent recovery and further engagement with animation in CAT.

Re-animating

With a few weeks to spare before the Level 2 Re-animation course commenced, I determined to write a reflective piece on how animation and CAT might sit together, some of which helped form this chapter. The course comprised a smaller group of just four participants, all health professionals, with varying levels of experience in animation. Mason and colleagues provided us with individual workstations where we could work on suggested exercises exploring the theme of well-being. We each progressed to producing our own independently created pieces before the conclusion of the two days.

The theoretical and discursive component drew heavily on occupational therapy models and practice, specifically the Model of Human Occupation (MOHO) developed in occupational therapy practice by Gary Kielhofner (see Taylor, 2017) and the Vona Du Toit Model of Creative Ability (see van der Reyden *et al*, 2019). There was also a focus on narrative and storymaking, and my recent immersion in Six-Part Story Method making was fresh and relevant.

Invitations to animate ranged from exploring the sensory manipulation of objects as forms of self-soothing, metaphors relating to identity, mandala-based work, and bringing to life the Kawa River, a culturally responsive model within occupational therapy practice (Iwama, 2006). I found this a particularly helpful exercise as it sat well with both CAT and my own personal challenges at that time. The Kawa model uses the metaphor of a river to help explore the flow of an individual's life, what obstructs this flow and what resources exist to help remove or manage these obstructions so that the individual's life force can flow more freely.

Altered Audrey

In the final self-directed exercise, I made use of a number of objects I'd brought which symbolized aspects of my cancer journey to date – traversing the shock of diagnosis, the impact of chemotherapy and how this manifested in embodied and cognitive ways. The following description is based on viewing the piece for the purposes of this chapter, more than a decade after it was made. At the time, I did not have a specific plan or storyboard for the action, but at some level I had made proactive choices about the materials brought for the trip.

Starting with a blank polystyrene head with a playful party wig and ribbons (carefree life before cancer), this changed into a hand-painted Audrey Hepburn mask, a personal artefact representing aspects of my younger, healthier self. The mask itself is exchanged for an accidentally distorted fabric print of the Audrey image, bringing in the notion of unintended, unanticipated change. A mix of headscarves, hats and wigs acquired over the period of my treatment moved on and off the head, interspersed with shreds of material obscuring features and particularly the eyes (as vitality, hope and possibility die away). The loss of hair, eyelashes and eyebrows represented some of the physical rigours of treatment, and a Spanish-style hand fan represented coping with the sudden violence and intensity of a chemically induced early menopause. The degraded aesthetic of 'Audrey' symbolized losses, fears and uncertainties about the future. In the concluding frames, the original Audrey mask is remounted and several of the elements used in the preceding action come to arrange themselves around it in a way that integrates the experience of cancer and regains a new aesthetic appeal. Audrey is forever altered but not forever damaged and beleaguered.

In his chapter on stop-frame animation with trauma and chaos narratives (Gammidge, 2021), art therapist Tony Gammidge, another pioneer in using animation as a therapeutic tool, draws on the ideas of Arthur Frank on illness narratives. He proposes how in both chaos narratives and trauma there is a lack of narrative progression when 'Life is reduced to a series of present-tense assaults' (Frank, 2013, p.xv). Gammidge suggests 'through the very gradual, methodical, frame-by-frame telling of a story allowed by stop-frame animation a way of ordering and progressing becomes possible. Reflection and distance from the chaos emerges (Gammidge, 2021, p233).

At that time, I could not have put into words exactly what this story was telling, nor could I have described verbally in a coherent way in a talking therapy what was happening for me. However, the non-verbal, right-hemisphere nature of this immersive two hours spent animating provided a valuable form of self-to-self 'voice'. Watching and reflecting now on the resulting forty-five-second-long piece helps me appreciate it as an important artefact of the journey of recovery I was on, personally, creatively and professionally. It formed an important timestamp in my recovery process, beyond the 'present-tense assaults' of illness and its repercussions. Illness both stops us in our tracks but invites and engenders growth. Altered Audrey helped me grasp my own sense of 'unfinaliseability' and tentative optimism for the future.

Taking the personal into the professional

After completing that second level training, I was keen to practice facilitating others' use of animation in a context of well-being. However, I was not in a position to invest in further training, qualification or specialist supervision in creative therapies. Nor did I feel confident to use these techniques safely in the context of others' psychological distress. An invitation to fellow CAT therapists through local channels didn't enlist volunteers to spend time experimenting as subject-participants for well-being purposes. In retrospect, the promise of a minute's worth of finished animation for several hours of experimental play can't have seemed too attractive. However, pushing where it moved, a few friends volunteered themselves and together we experimented with self-chosen themes such as a transnational migration story and a Kawa River consideration of work/life balance.

An opportunity to produce a solo piece arose when artist Paul Harfleet and I delivered a shared workshop at the 2014 ACAT annual conference in Liverpool, on 'Quiet Resistance and Conceptual Shields: A CAT Journey Alongside the Pansy Project'. I made a two-and-a-half-minute animation depicting my journey towards this collaboration since initially hearing about Paul's work challenging homophobic abuse through the Pansy Project (https://thepansyproject.com/). I narrated this live, using the action of two-dimensional cutout images moving around a street map to represent the timeline of connections with Paul and his work. This felt like a justifiable departure from a more traditional presentation given the workshop topic and was the first time I'd created an animation with the sole intention of conveying meaning to an audience. It was aesthetically very rudimentary and contrasted sharply with the striking beauty of Paul's photographic images of pansies planted at geographical locations of abuse and assault.

Animation really came to life for me in collaboration with others as preparation for ACAT's 2018 conference in Keele, on the theme of 'Therapist authenticity, creativity and use of positive resources in cognitive analytic therapy'. The organizers, Alison Jenaway, Carole Gregory and Rosemary Parkinson invited ten-minute 'culture shots' illustrating examples of creativity outside of one's immediate work role. This presented a perfect opportunity to bring together the many strands and connections made around animation over the preceding years. Regine Blattner, Ella Knight and I tentatively proposed a culture shot on 'Bringing our stories to life: animation in CAT'. We committed to creating two brief animations of two to three minutes each, illustrating how this medium might enhance and work with narrative. Regine and I worked together on one project in Manchester while Ella worked on her own piece in London.

Defining and developing our task: a story emerges

Regine and I reconvened our CPD meetings with a specific focus on this task. We initially identified a shared struggle with which we both identified, recalling that, in a very early practitioner training day pairs exercise, we described and mapped a problem procedure. At that time, we'd confided how we both accumulated untidy matter of one sort or another in our home environments. As the years had progressed, our families had grown, and work and other responsibilities dominated, we identified how close others complained about piles of stuff that had no apparent home. Initially discussing this with some mirth and levity, we recognized that, apart from the inconvenience and irritation this caused others, having mess and disorder in our domestic environments was a source of significant continued stress for ourselves too. It could lead to feelings of being anxious, overwhelmed, out of control and ashamed.

We tried to describe the problem in CAT terms, writing a description and mapping the pattern. Considering how this might translate to an animation, we initially contemplated storyboarding a procedural description or illustrating the Reciprocal Roles and emotional states evoked. However, we quickly moved away from the procedural, into a more spontaneously playful and creative approach to our task. Leaning into our shared interest in six-part stories, we began to imagine a parallel story, characters and a setting. In a short space of time, with surprising ease and spontaneity, we generated the outline of the story of 'Pilemonster and his Garden Friends'.

Bringing our animation to life

At later meetings, we imagined rough storyboards depicting the main scenes and how the action might move from one scene to the next. We transposed a summary outline into a narrator's script (provided at the end of this chapter). Next, we needed to create the characters we'd imagined: Pilemonster, Squirrel, Mole and Hedgehog. There were also a number of other elements to find or create, including a family, their domestic scene, a garden, and various other objects not yet anticipated.

Perhaps the longest part of our joint activity was sifting through boxes of accumulated crafting materials in order to create the characters and other props. Others experienced in this type of work may use characters created in simple ways from two-dimensional paper or cardboard cutouts, laid out on a flat background and filmed from above to simulate movement. Alternatively, simple plasticine or clay characters may be created for three-dimensional capture, standing up or supported against a vertical background. We used a mix of plasticine, pen and paper, small toys, ornaments and other objects including a scrubbing brush, firewood and bunting. The character of Pilemonster was constructed from the base of a paper spike with many scraps of paper which could be reduced and deconstructed as he shrank in size and shape over the course of the action.

Creating our 'cast' and props seemed to take us a long time and threatened to interrupt our creative flow. Had we been facilitated by a more experienced other, I imagine we may have been encouraged to keep our creations, or our story, more simple. But eventually we had made, or found, what we wanted. Another gift of my health challenges was deciding to prioritize creativity, and I was lucky to have secured a small, shared studio space with a friend. This became the venue for the majority of filming. Given our limited experience and confidence, our progress was gradual, and it was helpful to have the facility to return to a set undisturbed between sessions.

Two volunteers kindly stepped forward to act as narrators, and the younger one (favouring anonymity) was selected on the basis that a child's voice was more in keeping with the nature of the story.

We now had almost everything we needed. The majority of scenes were filmed, the voice-over was complete, and the two were ready to be edited together. At that stage, our enthusiasm for the project was overtaken by the technical challenges of merging audio and visual components. We realized that while we had sufficient capability for many components of the venture, the technicalities of editing and post-production were clearly beyond our ZPD.

Luckily, along with Ella Knight, we enlisted the support of Tony Gammidge in an intensive weekend gathering, who helped us complete the final stages of our respective projects. To this day, I am not sure how Tony worked his editorial magic to bring the Pilemonster story piece to completion but remain very grateful to him for doing so.

Our finished animation was certainly not polished, but a bit like the occasional jewels discovered in Pilemonster's sorted piles, it had a value. In terms of therapeutic impacts of engaging so deeply with the themes in our co-creation, we each experienced change, but in different directions. Regine found renewed energy for managing the build-up of objects in her home and at work, so change for her was more behavioural. Mine was more affective in that I felt less shame about those piles of things that remained in my world. My own personal Pilemonster continues to exist day-to-day, but I'm aided by the Squirrel's friendly energy, optimism and encouragement rather than oppressed by a more condemnatory Reciprocal Role.

Self-to-other

We showed 'Pilemonster and His Garden Friends', as planned, at Keele in July 2014. The three-minute run time did not reflect the hours of work that had gone into making it, and by this measure, the ends may not seem to have justified the means. It was followed by Ella Knight's much more emotive and haunting production 'Things That Happened When You Were Not There'. We took up a second opportunity to share it, accompanied by a little more context and explanation of our process, at the Catalyse 'Celebrating twenty-five years of CAT Practitioner Training in the North' conference in May 2019.

Integrating animation and CAT?
Reformulation

Given the brevity and structure of individual CAT, it would take a big shift in the model in order to incorporate creative animation techniques in the reformulation phase, unless the therapist was sufficiently skilled and proficient in animation, using unobtrusive technology or equipment. For example, a small and simple animation could be made representing a specific problematic pattern sequence and the dynamic movement between affect, aim, belief, action and consequences. Pen and paper mapping as in standard CAT may of course suffice for this purpose. What is quickly sketched out between therapist and client on paper could however act as preparation for potential later work. For example, during the mapping process, the therapist could additionally invite the client to elaborate a description of points in the procedure with more visual imagery or other sensory aspects of experience, forming a basis for visualizing and storyboarding a later animation, if helpful.

Where it may have other value is in the collaborative construction and re-authoring of a personal history and timeline to set in context the survival strategies which developed. The nuance of social and cultural influences may be more easily and dynamically represented through animated means. However, again within the tight timeframe of the reformulation period and other tasks therein, it is hard to see where this could fit without either a high level of facilitative skill on the part of the therapist, or the work being quite a different version of CAT. Colleagues who have found ways to integrate CAT and art therapy, such as John Hosie, who terms this 'CART' (personal communication, 26 April 2022), may have more thoughts to offer on this.

The middle part of CAT and emerging exits

As described earlier, animation may be particularly helpful where there is a need to slow down and engage with an aspect of experience, for example in trauma work. Gammidge (2016; 2021) provides detailed examples of his work with people in forensic settings where there may be a high degree of both past trauma and current risk. He notes how engaging with the 'methodical, time-consuming and immersive' process seems to help the creator manage potentially overwhelming feelings while depicting and recalling traumatic events, maintaining a dual awareness of both task and content as they focus on directing the action under their own control (Gammidge, 2021, pp234-235). In the same chapter, he outlines how clients selecting and directing their animated stories has aided their re-authoring of personal histories, enabled the imagining of new endings, or at times helped enact revenge fantasies in safe and contained ways. A sense of personal power and control through such creative activity may be boosted for people existing in social environments or service contexts where this is limited. CAT practitioners strive to collaborate in a doing-with rather than doing-to manner with clients, and animation might offer a further angle on this as therapy proceeds.

As in Richard's story, or the Pilemonster story, externalizing aspects of a problem or a part of the self can enable engagement with them in a less threatening way. Dream material might be represented and worked with, perhaps with a view to creating new endings. Animation may fruitfully develop and work with exit-related metaphors emerging through the therapeutic dialogue. Characters created through imaginative processes can assume a life of their own and surprise us. Or they may represent new or previously silenced aspects of the self who can strengthen their voice or sense of legitimacy. Like the Jet or Squirrel characters, they may become allies in change, or offer a new Reciprocal Role.

Endings

In my own personal animation work, loss, endings, and transition were strong themes, also evident in the couple of small pieces of work I helped facilitate. When a friend contacted me in distress about a family loss during the pandemic, we spoke about the potential for family members unable to attend the funeral because of restrictions to share images or ideas for an animated tribute, and she later contacted me to say that this idea had flown with the technical support of one of the younger family members who was able to weave such a thing together. The medium fits well with grief work through storytelling, memory, use of objects and images.

As a means of processing and summarizing therapy, a therapist skilled in collaborative animation might help to scaffold some form of joint story told through animated means, rather than (or building on) separate goodbye letters between therapist and client. This might focus primarily on exits emerging from the work, but could also depict moments of empathy, important enactments, or help work through feelings of abandonment or destructive impulses in ways that feel contained.

Imagining a group setting where creative approaches had already been introduced, perhaps earlier helping build group cohesion, a group animation might offer a way for all members to co-create a collective and lasting artefact of the group, giving space for different aspects of what can be taken away from it.

Given the time potentially involved, I wonder if animation work might more realistically be offered as a follow-up option after completing CAT, connected to it but outside of the initial therapy contract itself. This might be a way to consolidate, strengthen and help to maintain change going forward, as participants render their reflections on what they have learned and gained through therapy in a more durable manner.

Beyond therapy and self-to-other

If an animation has a primarily self-to-self function then, much like CAT maps, it could be expected that the content may not make full sense to an external viewer. However, there may be occasions where an individual or group wishes their story to be shared and understood by others. Gammidge (2016) gives a range of examples where animations have been shared by individuals with intention, for example to a team as an alternative to case notes, to a new clinician as part of communicating history or needs, or to family members as a way of helping them understand behaviours and events. Animations can convey expert-by-experience perspectives to professional education, training and conferences.

In an interesting paper, Gorman *et al* (2023) describe how participatively created animations on the experience of rare genetic diseases enabled helpful dialogue not just amongst participants in a qualitative research study, but between patients' families and clinicians. Used as part of medical student education, these helped students to 'reflect carefully on the importance of evaluating their language and thinking carefully and sensitively about how clinical terminology might be better explained. Others reflected on how animations revealed things they wouldn't normally see ... and gave them an appreciation of how and why patients may feel dismissed' (Gorman *et al*, pp15-16).

In this way, such materials may act as exits in themselves, as means of influencing, challenging, or communicating in new ways, of claiming a voice, campaigning or connecting with others who can act collectively towards a common goal. Gammidge (2016) cites several examples of clients in his animation sessions finding occupational and educational exits, going on to see themselves as artists and, in some cases, to train further in animation or other forms of further education where their creative skills flourished.

For teams and organizations, facilitated animation might be used with value for team building, shared consideration of key organizational issues, events, and perhaps critical incidents. A good example was the digitally illustrated account of the impact of the COVID pandemic on NHS staff, produced by Sara Casado and colleagues in the CAT Special Interest Group of Kent and Medway NHS and Social Care Partnership Trust. This pooled clinical experience and staff voices to share a diagrammatic reformulation of the impact of the pandemic on relationships at work, with a view to aiding dialogue and understanding within the workforce.

Walters *et al* (2023) share a case study describing how occupational therapists trained in the re-animation approach supported a co-produced participatory animation project in a locked secure inpatient hospital, which made it possible for patients to celebrate bonfire night on the fifth of November. Subject to leave restrictions and with no access to real fireworks on hospital grounds, fifty patients created their own firework display by combining a series of paper zoetrope animations depicting explosions and pyrotechnics. Edited together with music, it was projected onto a screen for a large group viewing and shared on DVD for those who could not attend this screening. This proved so popular that it became an annual event spanning five years. A CAT perspective on this example might describe the initiative as a service-wide opportunity to enrich the autonomy and self-determination of service users in an environment which has the potential to limit both, countering restrictive Reciprocal Roles such as excluding to excluded, and powerfully controlling to powerlessly controlled.

Accessibility considerations

One of the initial obstacles to my engagement with animation was the cost and complexity of understanding the technical kit required to make it happen. As technology has moved on, animation has become far more accessible to all through, for example, free or affordable apps for mobile phones. In Gorman *et al*'s (2023) study, participants were sent a kit of simple and easy-to-use equipment, and training workshops using these in tandem with a free animation app were successfully offered online as a means of scaffolding the further work. Undisturbed space for set-building was an important resource for making the Pilemonster piece possible, and one to which not all have easy access in their domestic spaces or indeed in health-service settings. As I did not attempt any animation work within an NHS setting, I am not sure whether there would be specific obstacles related to IT and information governance, but I imagine that this could be a potential issue.

As animation is largely a visual craft, people with sensory difficulties such as visual loss could well engage with the process of making animation through embodied activity (with adaptations and specific scaffolding to make this possible) but may be less easily able to appreciate the finished outcome.

While I have no experience of animation work in other languages, I expect that this would be very possible and am aware that both Gammidge and Mason have worked with refugee and displaced communities in the UK and abroad. A 'show, don't tell' principle helps to invite action or symbolic representation where language struggles. Fair representation of minoritized people and communities is entirely possible in animation, as characters and settings can be created and depicted as wished. No prejudice, obstacles or glass ceilings exist beyond the imagination of the maker. Scenes can easily include signs and symbols relevant to a specific socio-cultural context.

Younger people growing up alongside more advanced technology and with high exposure to forms of visual social media may be more at ease with animation than those in other cohorts lacking such exposure and familiarity. As a playful and non-threatening activity, it may be particularly helpful for children, and Mason (2009) gives many examples of its application with young people and their families.

Because of the many points of easy entry into animation activity, whether model making, drawing, creating sets, devising stories, narrating, moving objects, positioning a phone or webcam, or pressing buttons on a keyboard to operate software, engagement in the process can be supported for a wide range of people. With the right support and scaffolding, physical, sensory, learning or developmental disabilities, including cognitive decline, should not be obstacles to animating. The worst of my cognitive compromise was behind me by the time I attended my Level 2 training, but it was certainly not absent. Animation still gave me ways to engage with meaningful and transformative activity-based work which helped me process trauma and grief and move on with my 'new normal'.

For people with neurodiversity who may struggle with verbal therapies, or with sequencing and aspects of executive function, the clearly delineated steps and many options in animation-based work may provide a helpful framework, again with adaptation by the facilitator to ensure that any activity is suited to the individual's capabilities and ZPD.

Conclusions

Gorman *et al* (2023) suggest that arts-based methods may lack support because they are deemed 'frivolous' (p17). Through personally engaging with both the purely frivolous and quite profoundly transformative aspects of the medium, I feel that it has much potential as an adjunct or integrated aspect of CAT practice. While the acronym 'CANT' would match the terminology it would certainly misrepresent the spirit, given that animation makes many things more, not less, possible.

I encourage colleagues to research it further, to explore opportunities for hands-on experiential learning, and potentially connect with animators or creatives who may support and collaborate on developments in their localities. Thankfully, within the diversity of the CAT community, a range of professions are represented, including colleagues with a core training in occupational therapy and also those who have before or since trained as arts and creative health professions. I hope that this act of imagining animation in CAT may lead to more shared conversations, experimentation, consultation, supervision and support to help develop this rich and promising practice.

The Pilemonster

- Once upon a time there was a Pilemonster. He was very large and messy and took up far too much space. People in his home became cross with him quite often. He didn't quite fit anywhere and even when he breathed in tightly, he couldn't find a comfortable place where he wasn't in the way. He tried to sit down and relax with the family in his home, but it was a big squeeze for everyone.

- One day he felt very bad about himself, so ashamed and awful that he wanted to get out of the home that couldn't contain him any longer. He took himself out into the fresh air of the garden. He was very cross with himself and all he could think about was how useless and ugly and rubbish he was. He wondered if he should just climb into the bin and be done with it.

- He sat in the garden and cried, feeling very lonely and bad. Then some small animals heard his sobbing and came to join him on the grass. First a Squirrel darted over and looked brightly at the Pilemonster. Then a Hedgehog snuffled towards them. Next, a little mound of earth appeared and a Mole pushed his head up next to them.

- The animals asked him why he was crying, and he explained that he'd become far too big to stay in the house; everyone inside was cross with him.
- The animals said they would help and Pilemonster sat still while they started to pull away at his messiness. The Squirrel climbed over him, gradually pulling out things like old receipts, important letters, very interesting books and articles, and many small scraps of paper with really good ideas on them.
- Some of these had beautiful jewels attached which glinted even more brightly once they were out in the sunshine.
- The Hedgehog stayed still while the Squirrel darted up and down, bringing things and sorting them out on his spikes.
- The Squirrel took some of what was being sorted away to his hole in a tree, to make sure it was safe and dry and could be found when it was needed later.
- He took quite a lot of things that didn't seem to have a purpose to the bins outside the house. The Mole took some of the other things that didn't seem needed to shred up and make a warm bed for him and his family.
- Many jewels were found and the glinting lights from these lit up the garden and shone on Pilemonster. He quite liked what he now saw in himself. Rather than feeling ashamed, he felt good that he had in fact been holding on to quite a lot of valuable things, keeping them safe and not lost after all. He put them safely in a box.
- As the sun became low in the sky, the busy activity slowed and came to a stop. The animals sat awhile with Pilemonster, chatting, playing and relaxing, until it was time for them to go home. They were all tired but happy after such a busy and productive day.
- Pilemonster went back into the house with his box of precious things and squeezed himself onto the sofa with his house-people. He found it wasn't such a squeeze after all. They were pleased to see him and were delighted with the contents of his box. They all relaxed and had a happy evening together. From that day on, whenever Pilemonster started feeling bad he would remember his Garden Friends and their special day and remind himself to be his own Squirrel.

Chapter 16: Well-being workshops for CAT therapists

Steve Potter, in conversation with Annalee Curran and Elizabeth Wilde McCormick

In this chapter, Annalee Curran, Elizabeth Wilde McCormick and Steve Potter reflect on a series of one-day workshops on self-care for CAT therapists that Annalee and Liz have run over the past two decades. Their discussion was recorded, and has been edited into a dialogue between the authors with the creative aspects at the heart of CAT in mind.

Steve: You two have delivered one-day workshops on the theme of self-care for CAT therapists in Scotland, England and Finland a number of times over the years. It involved a lot of creativity.

Liz: The workshop was designed to offer the opportunity for participants to address the question: what is it about ourselves that gets left behind when we become a therapist?

Annalee: Our focus was on the therapists' own nourishment in whatever form it might arise and not about sorting patient problems. In the background is a question about what happens when one focuses on and throws one's whole being into the therapy and the role of therapist. We described the workshops as an opportunity to find a part of ourselves that hasn't had much of a voice in the everyday life of being a therapist.

Steve: You are suggesting that these overlooked parts need a voice if we are to bring out the best of ourselves as therapists. It is good for our own well-being and self-care, but it is good for the art of being available to clients. How did the day get structured? I am imagining not too tightly. Just enough to shape to scaffold the journey for each individual and for the group as a whole.

Annalee: The workshop ran from about 10.00am until 4.30pm. To begin, we outlined the format of the day, the importance of holding a safe place and it being a container for whatever might arise. We invited the group to experience the day at their own pace, and in safety, emphasizing that there were no hurdles to jump through!

Liz: We started with a simple mindfulness of breathing for a minute or two before everyone was invited to say their name and anything they would like to add such as: 'what has encouraged you to come today?' Annalee and I shared some thoughts about what being therapists demands of us and what of ourselves might get overlooked and deprived.

Annalee: Once there was some sense of community and trust, we asked them to work on a personal lifeline and to do it in a creative, multimedia way. Our aim was to get them to let go and play and, in so doing, to see their path in a new way, signposting important influences that had led them into the therapy path and also getting a sense of which part of themselves might have been left behind. And the feelings and images which arose in the process.

Steve: You weren't saying look for Reciprocal Roles or anything CAT-like?

Annalee: Not specifically, but the CAT therapists in the group could readily come to see those at play. We invited them initially to make the lifeline as if going back over a journey of their work life and to do this creatively in their own individual way. We encouraged this to be a playful and creative process, people often on hands and knees, creating their pictures or collages or whatever on the floor. There was a sense of the group setting enabling everyone to witness each other's emerging images, while still respecting their privacy if that is what was wanted.

Liz: We used creative art materials for drawing – coloured paper and crayons; coloured stickers, pompoms and sparkles and people could cut pictures out of cards we had collected for this workshop.

Annalee: We had many different things that could be invited in to help them so that they could create quite an elaborate collage with which they were in in dialogue.

Liz: They could create images on paper that might not be fully understood; but they often became aware, in the process of creating these images, that they were really important in some way. By the end of the day, they were in a new conversation with their creation and gathering new insights because of it. Like the star on paper coming to stand for the star I have been following, or it reminds me of the first therapist I met.

Steve: So, the pompoms and the stars and the paper and the colours are all ways of bringing this out in a multisensory conversation. Links and associations are being made but the structure or scaffolding of the creative materials is not intrusive or proscribing a particular path. It is like creating an external, even projective space, to recover a lost or overlooked dialogue between me the professional and me the human being. It is mapping out a journey, but very loosely. I like the idea that people are in and around each other not so much one-to-one but aware of the atmosphere of creative reflection and discovery in the room. In the air, so to speak.

Liz: We offered a lot of time for them to talk about it in pairs so that they could really articulate it for themselves. When they share in pairs, they go to different areas because we had a big room space usually, so they can be private and experiment together and name things and ask each other what this or that might mean or feel like. In Finland, they went out under the silver birch trees.

Annalee: There was no pressure or expectation to share details, but the invitation was to share as much as you want to and be open to what emerges in the conversation with your partner. We were inviting people to stumble upon metaphors which they maybe didn't fully understand at first but then helping them see that metaphor has wisdom.

Steve: It sounds like an open, unformulated but highly relational process allowing the disavowed, bypassed or unconscious voices to also speak. I imagine CAT as a model and the NHS and similar health services around the world can sometimes be over-organizing or structured and too formulation-driven, and this workshop offered an under-formulating, gently unravelling, playful and relational process. Less head and more heart.

Liz: We invited participants to work on large sheets of coloured paper which invited letting go of the professional stance if you like. People are either on the floor or standing or leaning against the wall or doing things like that rather than sitting in the chair like the therapist would. It was playful, almost a dance we do together. I remember one person stood up and she'd written a poem and she said, I feel I'm finding my voice, my own voice. It was so beautiful. And everybody was in tears.

Annalee: A sudden moment of liberation.

Liz: Obviously, it is a safe group and it's honouring the emotional experience. She was so surprised that the voice of the poet – it was a rhyme or music – came out of her. It was something that she could move to with her body, and she said something like, 'I'm going to say this to myself each day and to read this each day. It's found me.'

Steve: It sounds important that in that example there was a moment of meeting in that she had no idea what was going to happen until it happened. It was unrehearsed and spontaneous and presumably freeing for others.

Annalee: Yes. Unprepared, spontaneous. Totally and very precious. We were making it safe for people to open up to real emotional experience. They weren't just observing their life as a therapist from the outside in. They were also feeling what that meant for their full self. And they were engaged with it. We weren't trying to analyse. Through the combined creativity of the group and the activities, they're having the healing experience in the room through sharing it throughout the day.

Liz: We'd also have a walking meditation just before lunch. This helps keep the focus on the more heartfelt and holistic experience because it wasn't going back to theorizing or being cognitive.

Steve: It was finding ways to be in dialogue. And so, you're not over-finalizing or sorting it. The participants are going away with memories and connections that they can process later on. Can I ask? There's something important about how you both co-facilitated this. There is something creative and heartfelt in your relationship.

Liz: Annalee and I met right at the beginning of the brief therapy project in 1984, and we immediately had a lot in common. We also enjoyed a lot of creativity. Both of our backgrounds included working creatively. Annalee had had years in general practice and also with pregnant mothers. My background was in transpersonal, humanistic psychology and social psychiatry. We just found we were naturally able to work together in a very organic way. There were a number of people who were very dismissive about the idea that we could include words like 'heart' in relation to working in CAT. I wrote a paper called 'Does CAT have a heart? And if it does, does it make it soft and wet?' It is available in *Reformulation* (1993) and on the ACAT website online library.

Steve: This could be a separate talk: how you brought out Tony Ryle's implicit heart. Or how you brought the heart out in CAT, which was there, but not there. But, for how you co-facilitate, I think it's crucial not just that you trusted each other but were able to play with each other.

Annalee: Trust was the word that came to my mind first; we knew we could trust each other, that we were going in the same direction, but we hadn't planned the choreography step by step with each other because each of us was open, I think, to whatever came to us in the moment. We hadn't rehearsed it off pat at all. We were indeed playing with each other, like musicians jamming together.

Steve: Both of you loved doing these workshops because you knew you would get something from them for yourselves.

Annalee: Oh, yes, definitely.

Liz: Truly, absolutely.

Steve: So, next question about the detailed flow of the day is: you've had lots of ways of helping people be in dialogue within themselves and between each other but another one of them was the guided imagery to find fresh perspectives and emotions and a journey through obstacles. Could you say a bit about that, Liz?

Liz: This was a guided imagery that I had done at the Centre for Transpersonal Psychology a number of times. An imaginative journey to find the wellspring of fresh water. We did this lying down and using active imagination. You would begin by imagining yourself standing in the middle of in a field. In this place, you ask for three gifts to take with you. You are then invited to cross the field to find the path that will lead to the wellspring. On this path you will meet three obstacles. At each obstacle you invite one of your gifts to come forward to help you. You had to go into a wood, then you came to a stream, and you had to cross the stream; if there was no means of crossing it, you were confronting the first obstacle.

Annalee: You didn't specify what the obstacles were. So, for different people, that would be different things. And do you remember one person plunged into water, but her gift was a singing voice, and she sang, which lifted her out of the water, and then she walked on.

Liz: When you came to the wellspring, you just drank from the fresh water, or you bathed yourself, whatever you would like – but it's this fresh water of the wellspring. And then you bring it back with you safely to the field, and you stand in the field, and say your thanks and your gratitude, bringing the fresh water with you and also knowing you've overcome three obstacles.

Steve: Guided imagery is a scaffolding for people to go on their own journey. And have their own moments. What else did you do?

Annalee: So, there was a letter to themselves towards the end, in the light of everything that had emerged during the day and that sense of looking at themselves as a whole person and recognizing the value and fulfilment they got in their therapeutic work. But also taking on board the pressure or overwork and, in most cases, I think what bits of themselves got left behind. And often that would be to do with their more creative self. We would get them to write a letter, you know, kind of without being too specific, from a wise self to the self-who's carrying that life of the moment. And we would send them off to write the letter and give them the option of reading it out to each other. But if people didn't want to read it to someone else, they could go out into the garden or something and read it out loud. We really encouraged them that they had to hear their own voice saying it, wherever they might choose to do so. I remember there was one woman, Liz, who went to the mirror in the wall somewhere in the garden where we were working. And so she read it to herself in the mirror, which I thought was wonderful. Yes.

Steve: Why was that wonderful, looking in the mirror?

Annalee: Because she needed to hear it herself. And she needed to see herself speaking and so really inhabiting that dialogue with self.

Liz: I think that the final point of the day is a ritual ending where you step forward and say what you're leaving behind and what you're taking away.

Steve: Say what you're taking. Was it both taking and leaving behind? Yes. Can you say more about that?

Liz: Well, people would leave something behind which they had written on a bit of paper or that was symbolic; they'd leave it in the middle. And then, as Annalee said, they would say what they were taking with them. One time, in the winter, we had a fire. And if they needed to put something on the fire, then they could put it on the fire at the end. After that they would say what they were taking with them – 'And I take with me my warm heart' or whatever it is, whatever they felt.

Annalee: Yes, but we invited everyone to do it; it wasn't a case of if you feel like it. Liz and I did it too. Everybody left something behind and stepped forward and put that either in the fire or I think we might have had a basket or something once in Finland or something, and then they would step back, saying what they would take away with them. So, they'd have one piece of paper from which they would read what they were leaving and put that in the middle of the circle and then they would read out the positive thing they wanted to take with them. and step back into the circle, holding that piece of paper to their heart. And I remember we always waited so that people could spontaneously take their turn. We didn't go round in the circle where everybody had to do it in order. We were just in a wonderful sort of still space, wasn't it, as we drew things together. Yes. And just in that stillness, people knew when the moment was right for them to do their little two steps forward, two steps backwards. And it was an incredibly quiet way of ending. It came about because when we were planning the first of these days, we were wondering, how shall we end it? And we came up with that idea,

Steve: This is a wonderful workshop, and I can see that people will want you to do it again. Which you may. But if you were to advise people how to do a workshop like this what is the key advice you'd give or what would they need?

Liz: They need trust; to have trust, playfulness.

Steve: You need to do all the exercises yourself.

Annalee: Exactly. You need to participate, while holding the safe space.

Steve: Yes. And you need to be. You need to be brave. Because I think you two being good. ... like, who knows what the words are ... maternal or containing figures. I think a lot of therapists might be a bit scared of doing stuff like this. It's too open and messy. But you don't seem to be scared. Say a bit about how you need to be able to have a capacity to let people get emotional and create a mess. Or is that not true?

Annalee: Yes, exactly. Part of it is therapeutic. Creating a safe space and being able to hold whatever emerges. So that I think if one's running a workshop like this or if one's in a therapy session with a client, you know, you do have that sense of holding them safe, whatever might happen. And I can't remember if we had anybody who couldn't participate in any of the exercises. But you would give them that option not to participate in a particular exercise. There was actually one person once, Liz, I can't remember where, who kind of went back into the house to have a cup of tea while we did one of the activities, because something quite raw had happened in her life and it didn't feel comfortable. You have to be very finely tuned: I think when you're doing this, your antennae need to be finely and compassionately tuned to hold it safe.

Liz: You're saying to people, go at your own pace, own your own journey. Go where you want to go. Yes, that's implicit.

Steve: Do you want a final word?

Annalee: It's very lovely talking about this and bringing it alive again. If it opens the door for people to take care of themselves in a dialogic way, using imaginative, metaphorical, image-based ways of doing that, then it is worthwhile.

Liz: It was creative and nourishing for us too.

Annalee: Yes, very much so.

Steve: Do you miss it? Would you do it again?

Annalee: In theory, yes, I would definitely do it again.

Liz: I agree.

Steve: Well, this conversation was guided by the following points. How we use ourselves as we become therapists – what aspects of our full selves get left behind, and the risk of getting drained. We explored creative ways to be in dialogue through guided imagery to find energy and address obstacles. You ended the workshop with a letter to themselves and with a ritual of participants stepping forward and saying what they are leaving behind and then stepping back into the circle saying what they want to take with them into the future. All good steps in creative self-care I would say.

'The Jigsaw aka The Battle of Humpty'

Louise Yorke

The story of 'The Jigsaw aka The Battle of Humpty' (Yorke, 2018) was presented during a CAT psychotherapy training workshop. As the poem was read aloud, and proceeded through the 3Rs of CAT, the presenters took pieces of paper and 'put together' a pre-drawn jigsaw image of Humpty Dumpty. The creative session was a helpful method through which to process some of the teachings and emotions around trauma as well as a means by which to share clinical ideas.

'The Jigsaw aka The Battle of Humpty'
…How do we find peace in this life?
Is there ever an ending to
 our trauma and strife?
Can we put ourselves back-together
 when we stumble and fall
Can we find the path? Hear the CAT call?

'Reformulation….'
Words first heard in the nursery
Can take hold in the mind.
Such damaging procedures
In those sayings and rhymes.
… In the long battle of Humpty
The war rages on.
Unbearable terror, never forgotten.

'Recognition …'
For those caught in the conflict
Every man woman and child.
Come to know the peace process
Reflect – You could find
This life – can we fix-it?

Ask a question so strange.
Is there ever an exit?
Puzzle pieces rearranged.

'Revision …'
Now the Battle of Humpty
On some far distant field.
Snags, traps and dilemmas
Over time they are healed.
Hear these words now re-spoken
Bringing hope from the pain.
Change your lives by this token
Meaning found in refrain:
Reciprocal voices,
Mapped with the therapy pen
Could put Humpty together again.

Louise Yorke (2018). The Jigsaw aka The Battle of Humpty. *Reformulation*, Winter, p43

Afterword

Yvonne J. Stevens

This has been a personal project for all involved, and drawing on these creative techniques necessarily brings the intimacy of our self-self relationships into the self-other relationships in the therapy room. We need to stay in the present moment to constantly renew and remember how we nurture ourselves (and our colleagues) and stay connected to ourselves and so to others. This enables a particular authenticity in the therapy room of openness and intersubjective connection. There are reflections in these pages on the well-being of the integrated and creative CAT therapist, and there is plenty more to say about how we sustain this, our communities and our environment.

The ICATA CAT Climate Special Interest Group has been exploring how we find creative responses through the dialogue and relationality of CAT to the climate crisis. Robert McFarlane's beautiful and haunting book, *Lost Words* (2017), evokes estranged parts of the self, on precious connections with nature we have lost or forgotten. Carl Rogers described our need for authenticity and congruence in our lives (Rogers, 1961) and we will need both to find the creativity needed to move us into the next age that is not dependent on fossil fuels; you cannot create a new future without an authentic, meaningful vision.

I am leaving the last word to Kurt Vonnegut, one of the most imaginative minds of the twentieth century, who wrote about our deepest fears of guilt and annihilation, and of our most passionate hatreds and loves, like no other author. From his final published work *A Man Without a Country* (2005):

> 'Practicing an art, no matter how well or badly, is a way to make your soul grow, for heaven's sake. Sing in the shower. Dance to the radio. Tell stories. Write a poem to a friend, even a lousy poem. Do it as well as you possibly can. You will get an enormous reward. You will have created something.'

Glossary of CAT terms

CAT framework/scaffolding: the containing structure of CAT having a beginning, middle and end phase, that supports the client and the therapist in the therapeutic relationship.

- Beginning phase: identifying TP's, TPP's, RRP's and aims for therapy; psychoeducation; reformulation both prose and diagrammatic.
- Middle phase: scaffolding for change-focused or trauma-focused work; use of other models of therapy such as body work, mindfulness, emotion focused work, CFT.
- Ending phase: working with endings, loss, abandonment, disappointment and rejection; valuing what has been shared and held.

core pain/chronically endured pain: early loss, deprivation, unmet need, sadness, destructive feelings, the effects of which continue to be struggled with in the present.

countertransference: identifying and/or reciprocating with shared understanding of a person's affect or states from either one's own experiences or from a subjective empathic resonance.

dilemmas: as if choices of how to behave or relate to others are somehow limited or restricted.

exits: (revisions) are built on reformulation and recognition – not external solutions; noticing and naming, expressing feelings, processing trauma, changing behaviour, expression of feelings, challenging negative thinking.

dialogism: Mikael Bakhtin's philosophy and theory relating to language and cultural and social discourse; the self is relational, the multiplicity of selves is in constant dialogue with self and others, every thought and utterance is dialogical and has an addressee.

enactment: when state shifts occur, when there is pressure on the therapist to reciprocate, including when feelings are cut off or avoided; based on the psychodynamic ideas of transference and countertransference that relational patterns from the past will be repeated within therapy.

goodbye letters: exchanged at the end of therapy by the therapist and client; the therapist describes what has been shared, what has been gained and what has not, naming both the gratitude and disappointment and the feelings about loss and ending.

- Brief description of original difficulties and presenting problems
- Challenges to therapy: non-attendance, withholding, overwhelmed
- Summary and reminder of the reformulation
- Accurate, plain description of what has been achieved and what remains to be done
- Naming and expression of feelings, including regarding loss and endings
- Reminder of the new skills and conceptual tools developed during therapy
- Positive achievements and mutual work achieved in the relationship

healthy island: a place on the person's map or diagram that describes hopeful aims and goals and positive self-states.

mapping: the process of co-creating diagrams in therapy, drawing out procedures and reciprocal roles (see Appendix 6).

Multiple Self States Model (MSSM): the MSSM is a trauma model of structural dissociation resulting in a multiplicity of self-processes, through this model previously dissociated and disconnected and more or less distinct parts of the self can be identified, named and filled out, brought into the conscious mind for scrutiny and description, so that they become known and connected through understanding their roles to each other and promote a more integrated sense of self.

Object Relations theory: developed by Klein – offers an account for different parts of the self, describes unconscious processes of projection and projective identification.

The Psychotherapy File: a self-report therapy inventory developed by Ryle and used at the beginning of a CAT therapy outlining descriptions of procedures and self-states to enable an early conversation to identify the focus for therapy and the beginnings of a shared language and encouragement to reflect on the self (see Appendix 1).

Procedural Sequence Object Relations Model: the basic unit of CAT, describing aim-directed relational activity combining in sequence: intention or perception, appraisal, plans, actions, the consequence of acting, confirmation or revision of the procedure. Procedures can be restrictive and maladaptive resulting in maintenance of distress.

"push where it moves": almost anything that moves the therapy along and engages the active participation of the person in the present, tasks that may keep the person in touch with therapy and can offer containment over the week or during breaks, custom designed to fit the needs of the client.

3R's: recognition/reformulation/revision – the three stages of a CAT therapy.

reciprocal roles: relational roles that can be understood as parent-derived upper role and child-derived lower role relational patterns, and that can be recognised from descriptions of early relationships, descriptions of current relationships, descriptions of difficulties, "In the room" transference / countertransference, and from embodied actions or CT responses.

reciprocal role procedures: jointly agreed descriptions of one's self- self/self-other relational repertoire arising from early relational experiences, current life and arising in the therapy relationship. The RRP has two components: the individual's experience in relation to the other and how the other was experienced e.g. critically rejecting to criticised, rejected and humiliated.

reflexivity: the self-reflective capacity to think about the self, which for some people, due to traumatic experiences, may have been restricted or distorted (see Appendix 3).

reformulation: a narrative and diagrammatic process in CAT that is integrative and collaborative naming painful unmet needs from childhood experiences and linking these to the development of unhelpful procedures and reciprocal role repertoires, and outlining potential aims for therapy. Reformulation links past relational patterns (procedures) to present problems and future exits. Reformulation is an open, collaborative process involving shared CAT tools such as letters and maps.

reformulation letter: a jointly created prose narrative letter, usually read by the therapist to the client by session 4-6. It incorporates descriptions of childhood and chronically endured pain arising from neglect, abuse or deprivation and naming early self-management and relational role strategies developed to cope or survive and so integrating previously discontinuous, disconnected fragmented experiences of the self. The written reformulation seeks to place the person's narrative and in particular the trauma they have experienced in the context of their environment, identity and culture in their past and their present life. Aim of the letter is to give high level accurate descriptive account of patient's suffering and their survival/ coping strategies and provide a focus and the aims for therapy in the context of the therapeutic relationship.

self-states: a distinct, separate, sense of oneself in relation to other distinct self-states, describing how one is feeling, acting, and being with self and others, and may be described as one pole of a reciprocal role procedure.

sequential diagrammatic reformulation: at the centre of CAT is the development of the SDR, integrating the power of the mapping diagram to bring together previously experienced disconnected and sometimes hidden parts of the self in relation to self to self and self to other procedures. The SDR incorporates the RRs and RRPs. This is a schematic diagram with the individual's reciprocal role procedures, states and patterns which offers a meta-perspective of self-self and self-other enactments though the inclusion of the 'observing eye'. This becomes the vehicle for recognition and subsequent revision (see Appendix 6).

snags: subtle negative aspects of gains – undermining beliefs about the self, and the feared responses of others, leading to undoing or sabotaging good things.

target problems: brief descriptions of the focus of therapy negotiated between the therapist and patient as problems requiring revision, that they will be working on together in therapy, which may be interpersonal, intrapersonal or symptomatic in origin.

target problem procedures: patterns of thinking, feeling, and behaving which we use to achieve an aim or respond to an event, and which underpin and maintain the target problem. Individuals seeking help usually deploy a sequence of self-self/self-other behaviours in specific situations identified as Target Problems (TPs) and Target Problem Procedures (TPPs). Procedures can be restrictive and maladaptive resulting in maintenance of distress.

therapeutic change in CAT: the creation and maintenance of a non-collusive and respectful relationships, the collaborative creation of mediating tools (descriptions, diagrams) which make the patient's specific problem procedures and structures available for conscious reflection, movement through the stages of reformulation, practice in recognition and the process of revision or replacement of problematic procedures.

traps: negative beliefs about the self, leading to negative choices of behaviour or avoidance with negative consequences confirming negative beliefs about the self.

zone of proximal development (ZPD): from Vygotsky, learning and growth takes place within the ZPD – the difference between where the client is today and where they could be with the therapist's help. It is the responsibility of the therapist to keep within the ZPD of the client and to be responsive to the different starting and finishing points of each client, that is neither within the core competence nor beyond the competence of the person. 'What the child does with an adult today he/she will do by her/himself tomorrow.' – Vygotsky.

Appendices

Appendix 1: The Psychotherapy File

We have all had just one life. What has happened to us, and the sense we made of this, colours the way we see ourselves and others. How we see things is, for us, how things are, and how we go about our lives seems 'obvious and right'. Sometimes, however, our familiar way of understanding and acting can be the source of our problems. In order to solve our difficulties, we may need to learn to recognise how what we do makes things worse. We can then work out new ways of thinking and acting.

These pages are intended to suggest ways of thinking about what you do. Recognising your particular patterns is the first step in learning to gain more control and happiness in your life.

Keeping a diary of your moods and behaviour

Symptoms, bad moods, unwanted thoughts or behaviours that come and go can all be better understood and controlled if you learn to notice when they happen, and what starts them off.

If you have a particular symptom or problem of this sort, start keeping a diary. The diary should be focused on a particular mood, symptom or behaviour, and should be kept every day if possible. Try to record this sequence:

1. How you were feeling about yourself and others and the world before the problem came on.
2. Any external event, or any thought or image in your mind that was going on when the trouble started, or what seemed to start it off.
3. Once the trouble started, what were the thoughts, images or feelings you experienced.

By noticing and writing down in this way what you do and think at these times, you will learn to recognise, and eventually have more control over, how you act and think at the time. It is often the case that negative feelings like resentment, depression or physical symptoms are the result of ways of thinking and acting that are unhelpful. Diary keeping in this way gives you the chance to learn better ways of dealing with things.

It is helpful to keep a daily record for 1-2 weeks, and then discuss what you have recorded with your therapist or counsellor.

Patterns that do not work, but are hard to break

There are certain ways of thinking and acting that do not achieve what we want, but which are hard to change. Read through the lists on the following pages and mark how far you think they apply to you.

Applies strongly ++   Applies +   Does not apply 0

1. Traps

Traps are things that we cannot escape from. Certain kinds of thinking and acting result in a 'vicious circle' when, however hard we try, things seem to get worse instead of better. Trying to deal with feeling bad about ourselves, we think and act in ways that tend to confirm our badness.

Examples of traps

1. **Fear of hurting others trap**

Feeling fearful of hurting others* we keep our feelings inside, or put our own needs aside. This tends to allow other people to ignore or abuse us in various ways, which then leads to our feeling, or being, childishly angry. When we see ourselves behaving like this, it confirms our belief that we shouldn't be angry or aggressive and reinforces our avoidance of standing up for our rights.

++	+	0

* *People often get trapped in this way because they mix up aggression and assertion. Mostly, being assertive - asking for our rights - is perfectly acceptable. People who do not respect our rights as human beings must either be stood up to or avoided.*

2. **Depressed thinking trap**

Feeling depressed, we are sure we will manage a task or social situation badly. Being depressed, we are probably not as effective as we can be, and the depression leads us to exaggerate how badly we handled things. This makes us feel more depressed about ourselves.

++	+	0

3. **Trying to please trap**

Feeling uncertain about ourselves and anxious not to upset others, we try to please people by doing what they seem to want. As a result:

1. We end up being taken advantage of by others which makes us angry, depressed or guilty, from which our uncertainty about ourselves is confirmed; or
2. Sometimes we feel out of control because of the need to please, and start hiding away, putting things off, letting people down, which makes other people angry with us and increases our uncertainty.

++	+	0

4. **Avoidance trap**

We feel ineffective and anxious about certain situations, such as crowded streets, open spaces, social gatherings. We try to go back into these situations, but feel even more anxiety. However, by constantly avoiding situations our lives are limited and we come to feel increasingly ineffective and anxious.

++	+	0

5. Social isolation trap

Feeling under-confident about ourselves and anxious not to upset others, we worry that others will find us boring or stupid, so we don't look at people or respond to friendliness. People then see us as unfriendly, so we become more isolated from which we are convinced we are boring and stupid - and become more under-confident.

++	+	0

6. Low self-esteem trap

Feeling worthless we feel that we cannot get what we want because:

1. We will be punished.
2. Others will reject or abandon us.
3. Anything good we get is bound to go away or turn sour.
4. Sometimes it feels as if we must punish ourselves for being weak.

From this we feel that everything is hopeless so we give up trying to do anything, which confirms and increases our sense of worthlessness.

++	+	0

2. Dilemmas (False choices and narrow options)

We often act as we do, even when we are not completely happy with it, because the only other ways we can imagine, seem as bad or even worse. Sometimes we assume connections that are not necessarily the case - as in "If I do 'x' then 'y' will follow". These false choices can be described as either/or, or if/then dilemmas. We often don't realise that we see things like this, but we act as if these were the only possible choices.

Do you act as if any of the following false choices rule your life? Recognising them is the first step to changing them. Choices about myself: I act AS IF:

Appendix 1: The Psychotherapy File

		++	+	0
1	Either I keep feelings bottled up or I risk being rejected, hurting others, or making a mess.			
2	Either I feel I spoil myself and am greedy or I deny myself things and punish myself and feel miserable.			
3	a) If I try to be perfect, then I feel depressed and angry;			
	b) If I don't try to be perfect then I feel guilty, angry and dissatisfied.			
4	If I must then I won't. It's as if when faced with a task I must either 1) gloomily submit or 2) passively resist. Other people's wishes, or even my own, feel too demanding, so I put things off or avoid them.			
5	If I must not then I will. It's as if the only proof of my existence is my resistance. Other people's rules, or even my own, feel too restricting, so I break rules and do things which are harmful to me.			
6	If other people aren't expecting me to do things for them or look after them, then I feel anxious, lonely and out of control.			
7	Either I get what I want and I feel childish and guilty; or I don't get what I want and feel frustrated, angry and depressed.			
8	Either I keep things (feelings, plans) in perfect order, or I fear a terrible mess.			

Appendix 1: The Psychotherapy File

		++	+	0
1	Either I'm involved with someone and likely to get hurt or I don't get involved and stay in charge, but remain lonely.			
2	Either I stick up for myself and nobody likes me, or I give in and get put upon by others and feel cross and hurt.			
3	Either I'm a brute or a martyr (secretly blaming others).			
4	a) With others either I'm safely wrapped up in bliss or I'm fighting			
	b) If I'm fighting then I'm either a bully or a victim.			
5	Either I look down on people, or I feel they look down on me.			
6	a) Either I'm made happy by the admiration of others whom I admire, or I feel vulnerable.			
	b) If I feel vulnerable, either I put others down or I put myself down.			
7	Either I'm involved with others and feel taken over or smothered, or I stay safe and uninvolved but feel lonely and isolated.			
8	When I'm involved with someone I care about then either I have to give in or they have to give in.			
9	When I'm involved with someone I depend on then either I have to give in or they have to give in.			
10	Either I have to do what others want or I stand up for my rights and get rejected			
11	Either I can't have any feelings or I am an emotional mess.			

3. Snags

Snags are what is happening when we say "I want to have a better life, or I want to change my behaviour but..." Sometimes this comes from how we or our families thought about us when we were young, such as "she was always the good child", or "in our family we never..." Sometimes the snags come from the important people in our lives not wanting us to change, or not able to cope with what our changing means to them. Often the resistance is more indirect, as when a parent, husband or wife becomes ill or depressed when we begin to get better.

In other cases, we seem to 'arrange' to avoid pleasure or success, or if they come, we have to pay in some way, by depression, or by spoiling things. Often this is because, as children, we came to feel guilty if things went well for us, or felt that we were envied for good luck or success. Sometimes we have come to feel responsible, unreasonably, for things that went wrong in the family, although we may not be aware that this is so. It is helpful to learn to recognise how this sort of pattern is stopping you getting on with your life, for only then can you learn to accept your right to a better life and begin to claim it.

You may get quite depressed when you begin to realise how often you stop your life being happier and more fulfilled. It is important to remember that it is not being stupid or bad, but rather that:

a) We do these things because this is the way we learned to manage best when we were younger.

b) We don't have to keep on doing them now we are learning to recognise them.

c) By changing our behaviour, we can learn to control not only our own behaviour, but we also change the way other people behave towards us.

d) Although it may seem that others resist the changes we want for ourselves (for example, our parents, or our partners), we often underestimate them; if we are firm about our right to change, those who care for us will usually accept the change.

Do you recognise that you feel limited in your life:

Appendix 1: The Psychotherapy File

		++	+	0
1	For fear of the response of others, for example, I must sabotage success, a) as if it deprives others,			
	b) as if others may envy me			
	c) as if there are not enough good things to go around.			
	d) There may be other concerns you have about how others will react if you change – write them here			
2	Because of something inside yourself: e.g. I must sabotage good things a) as if I don't deserve them.			
	b) There may be other examples of things (beliefs, expectations) inside yourself that make it hard to change – write them here			

4. Difficult and unstable states of mind

Some people find it difficult to keep control over their behaviour and experiences because things feel very difficult and different at times. Indicate which of the following, if any, apply to you:

		++	+	0
1	How I feel about myself and others can be unstable; I can switch from one state of mind to a completely different one.			
2	Some states may be accompanied by intense, extreme and uncontrollable emotions.			
3	Others by emotional blankness, feeling unreal, or feeling muddled.			

		++	+	0
4	Some states are accompanied by feeling intensely guilty or angry with myself wanting to hurt myself.			
5	Some states are accompanied by feeling that others can't be trusted, are going to let me down, or hurt me.			
6	Some states are accompanied by being unreasonably angry or hurtful to others.			
7	Sometimes the only way to cope with some confusing feelings is to blank them off and feel emotionally distant to others.			
	There may be other things you have noticed about difficult and unstable states of mind. Write down anything else that you want to share with your therapist.			

Different States

Everybody experiences changes in how they feel about themselves and the world. But for some people these changes are extreme, sometimes sudden and confusing. In such cases, there are often a number of states that re-occur. Learning to recognise them and shifts between them can be very helpful.

Below are descriptions of such states. Please tick those that you experience. You can delete or add words to the descriptions. At the end of the list you can add any descriptions that are not listed but apply to you.

1	Zombie. Cut off from feelings, cut off from others, disconnected.
2	Feeling bad but soldiering on, coping
3	Out of control rage
4	Extra special. Looking down on others.
5	In control of self, of life, of other people.
6	Cheated by life, by others. Untrusting.
7	Provoking, teasing, seducing, winding up others.
8	Clinging, fearing abandonment.
9	Frenetically active. Too busy to think or feel.
10	Agitated, confused, anxious.
11	Feeling perfectly cared for, blissfully close to another.
12	Misunderstood, rejected, abandoned.
13	Contemptuously dismissive of myself.
14	Vulnerable, needy, passively helpless, waiting for rescue.
15	Envious, wanting to harm others, put them down, pull them down.
16	Protective, respecting of myself; of others.
17	Hurting myself, hurting others.
18	Resentfully submitting to demands.
19	Hurt, humiliated by others.
20	Secure in myself, able to be close to others.
21	Intensely critical of self, of others.
22	Frightened of others.

Appendix 2: Describing self-states

(with thanks to Hilary Beard)

Self-states questions

Try to identify the distinct different states and give each one a name (e.g. rose-coloured spectacles, lost boy etc.).

For each state list:

a) How I feel for others in this state.

b) How I feel inside myself.

c) How I feel others feel about me.

d) How I feel or judge myself in this state.

e) Bodily feelings.

f) What I tend to do in this state.

g) How I try and avoid this state.

h) How I comfort myself in this state.

i) How I get myself out of this state.

Appendix 3: Restrictions on capacity for reflexivity

> From Ryle (1984) *Consciousness and Psychotherapy.* (abridged). (pp120-121)
>
> 1. **Restricted experience.** The roles enacted in a given family may be narrow or culturally inappropriate, family myths may impose particular demands or restrictions.
> 2. **Restricted self-reflection.** The child will learn to display, perform or obey but may gain little or no awareness of their subjective experience shaped by the kind of reflection offered in the family.
> 3. **Disjointed self-reflection.** Inconsistent parenting, where neglect or abuse occur, with incoherent or distorting accounts. The result is the persistence of more-or-less dissociated 'sub-personalities', each with a partial procedural repertoire.
> 4. **Errors of attribution.** Pursuing aims, which, in childhood, were perceived to be dangerous or forbidden, will be abandoned and replaced by others, often avoidant, submissive or symptomatic.
> 5. **Unmanageable experiences.** Extreme experiences may overwhelm the capacity of an individual to feel, think or act.
> 6. **Silencing.** Discrepancies between an experience and the account given of it by others, especially when accompanied by threats, as in the sexual abuse of children, becoming unsayable and in due course unrecallable.
> 7. **Defensive anxiety reduction.** Critical, prohibiting responses from parents, in relation to personally felt desires, can evoke anxiety of an intolerable degree, then avoided by denying the desire or the possibility of pursuing it.

Ryle suggested that "these forms of restrictions on the capacity for reflexivity are derived from both trauma and deprivation, and frequently co-exist. The therapeutic task is to describe and name these restrictions on the capacity to reflect on the self in the reformulation letter and map and address them through the therapeutic relationship and through the creation of alternative narratives and 'targeted interpersonal activity'".

Appendix 4: The House of Self States template

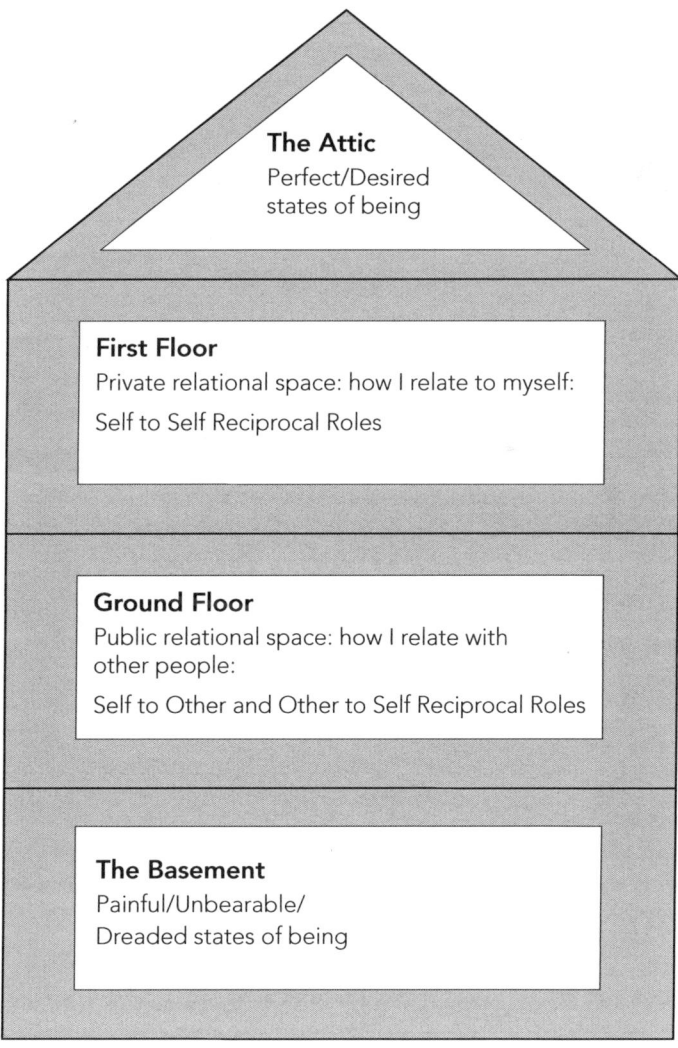

Hoss, Vicky Petratou, 2019©

Petratou, V. (2019) The House of Self States (HOSS): Using a creative integrative and containing mapping technique across the therapies. *Reformulation* **53** Winter 2019/20, pp6-9.

Appendix 5: Six-Part Story Method template

Main character & Setting	The Task	Who or what helps?
Who or what hinders?	What happens?	Consequences?

In the Six-Part Story Method the client is initially given progressive instructions to draw each part of a new, fictional story. At this stage, they do not respond verbally but just with sketched pictures. Once the sequence is complete, they are asked to tell the story right through without interruption. The client is asked to (1) create a main character (not necessarily human) in a fictional, fantasy or historical setting – i.e. as far away from 21st century real life as possible. The instructions lead the client/author on through (2) the creation of a task for the main character, (3) obstacles they encounter, (4) helpful factors, (5) the climax of the story and (6) its aftermath.

Dent-Brown, K., (2011) Six-Part Storymaking: a tool for CAT practitioners. Reformulation, Summer, pp.34-36.

Appendix 6: Reciprocal Roles – ways of relating to self and others

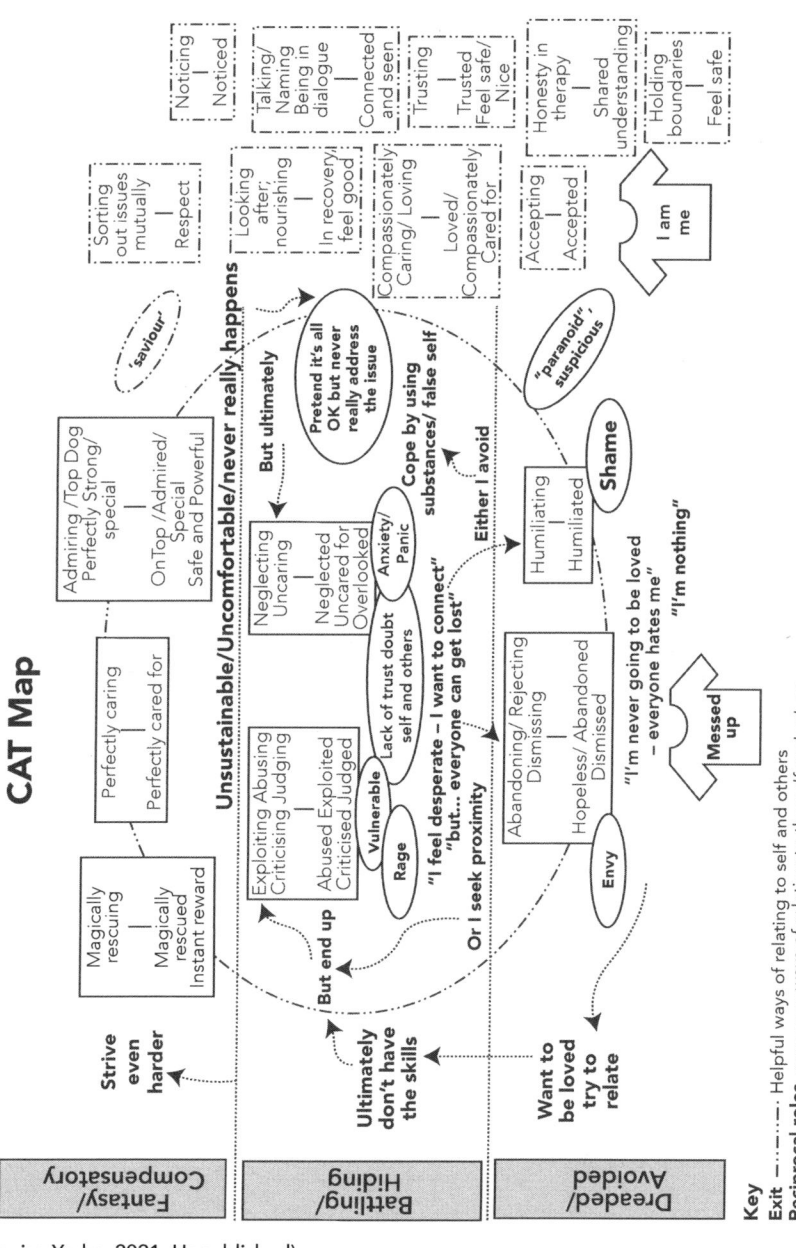

(Louise Yorke, 2021. Unpublished)
Printed with permission.

Appendix 7: Creative tasks for trainee therapists and clients

TASK 1
Getting creative early on

Draw your family tree with 3-4 generations, including any significant extended family members.

Write three descriptive adjectives next to each person.

Use coloured pens to indicate closeness, and tensions between family members, and dotted lines to indicate lack of contact or close groups in the family.

1. When you have finished take a few minutes to reflect on your position in the family, and how this might have shaped how you have developed your own relationships.
2. How do words you have chosen to describe family members reflect through the generations, and how these might be developed into inner-generational reciprocal roles?

TASK 2
Creative ways that you might depict your lifeline/timeline.

Draw a map of your life so far as a road, or mountain path or river

- Beginning with birth and extending to the present
- Show the good places (i.e. scenic or open road)
- .... And the bad places (bumpy road, steep incline, road works)

Compare your life's past course with your imagined future

- What has made the good spots?
- How do you avoid the detours and potholes?

TASK 3
Self-characterisation (after George Kelly (1955) Personal Construct Theory)

Write a description of yourself in the third person (about 200-400 words) as if:

- Either: as if written by a close friend who knows you well.
- Or: as if you were a character in a play, and you need to direct the actor playing you about your personality, the kind of person you are.

Reflections:

- Did you find it difficult to say positive things about yourself?
- How different would other people's view of you be?

TASK 4
Using objects to reflect on myself and others: self-self/ self-others.

Represent one of the following - you can use buttons, beads, stones, crystals, coloured crayons or pens, coins, small figures, Russian dolls, puppets etc.

a) Select an object that you feel represents you as you see yourself now, and a past or future self; or you in the different roles in your life.

b) Select an object that you feel represents yourself now, one that represents you as a child, and members of your family.

c) Select an object that you feel represents yourself, your supervisor, your manager, or your therapist.

Compare the qualities of the objects that you have chosen and write down the words that describe the similarities and differences that the objects represent.

- What do the objects reveal about the relationships you are reflecting on?

TASK 5
Using creativity to express feelings and "author my life."

Create one of the following:

- Letter to a younger me.
- My life story as a fairy-tale/film script/soap opera storyline.
- Create a picture or collage of my life now.
- Write a poem to myself.
- Any ideas of your own? (Remember only 20-30 minutes for this task).

References

Abbatielo, G. (2006) Cognitive Behavioural Therapy and Metaphor. *Perspectives in Psychiatric Care* **42** (3), pp208-211.

Adams, M.V. (1997) Metaphors in psychoanalytic theory and therapy. *Clinical Social Work Journal* **25** (1) pp27-39.

Aitken, K. A. & Trevarthen, C. (1997). Self/other organization in human psychological development. *Dev. Psychopathol.* **9**, 653–677. 10.1017/S0954579497001387,

Akande, R. (2007) A sign for the therapeutic relationship, *Reformulation* Winter 6-7.

Aldrich, V. (1968) Visual Metaphor. *Journal of Aesthetic Education* **2** (1) pp73-86.

Anderson-Warren, M. and Grainger, R. (2000) *Practical Approaches to Dramatherapy: The Shield of Perseus*, London: Jessica Kingsley

Animation Therapy HM (2013) *Richard's Story 2* [online]. Available at: https://youtu.be/6t7Ln_g4OJk?si=zceeWS8rUloz9_hI (accessed May 2024).

Armstrong C. R., Rozenberg M., Powel M. A., Honce J., Bronstein L., Gingras G. & Han, E. (2016) A step toward empirical evidence: Operationalizing and uncovering drama therapy change process. *The Arts in Psychotherapy* **49** 27-33.

Ashworth, J. & Mason, H. (2010) Animation in Therapy: The innovative uses of haptic animation in clinical and community therapeutic practice. *Society of Animation Studies*, Edinburgh, 2010. DOI:10.13140/2.1.1401.5367

Axline, V. (1964) *Dibs in Search of Self*. London: Pelican.

Bakhtin, M. (1984b) *Rabelais and His World*. Bloomington, IN: Indiana University Press.

Bakhtin, M. M. (1984a) *Problems of Dostoevsky's poetics*. (C. Emerson, Trans. & Ed.). Minneapolis, MN: University of Minnesota Press.

Bakhtin, M. M. (1986) *Speech genres and other late essays*. (trans. V. W. Maghee, eds. C. Emerson and M. Holquist). Austin, TX: University of Texas Press.

Bakhtin, M. M. (1990) Author and hero in aesthetic activity. In: M. M. Bakhtin, *Art and answerability: Early philosophical works*, Eds. M. Holquist and V. Liapunov, Austin Texas, University of Texas Press. (V. Liapunov Trans.).

Bakhtin, M.M. (1973) *Problems of Dostoevsky's Poetics* (R.W. Rotsel, Trans.). Ann Arbor, MI: Ardis.

Bakhtin, M.M. (1981). *The dialogic imagination: four essays*. Edited by M. Holquist. Trans. M. Holquist and C. Emerson. University of Texas Press.

Bakhtin, M.M. (1986) *Speech Genres and Other Later Essays* (trans. V.W. Magee, Eds.

Balch, O. (2024) 'As with a poem, each patient is unique': the cancer surgeon using poetry to help train doctors. *The Guardian* Saturday 17th February 2024 13.00 GMT. Available at: https://www.theguardian.com/science/2024/feb/17/joao-luis-barreto-guimaraes-cancer-surgeon-poetry-pessoa-prize.

Balmain, N., Melia, Y., John, C., Dent, H. and Smith, K. (2021) Experiences of receiving cognitive analytic therapy for those with complex secondary care mental health difficulties. *Psychology and Psychotherapy*, **94**(1),120-136.

Bandlamudi, L. (2015) *Difference, Dialogue, and Development: A Bakhtinian world*. Routledge.

Barker, P. (1985) *Using Metaphors in Psychotherapy*. Brunner/Mazel, New York

Barker, P. (1996) *Psychotherapeutic Metaphors: A guide to theory and practice*. New York Brunner/Mazel.

Barker, P. and Buchanan-Barker, P. (2005) *The Tidal Model: A guide for mental health professionals*. Bruner Routledge.

Barrault, J.L. (1962) *The Theatre of Jean-Louis Barrault*. London: Barrie and Rockliff.

Barresi, J. (2002) From 'The Thought is the Thinker' to 'the Voice is the Speaker': William James and the Dialogical Self. *Theory and Psychology* **52** pp1-26.

Bateson, G. (1972). *Steps to an ecology of mind*. Chandler Publishing.

Battino, R. (2002) *Metaphoria: Metaphor and guided metaphor for psychotherapy and healing*. Carmarthan: Crown House Publishing.

Bayne, R., & Thompson, K. L. (2000) Counsellor response to clients' metaphors: An evaluation and refinement of Strong's model. *Counselling Psychology Quarterly* **13** (1) 37-49. doi:10.1080/09515070050011051.

Bennett, D. and Ryle, A. (2005) The characteristic features of common borderline states: a pilot study using the states description procedure. *Clinical Psychology & Psychotherapy: An International Journal of Theory & Practice*, **12**(1), pp.58-66.

Bennett, D., & Parry, G. (2004). A measure of psychotherapeutic competence derived from cognitive analytic therapy. *Psychotherapy Research*, **14**(2), 176-192.

Berne, E. (1961) *Transactional Analysis in Psychotherapy*. New York. Grove Press, Inc

Billow, RM. (1977) Metaphor: A review of the psychological literature. *Psychological Bulletin*, **84** (1), 81.

Bird, D. (2019) A Heuristic model of supervision using small objects to develop the senses. *Online Journal of Complementary and Alternative medicine* pp1-8.

Birtchnell, J. and Evans, C. (2004) The persons relating to others questionnaire. *Personality and Individual Differences* **36** pp125–40

Birtchnell, W. (2020) *Proq2 online scoring tool* available at: https://willbir.github.io/proq-creoq/ (accessed on 20/06/2024)

Black, M. (1998) More about Metaphor. In: A. Ortony (Ed.), *Metaphor and Thought* (2nd Edition.). Cambridge: Cambridge University Press.

Blatner, A. & Glass, Collins J. (2008) Using psychodrama and dramatherapy methods in supervising dramatherapy practicum students. In P. Jones & D. Dokter (eds) *Supervision of Dramatherapy*. East Sussex Routledge

Bloch, S., Orthous, P., & Santibazez, H. (1995) Effector patterns of basic emotions: A psycho-physiological method for training actors. In: B. Zarrilli. *Acting reconsidered. Theories and Practices*. London: Routledge

Boal, A. (1995) *The Rainbow of Desire: The Boal method of theatre and therapy*. London: Routledge.

Boal, A. (2006) *The Aesthetics of the Oppressed*. London: Routledge.

Boik, B., Labovitz, A. & Goodwin, E. (2000) *Sand Play Therapy: A step-by-step manual for psychotherapists of diverse orientations*. New York, WW Norton & Company.

Boterhoven de Haan, K.L., Lee, C.W., Fassbinder, E., van Es, S.M., Menninga, S., Meewisse, M-L., Rijkeboer, M., Koesmaker, M., Arntz, A. (2020) Imagery rescripting and eye movement desensitization and reprocessing as treatment for adults with post – traumatic stress disorder from childhood trauma: randomised clinical trial. *British Journal of Psychiatry*, **217**(5):609-615.

Botha, M., Chapman, R., Giwa Onaiwu, M., Kapp, S. K., Stannard Ashley, A., and Walker, N. (2024) The neurodiversity concept was developed collectively: An overdue correction on the origins of neurodiversity theory. *Autism*, **28**(6), 1591-1594.

Bradshaw, J. (1990) *Home Coming: Reclaiming and championing your inner child*. London: Bantam Books.

Bravesmith, A. (2008) Supervision and Imagination, *Journal of Analytical Psychology*, vol: **53**, Issue 1, 101-117.

Brede, J., Cage, E., Trott, J., Palmer, L., Smith, A., Serpell, L., & Russell, A. (2022) 'We Have to Try to Find a Way, a Clinical Bridge' – autistic adults' experience of accessing and receiving support for mental health difficulties: A systematic review and thematic meta-synthesis. *Clinical Psychology Review* **93** 102131.

Bristow, J. (2006) Change of state: learning how to manage unmanageable feelings and states. *Reformulation*, Summer, pp.6-7.

Bristow, J. and Reason, A. (2010) Therapeutic Change that is Dialogically Structured, Mediated by Signs, and Enabled by a Relationship – A Case Example. *Reformulation*, Summer, pp31-33.

Brummer, L., Cavieres, M. & Tan, R. (Eds.), *Oxford handbook of cognitive analytic therapy.* Oxford University Press

Campbell, N.C., Murray, E. and Darbyshire, J. (2007) Designing and evaluating complex interventions to improve health care. *British Medical Journal* **334** pp455–9.

Capacchione, L. (1991) *Recovery of Our Inner Child: The highly acclaimed method for liberating your inner self.* New York: Simon and Schuster.

Capacchione, L. (2015) *The Creative Journal: The art of finding yourself.* Ohio: Ohio University Press.

Capacchione, L. (2017) *Hello, This is Your Body Talking: A draw-it-yourself coloring book.* Ohio: Ohio University Press.

Cassidy, S., Gumley, A. and Turnbull, S. (2017) Safety, play, enablement, and active involvement: Themes from a Grounded Theory study of practitioner and client experiences of change processes in Dramatherapy. *Arts in Psychotherapy* **55** pp174-185

Charles, A., & Felton, A. (2020) Exploring young people's experiences and perceptions of mental health and well-being using photography. *Child and Adolescent Mental Health* **25** (1) 13-20. doi:10.1111/camh.12351.

Chesner, A. & Zografou, L. (2014) *Creative Supervision across modalities: Theory and applications for therapist, counsellors and other helping professionals.* London: Jessica Kingsley.

Chesner, A. *Psychodrama: A Passion for Action and Non-action in Supervision.* In R. Shohet Passionate Supervision, London Jessica Kingsley, 132-149.

Chorlton, E. (2023) Reflections on using CAT for people recently diagnosed with autism. *Reformulation* **56** 21-25.

Clark, K. & Holquist, M. (1984). *Mikael Bakhtin.* Cambridge: Harvard University Press

Clarkson, P. (2003) *The Therapeutic Relationship.* New Jersey, Wiley-Blackwell.

Clarkson, P. and Mackewn, J. (1993) *Key Figures in Counselling and Psychotherapy.* Fritz Perls. Sage Publications.

Clayton, P. (1999) *The Psychotherapy File Adapted for People with Learning Disabilities.* Calderstones, NHS Trust.

Compton Dickinson, S. (2006) Beyond body, Beyond words: Cognitive Analytic Music Therapy in forensic psychiatry–new approaches in the treatment of personality disordered offenders. *Music Therapy Today* **7** 4.

Compton Dickinson, S. J. (2015) *A Feasibility Trial of Group Cognitive Analytic Music Therapy in Secure Hospital Settings.* Unpublished manuscript. Anglia Ruskin University.

Compton Dickinson, S. J. & Hakvoort, L. (2017) *The Clinician's Guide to Forensic Music Therapy: Treatment manuals for group cognitive analytic music therapy and music therapy anger management.* London, UK: Jessica Kingsley Publishers.

Compton Dickinson, S.J. (2006) Beyond body, beyond words: cognitive analytic music therapy in forensic psychiatry – new approaches in the treatment of personality disordered offenders. *Music Therapy Today* **7** (4) pp39–75.

Compton Dickinson, S.J. (2013) A case of work, rest and play: Music therapy in Early Onset Psychosis pp89-104 IN: S. Compton Dickinson, H. Odell-Miller and J. Adlam, eds. (2013). *Forensic Music Therapy: a 261 treatment for men and women in secure hospital settings.* London: Jessica Kingsley Publishers

Compton Dickinson, S.J. (2021) Finding an authentic voice music therapy in multi-disciplinary psychiatric treatment. In: Parker, I., Schnakenberg, J., Hopvenbeck, M. *The Practical Handbook of Hearing Voices: therapeutic and creative approaches* pp384–395. PCCS Books UK

Compton Dickinson, S.J. & Jolliffe, D. (2021) Enhancing empathy amongst mentally disordered offenders with music therapy. In: Jolliffe, D. & Farrington, D.P. (Eds) *Empathy Versus Offending, Aggression and Bullying: Advancing knowledge using the basic empathy scale,* pp142- 155. Taylor & Francis.

Coombes, J. (2024) Bridging the theory to practice gap. In Laura Brummer, L., Cavieres, M. & Tan, R., (Eds) (2024) *The Oxford Handbook of Cognitive Analytic Therapy*, pp 748-749 Oxford University Press.

Corbridge, C., Brummer, L., & Coid, P. (2018) *Cognitive Analytic Therapy. Distinctive Features*. New York. Routledge

Coulter, N. & Rushbrook, S. (2010) Playfulness in CAT. *Reformulation*, Winter, 35 pp24-27.

Cozolino, L. (2016) *Why Therapy Works: Using our minds to change our brains*. W. W. Norton & Company.

Daley, P. (2023) 'Pushed into humanity': Can learning about storytelling make better doctors? *The Guardian* 11th June. Available at: www.theguardian.com/australia-news/2023/jun/12/narrative-medicine-doctors-gps-learning-about-storytelling-communication-skills?CMP = Share_iOSApp_Other (accessed May 2024).

Daly, A-M., Llewellyn, S. and McDougall, E. (2010) Rupture resolution in the Cognitive Analytic Therapy for adolescents with borderline personality disorder. *Psychology and Psychotherapy: Theory, Research and Practice* **83** 273-288.

Darongkamas, J., Kiely, B., Walker, M. J. (2016) A CAT envelope to deliver EMDR: Cognitive Analytic Therapy around Eye Movement Desensitization and Reprocessing. *Psychotherapy Integration* **26** 462-477.

Dent-Brown, K. (2011) Six-Part Storymaking – a tool for CAT practitioners. *Reformulation*, Summer, pp34-36.

Dent-Brown, K. (2024) Adapting the six-part story method to CAT. In: In L. Brummer, M. Cavieres, & R. Tan (Eds.), *Oxford handbook of cognitive analytic therapy*. 687-701.

Dent, C. and Rosenberg, L. (1990) Visual and Verbal Metaphors: Developmental Interactions. *Child Development* **61** 983–994. doi: 10.1111/j.1467-8624.1990.tb02836.x.

Dickens, C. (2003) *Great Expectations*. Penguin Classics

Domino,G., Affonso, DA., and Hannah, MT. (1992) Assessing the imagery of cancer: the cancer metaphor test. *Journal Psychosocial Oncology* **9** (4) 103–21.

Donaldson Trust (2024). *Donaldsons.org.uk/neurodiversity*.

Dower, C. (2014) Bringing bodies into dialogue, *Reformulation* **43** 15-21.

Edwards, D. (2010) Play and metaphor in clinical supervision: Keeping creativity alive. *The Arts in Psychotherapy* **37** pp248–254.

Ehlers, A. and Clark, D.M. (2000) A cognitive model of post-traumatic stress disorder. *Behaviour Research and Therapy* **38** 319-345.

Elia, I. and Jenaway, A. (2007) You are driving me insane: Literature, Lyrics and Drama through CAT eyes for clients and students. *Reformulation*, Summer, pp43-44.

Emerson, C. & Holquist, M. Austin. Texas University. Texas Press.

Emunah, R. (1994) *Acting for Real: Drama Therapy Process, Technique, and Performance*. New York: Brunner-Routledge.

Eynon, T. (2002) Cognitive linguistics. *Advances in psychiatric Treatment* **8** 399-407

Fainsilber, L., & Ortony, A. (1987) Metaphorical use of language in the expression of emotion. *Metaphor and Symbolic Activity* **2** 239-250.

Feltham, C. and Dryden, W. (1993) *Dictionary of Counselling*. London. Whurr publishers.

Fletcher, H.K. (2016) *Attachment in Intellectual and Developmental Disability: A clinician's guide to practice and research*. Wiley, New Jersey.

Forceville, C. (2008) Metaphor in Pictures and multi modal representations. In: R.W. Gibbs (2008). *The Cambridge Handbook of Metaphor and Thought*. Cambridge: Cambridge University Press.

Foulkes, S.H. (1983). Introduction to Group-Analytic Psychotherapy. London, Routledge.

Francis, D., Kaiser, D. and Deaver, S. (2011) Representations of attachment security in the bird's nest drawings of patient with substance abuse disorders. *Journal of the American Art Therapy Association* **20** 3 125-137.

Frank, A. (2013) *The Wounded Storyteller: Body, illness and ethics*. 2nd edn. Chicago: University of Chicago Press.

Frank, R. (2023) *The Bodily Roots of Experience in Psychotherapy*. London Routledge.

Fraser, E (1998) The Use of Metaphors with African-American Couples. *Journal of Couples Therapy* 7 3 137-148.

Freeman, A and Dattilio F.M. (1992) *Comprehensive Casebook of Cognitive Therapy*. Plenum Press.

Freeze the Fear with Wim Hof (2022) Series 1, Episode 6, 12:46, Directed by Sabeh Bali, Alex Reynolds and Ben Roe, written by Dawson Bros, British Broadcasting Corporation (BBC). Online]. Available at: www.bbc.co.uk/iplayer/episode/m0017g60/freeze-the-fear-with-wim-hof-series-1-episode-6 (accessed May 2024).

Freud, S. (1962) *Two Short Accounts of Psycho-Analysis: Five lectures on psycho-analysis and the question of lay analysis*. J Strachey (ed.) p 33. England: Penguin Books.

Freud, S. (2010) *The Interpretation of Dreams. The Illustrated Edition*. Sterling Press.

Gammidge, T. (2016) Story To Tell: Stories from animation projects in secure and psychiatric settings. In: Rothwell, K. (ed.) *Forensic Arts Therapy, Anthology of Practice and Research*. pp199-216. London: Free Association Books.

Gammidge, T. (2021) Frame by Frame: Stop-frame animation with trauma and chaos narratives. In: West, J. (ed.) *Using Image and Narrative in Therapy for Trauma, Addiction and Recovery* (pp229-245). London: Jessica Kingsley Publishing.

Gendlin, E. (2003) *Focusing: How to gain direct access to your body's knowledge*, 25th Anniversary Edition. London: Rider.

Gentile, M. (Ed.). (1997). Functional visual behaviour: A therapist's guide to evaluation and treatment options. *American Occupational Therapy Association*.

Georgaca, E. (2001) Voices of the self in psychotherapy: a qualitative analysis. *British Journal of Medical Psychology* 74 (2) pp224.

Gersie, A., & King, N. (1990). *Storymaking in education and therapy*. Jessica Kingsley Publishers; Stockholm Institute of Education Press.

Gibbs, R. W. (2019) Metaphor as Dynamical–Ecological Performance. *Metaphor and Symbol* 34 (1) 33-44. doi:10.1080/10926488.2019.1591713.

Gilbert, M. C. & Evans, K. (2000) *Psychotherapy supervision: An integrative relational approach to psychotherapy supervision*. Open University Press.

Gilbert, P. (2003) Working with Shame. *Reformulation*, Summer, pp.13-15.

Gilbert, P. (2009) *The Compassionate Mind*. Robinson.

Glucksberg, S. and Keysar, B. (1990) Understanding metaphorical comparisons: Beyond similarity. *Psychological Review* 97 (1) 3-18. doi: 10.1037/0033-295X.97.1.3

Gorman, R., Farsides, B. & Gammidge, T. (2023) Stop-motion storytelling: Exploring methods for animating the worlds of rare genetic disease. *Qualitative Research* 23 (6) pp1737-1758. doi: https://doi.org/10.1177/14687941221110168

Green, M. (2015) *Aftershock: The Untold Story of Surviving Peace*. Portobello Books

Gregory, C. (2020) Therapeutic Creativity and the Therapist's Zone of Proximal Development. *Reformulation* 54 pp54-57.

Gregory, C. and Wilde McCormick, E. (2019) Poetry and Cognitive Analytic Therapy. *Reformulation*, Summer, pp33-35.

Gregory, C., Jenaway, A. and Lee, M. (2023) Integrating Ideas from Internal Family Systems Into Cognitive Analytic Therapy, *Reformulation* 56 pp4-10.

Hallett, S. and Crompton, C.J., (2018) Too complicated to treat? Autistic people seeking mental health support in Scotland [online]. *Autistic Mutual Aid Society Edinburgh (AMASE)*. www.amase.org.uk/mhreport.

Hawkins, P. & McMahon, A. (2020) *Supervision in the Helping Professions*. Open University Press. London.

Heiney, S. (1995) The healing power of story. *Oncology Nursing Society* **22** (6) pp.899-903.

Hepple, J. (2004) Ageism in psychotherapy and beyond. In: *Cognitive Analytic Therapy and later life. A new perspective on old age*. Eds. J Hepple and L Sutton. Hove & New York. Brünner-Routledge. 45-66.

Hepple, J. (2006) Developing a language for the psychotherapy of later life. *Reformulation* Winter 23-28 (p 25).

Hepple, J. (2009) Dialogue and Desire: Michael Bakhtin and the Linguistic Turn in Psychotherapy by Rachel Pollard. *Reformulation*, Winter, pp10-11.

Hepple, J. (2010) A little bit of Bakhtin – from inside to outside and back again. *Reformulation* **35** 14-15.

Hepple, J. (2012). Cognitive-analytic therapy in a group: Reflections on a dialogic approach. *British Journal of Psychotherapy*, **28**(4), 474-495.

Hepple, J. (2024) The 'D' in CAT. In: *The Oxford Handbook of Cognitive Analytic Therapy*, pp. 53-61 Eds. L. Brummer, M. Cavieres, and R. Tan. Oxford University Press.

Hepple, J. (Eds) Deborah Pick Vance (2013) *Cognitive Analytic Supervision: A relational approach*, London, Routledge.

Hepple, J. and Sutton. L. (Eds.) (2004) *Cognitive Analytic Therapy and later life. A new perspective on old age*. Hove & New York. Brünner-Routledge.

Herman, J. (1992) *Trauma and Recovery*. Basic Books

Hermans, H. J. M., & Kempen, H. J. G. (1993) *The Dialogical Self: Meaning as movement*. Academic Press.

Hermans, H., Rijks, T. & Kempen, H. (1993) Imaginal dialogues in the self: theory and method. *Journal of Personality* **61** (2) pp207-236.

Hermans, H.J.M. (2003) The construction and reconstruction of a dialogical self. *Journal of Constructivist Psychology* **16** pp89-130.

Hestbech, M.A. (2018) Reclaiming the inner child in cognitive-behavioural therapy: The complementary model of the personality. *American Journal of Psychotherapy* **1** 21-27.

Hillman, J. (2018) *The Dream and the Underworld*. Avon.

Hilton, M. (2006) Reflective Creativity: Reforming the Arts Curriculum for the Information Age. In: P. Burnard & S. Hennessy (eds) *Reflective Practices in Arts Education*. Dordrecht: Springer.

Holquist, M. (2003). *Dialogism: Bakhtin and his world*. Routledge.

Holquist, M. (2004) *Dialogism: Bakhtin and his world*. (Second Edition). London. Routledge

Hughes, H. (2007) An enquiry into an Integration of Cognitive Analytic Therapy with Art Therapy. *International Journal of Art Therapy:* Inscape. Summer edition.

Hull, L., Mandy, W., Lai, M.C., Baron-Cohen, S., Allison, C., Smith, P. and Petrides, K.V., (2019) Development and validation of the camouflaging autistic traits questionnaire (CAT-Q). *Journal of autism and developmental disorders* **49** pp.819-833.

International Society for the Study of Trauma and Dissociation (2011) Guidelines for treating dissociative identity disorder in adults (Third Revision). *Journal of Trauma and Dissociation* **12**(2) 115-187.

Iwama, M.K. (2006) *The Kawa Model: Culturally relevant occupational therapy*. Churchill Livingstone Elsevier.

Jacobs, L. & Hycner, R. (2008) *Relational Approaches in Gestalt Therapy* (2008) Routledge, Taylor & Francis.

James, W. (1890). *The principles of psychology*, 2 vols. Dover.

Janson, T. (1962) *Tales from Moominvalley*. Penguin Books.

Jaques, E. (1965) Death and the mid-life crisis. *The International journal of Psychoanalysis*, **46** (4) 502-14.

Jefferis, S. (2011) Memoirs, myths and movies: using books & film in Cognitive Analytic Therapy. *Reformulation*, Summer, pp29-33.

Jefferis, S., Fantarrow, Z. and Johnston, L. (2021) The torchlight model of mapping in cognitive analytic therapy (CAT) reformulation: a qualitative investigation. *Psychology and Psychotherapy: Theory, Research and Practice* **94**, pp.137-150.

Jellema, A. (2000) Insecure attachment states; their relationship to borderline and narcissistic personality disorders and treatment process in cognitive analytic therapy. *Clinical Psychology and Psychotherapy*, vol **7**, 138-154.

Jellema, A. (2003) *An animal living in the world of symbols: Attachment theory and Bakhtin in relation to CAT*. Paper presented at the first International CAT Conference, Valamo, Finland, 5-8 June.

Jenaway, A. (2016) Incorporating Eye Movement Desensitisation and Reprocessing (EMDR) into Cognitive Analytic Therapy – Reaching Reciprocal Roles that other therapies cannot reach. *Reformulation* **47** 21-28.

Jenaway, A. (2019) *A Letter to Cinderella* [online]. Available at: www.engage.acat.org.uk/a-letter-to-cinderella/ (accessed May 2024). CC BY-SA 4.0 Used with permission.

Jenaway, A. and 'Nick', Service User and Expert by Experience (2016) Incorporating eye movement desensitisation and reprocessing (EMDR) into cognitive analytic therapy – reaching Reciprocal Roles that other therapies cannot reach. *Reformulation* Winter 21-28.

Jennings, S. (1990) *Dramatherapy with families, groups and individuals*, London, Jessica Kingsley.

Jennings, S. (2002). *Neuro -Dramatic-Play(NDP) and Embodiment-Projection-Role (EPR)*. https://www.suejennings.com/eprndp.html.

Joey Essex Grief and Me (2021) 20:30, 44:16, Directed by Niamh Kennedy, *British Broadcasting Company (BBC)*, 3 June [Online] Available at: www.bbc.co.uk/iplayer/episode/p09hy0vh/joey-essex-grief-and-me (accessed May 2024).

Johnstone, K. (2018) *Impro: Improvisation and the Theatre*. Bloomsbury Publishing. (Originally published in 1979.)

Jones, P. (1996) *Drama as Therapy, Theatre as Living*. London: Routledge.

Jones, P. (2021) A*rts Therapies: A revolution in healthcare, 2nd Edn*. New York, NY: Routledge.

Jones, P. & Dokter, D. (2008) *Supervision of Dramatherapy*. Routledge.

Jung, C.G. (1902) 'A Case of Hysterical Stupor in a Prisoner in Detention'. In (Eds.) H. Read, M Fordham, G Adler and W Mcguire (eds.) *The Collected Works of C.G. Jung: Volume One, Psychiatric Studies IV* pp 265-303 (p293). England: Routledge Kegan Paul.

Jung, C.G. (1951) 'The Psychology of the Child Archetype'. In: H. Read, M Fordham, G Adler and W Mcguire (eds.) *The Collected Works of C.G. Jung: Volume Nine, Part One, Archetypes and the Collective Unconscious IV* pp 8263-8321 (p8284). England: Routledge Kegan Paul.

Jung, C.G. (1968) *Man and His Symbols*. Dell Publishing.

Jung, C.J. (1963) *Memories, Dreams and Reflections.* Pantheon Books

Kalff, D. M. (1980) *Sandplay, A Psychotherapeutic Approach to the Psyche*. Boston: Sigo Press.

Keijsers, G. P. J., Schaap, C. P. D. R., and Hoogduin, C. A. L. (2000) The impact of interpersonal patient and therapist behavior on outcome in cognitive-behavior therapy a review of empirical studies. *Behavior Modification* **24** (2) 264-297.

Kellett, S. (2005) The treatment of dissociative identity disorder (DIDS) with cognitive analytic therapy: experimental evidence of sudden gains. *Journal of Trauma and Dissociation* **6** (3) pp55–81.

Kellett, S., Hall, J. & Compton Dickinson, S. J. (2018) Group cognitive analytic music therapy: a quasi-experimental feasibility study conducted in a high secure hospital. *Nordic Journal of Music Therapy* **28** 224-255.

Kerr I. B. and Beard, H. (2024) The evolving CAT model and its current core features. In L. Brummer, M. Cavieres, & R. Tan (Eds.), *Oxford handbook of cognitive analytic therapy*. 15-32.

Khan, H.K. (1988) *The Music of Life : The inner nature and effects of Sound from the Teachings of Hazrat Inayat Khan*. Omega Books, London.

King, R. (2005) CAT, the Therapeutic Relationship and working with People with Learning Disability. *Reformulation*, Spring, pp.10-14

Klein M. (1955). The psychoanalytic technique through play: its history and significance, in: *New Directions in Psychoanalysis*, eds Klein M., Heimann P., Money-Kyrle R. E. (London: Tavistock Publications Limited), 25–48.

Klein, M. (1988). *Envy And Gratitude and Other Works* 1946-1963. Virago Press

Knox, J. (2011) *Self-Agency in Psychotherapy, Attachment, Autonomy, and Intimacy*. Norton Series on Interpersonal Neurobiology IPNB Series.

Kohut, H. (1971) *The Analysis of the Self: A systematic approach to the psychoanalytic treatment of narcissistic personality disorders*. University of Chicago Press.

Kok, J.K., Lim, C.M., and Low, S.K. (2011) *Attending to metaphor in counselling*. In 2011 International Conference on Social Science and Humanity (Vol. 5, pp. V1-54).

Kopp, R. R. (1995 and 2013) *Metaphor Therapy: Using patient generated metaphors in psychotherapy*. Brunner, New York.

Lacroix, L., Peterson, L and Verrier, P. (2011) Art Therapy, Somatizatrion, and narcissistic Identification. *Journal of the American Art therapy Association* **18** (1) 20-26.

Lahad, M. (1992) Story-making in assessment method for coping with stress. In: Jennings, S (ed.) *Dramatherapy Theory and Practice*, 150-163. London: Routledge.

Lahad, M. (2000) *Creative Supervision: the use of expressive arts methods in supervision and self-supervision*. London: Jessica Kingsley Publishers.

Lahad, M., & Ayalon, O. (1993). *BASIC Ph - The story of coping resources, Community stress prevention* (Vol. II). Kiryat Shmona, Israel: Community Stress Prevention Centre.

Lai, M. C., Kassee, C., Besney, R., Bonato, S., Hull, L., Mandy, W., Szatmari, P., & Ameis, S. H. (2019) Prevalence of co-occurring mental health diagnoses in the autism population: a systematic review and meta-analysis. *The Lancet Psychiatry* **6** (10) 819-829.

Laing, R.D. (1960). *The Divided Self*. Penguin.

Lakoff, G. and Johnson, M. (1980) *Metaphors We Live By*. Chicago: University of Chicago Press.

Lakoff, G., and Turner, M. (2009) *More Than Cool Reason: A field guide to poetic metaphor*. University of Chicago Press.

Landreth, G.L. (2012) *Play Therapy: The art of the relationship (3rd ed.)* London: Taylor and Francis.

Landy, R. (2009) Role Theory and their role method of drama therapy. *Current approaches in drama therapy* **2** pp65-88.

Landy, R. J. (1983) The use of Distancing in Drama therapy. *The Arts in Psychotherapy*, vol **10**, 175-185.

Landy, R. J. (1993) *Persona and Performance*. London Jessica Kingsley.

Lawday, R. and Compton, S.J. (2013). Integrating models for integrated care pathways. In: S. Compton Dickinson, H. Odell-Miller and J. Adlam, eds. (2013). *Forensic Music Therapy: a 261 treatment for men and women in secure hospital settings*. London: Jessica Kingsley Publishers. Ch.9.

Lee, C. A. (2016) *Music at the Edge : The Music Therapy Experience of a Musician with AIDS*. Routledge 2nd Edition. ISBN: 1138856576Maguire, A. (2020) *Music Therapy Conversations Épisode 44 British Association of Music Therapy* [online]. Available at www.bamt.org/DB/podcasts-2/alex-maguire-part-1 (accessed May 2024).

Leiman, M. (2002) Toward semiotic dialogism: The role of sign mediation in the dialogical self. *Theory & Psychology* **12** (2) 221-235.

Levine P. (2019) Trauma is playing out in the theatre of the body. *The Psychologist*, August (2019) British Psychological Society.

Levine, P. (2012) *In an Unspoken Voice: How the body releases trauma and restores goodness*. North Atlantic Books.

Levine, P. (2015) *Trauma and Memory: Brain and body in a search for the living past: A practical guide for understanding and working with traumatic memory*. Berkeley, CA: North Atlantic Books.

Lewis, J and Krippner, S. (2016) *Working with Dreams and PTSD Nightmares*. Praeger Publishers Inc.

Lloyd, J. & Clayton, P. (2013) *Cognitive Analytic Therapy for People who have an Intellectual Disability and Their Carers.* Jessica Kingsley.

Lloyd, J.(2019). Trauma, Trauma and More Trauma: CAT and Trauma in Learning Disability. *Reformulation*, Summer, pp.44-46.

Macfarlane, R. & Morris, J. (2017) *The Lost Words.* Hamish Hamilton. ISBN 9780241253588

MacIntyre, A. (1981) *After virtue.* London, UK: Duckworth and Co.

Mair, J.M.M. (1977). "The community of self." In *New Perspectives in Personal Construct Theory*, Edited by Bannister, D. London: Academic Press

Marks-Tarlow, T. (2012) Clinical Intuition in Psychotherapy. W. W. Norton & Company, Inc. and printed in: *American Journal of Play* **4** (3).

Marks-Tarlow, T., Solomon, M. and Seigel D. (2017) *Play & Creativity in Psychotherapy.* W. W. Norton & Company.

Martin, J., Cummings, A. and Hallberg, ET. (1992) Therapists' intentional use of metaphor: Memorability, clinical impact, and possible epistemic/motivational functions. *Journal of Consulting and Clinical Psychology* **60** (1) 143-145. doi: 10.1037/0022-006X.60.1.143.

Mason, H. (2009) Dare to Dream: The Use of Animation in Occupational Therapy. *Mental Health Occupational Therapy* **14** (3) pp11–115.

Mason, H. (2011) The re-animation approach: animation and therapy. *Journal of Assistive Technologies* **5** (1) pp40-42. doi: https://doi.org/10.5042/jat.2011.0102

Mcferran, K., Chan, V., Tague, D., Stachyra, K. & Mercadal-Brotons, M. (2023) A comprehensive review classifying contemporary global practices in music therapy. *Music Therapy Today Online Journal Proceedings of the 17th World Congress of Music Therapy* **18** (1) pp474-493.

McIntosh, P. (2010) The puzzle of metaphor and voice in arts-based social research. *International Journal of Social Research Methodology* **13** (2) 157-169.

McMullen, L.M. (2008) Putting It in Context: metaphor and psychotherapy. In: Raymond, W. Gibbs (Ed) *The Cambridge Handbook of Metaphor and Thought.* Cambridge University Press. 397-411.

Milton, D. E. (2012) On the ontological status of autism: the 'double empathy problem'. *Disability & Society*, **27**(6), pp883-887.

Naiman, R. (2017) Dreamless: The Silent Epidemic of REM Sleep Loss. *Annals of the New York Academy of Sciences* **1406** (1) 77-85.

National Institute for Health and Care Excellence (2010) NICE Clinical Guidance no.77. *Guidelines set to improve treatment and management of people with antisocial personality disorder.* available athttps://www.ncbi.nlm.nih.gov/books/NBK555205. Accessed on 18/06/2024

Nehmad, A. (1997). Narcissism destructive and disowned: Shakespeare's Troilus and Cressida. *Reformulation*, ACAT News, Winter, p.x.

Nordoff, P., and Robbins, C. (1985) *Therapy in Handicapped Children.* Orion Publishers Group.

Odell-Miller, H. (2013) Inside and outside the Walls: Music Therapy Supervision in Forensic Settings In: Compton Dickinson, S. J., Odell-Miller, H., & Adlam, J., eds. *Forensic Music Therapy: A treatment for men and women in secure hospital settings* (pp42–58) London: Jessica Kingsley Publications.

Ogden, P. (2006) *Trauma and the Body: A sensorimotor approach to psychotherapy.* Norton Series on Interpersonal Neurobiology

Ogden, P. (2018) Play, creativity, and movement vocabulary. In: Marks-Tarlow, T., Solomon, M., Seigel D. (Eds) *Play & Creativity In Psychotherapy.* W. W. Norton & Company.

Panhofer, H. Payne, H., Meekums, B. & Parke, T. (2011) Dancing, moving and writing in clinical supervision? Employing embodied practices in psychotherapy supervision. *The Arts in Psychotherapy* **38** 9–16.

Panksepp, J. (2012) *The Archaeology of Mind: Neuroevolutionary origins of human emotions.* New York: W. W. Norton & Company.

Parahoo, K. (1997) *Nursing Research: Principles, process, and issues.* London: Macmillan.

Parks, P. (1990) *Rescuing the 'Inner Child'*. London: Souvenir Press.

Parks, P. (1994) *The Counsellor's Guide to Parks Inner Child Therapy*. London: Souvenir Press.

Patterson, E. (2020) Reflect to Create – The Dance of Reflection for Creative Leadership, Professional Practice and Supervision. *Reflective Journal and Workbook*. IgramSpark

Pavlicevic, M., & Ansdell, G. (Eds.). (2004) *Community Music Therapy*. London: Jessica Kingsley Publishers.

Perls, F. (1969) *Gestalt Therapy Verbatim*. Moab. UT Real People Press.

Perls, F. (1973) The Gestalt Approach and Eyewitness to Therapy. Science and Behaviour Books.

Pernicano, P. (2010) *Metaphorical Stories for Child Therapy: Of magic and miracles*. Jason Aronson publishers (Lanham MD, IN, USA).

Perry, R. B. (1935) *The thought and character of William James: as revealed in unpublished correspondence and notes, together with his published writings. Vol. 1, inheritance and vocation; Vol. 2, Philosophy and psychology*. Little, Brown.

Petratou, V. (1994) The use of key working as a psychological bridge into group participation: A case report. *Therapeutic Communities: The International Journal for Therapeutic and Supportive Organisations*, Vol 15, No 3, 183-192.

Petratou, V. (2007) Bringing Drama to Dialogue: the use of Dramatherapy methods in Cognitive Analytic Therapy. *Dramatherapy Journal of the British Association of Dramatherapists* **29** 10-15. https://doi.org/10.1080/02630672.2007.9689710

Petratou, V. (2019) The House of Self States (HOSS): Using a creative integrative and containing mapping technique across the therapies. *Reformulation*, Issue 53, Winter 2019/20, 6-9.

Pollard, R. (2008) *Dialogue and Desire: Michael Bakhtin and the Linguistic Turn in Psychotherapy*. UKCP, Karnac Series.

Pollard, R. (2012) Great time: from Blade Runner to Bakhtin. *Reformulation*, Summer.

Pollock, P.H. (2001) Cognitive Analytic Therapy for Adult Survivors of Childhood Abuse: Approaches to treatment and case management, pp. 87-89. Michigan: Wiley.

Pollock, P.H., Broadbent, M., Clarke, S., Dorrian, A. and Ryle, A. (2001) The Personality Structure Questionnaire (PSQ): A measure of the multiple self-states model of identity disturbance in cognitive analytic therapy. *Clinical Psychology & Psychotherapy: An International Journal of Theory & Practice*, **8**(1), pp.59-72.

Porges, S. W. (2011) *The Polyvagal Theory: Neurophysiological foundations of emotions, attachment, communication, and self-regulation*. New York: W. W. Norton and Company.

Porges, S.W. (2001) The polyvagal theory: phylogenetic substrates of a social nervous system'. *International Journal of Psychophysiology* **42** (2) 123–146.

Potter, S (2010) Words with Arrows: The benefits of mapping whilst talking. *Reformulation*, April, pp 1-14.

Potter, S. (2010) Words with arrows: the benefits of mapping whilst talking. *Reformulation*, Summer, pp37-45.

Potter, S. (2013) The Helper's Dance List. In J. Lloyd & P. Clayton *Cognitive Analytic Therapy for People with Intellectual Disabilities and their Carers*. London: Jessica Kingsley, 89-121.

Potter, S. (2016) Negotiator's Mind. *Reformulation*, Summer, pp29-32.

Potter, S. (2019) *Dorset CAT Practitioner Training* 2017-2019.

Potter, S. (2020) *Therapy with a map a cognitive analytic approach to helping relationships*. West Sussex: Pavilion Publishing.

Potts, A., & Semino, E. (2019) Cancer as a metaphor. *Metaphor and Symbol* **34** (2) 81-95. doi:10.108 0/10926488.2019.1611723

Pugh, M. (2017) Pull up a chair: on the use and potential of chair work. *The Psychologist*, June 2017.

Raabe, S., Ehring, T., Marquenie, L., Arntz, A. and Kindt, M. (2022) Imagery rescripting as a stand-alone treatment for posttraumatic stress disorder related to child abuse: A randomized controlled trial. *Journal of Behavior Therapy and Experimental Psychiatry* **77** 101769 – 101781.

Randall, J. (2023) Neurodivergence Within the Therapy Room: CAT for Autistic People Presenting with Complex Trauma and Mental Health Difficulties. *Presentation at Gaining Ground: what's new on the CAT landscape*. 30th June. Manchester.

Reid, J.S. (2023) *Sound Therapy and Music Medicine -Biological mechanisms* with John Stuart Reid. Cymatics study of visible sound. Public lecture on 2.10.2023 for Cambridge Institute of Music Therapy Research (CIMTR).

Ribeiro, S. (2021) *The Oracle of the Night. The History of Science and Dreams*. Bantam Press

Riley, S.F. (2004) Reflections on reflecting art therapy team in education and treatment. *Journal of the American Art Therapy Association* **21** (2) 88-94.

Rogers, C.R. (1961) *On Becoming a Person: A Therapist's View of Psychotherapy*. Houghton Mifflin, Boston.

Rose, M. (2017) *Easy Read Cognitive Analytic Therapy Leaflet*.

Ryle, A. (1975) 'Self-to-Self, Self-to-Other: The World's Shortest Account of Object Relations Theory', *New Psychiatry*, April, pp 12-13.

Ryle, A. (1983) The value of written communications in dynamic psychotherapy. *British Journal of Medical Psychology* **56** 361-366 https://doi.org/10.1111/j.2044-8341.1983.tb01568.x

Ryle, A. (1985) Cognitive theory, object relations and the self. *British Journal of Medical Psychology* **58** 1-7 (p3).

Ryle, A. (1990) *Cognitive-Analytic Therapy: Active Participation in Change: A new integration in brief psychotherapy*, p52; p. 100. Chichester: Wiley.

Ryle, A. (1991) Object Relations Theory and Activity Theory: A proposed link by way of the procedural sequence object relations model. *Brit. J. of Medical Psychology* **64** 307-316.

Ryle, A. (1994) Consciousness and psychotherapy. *British Journal of Medical Psychology* **67** (Pt 2).

Ryle, A. (1997) *Cognitive Analytic Therapy and Borderline Personality Disorder: The Model and the Method*. John Wiley and Sons Inc.

Ryle, A. (1997) The Multiple Self States Model of Borderline Personality Disorder. In: *Cognitive Analytic Therapy and Borderline Personality Disorder: The Model and The Method*. Wiley & Sons, p26-42.

Ryle, A. (1997) The structure and development of borderline personality disorder: a proposed model. *The British Journal of Psychiatry*, **170**(1), 82-87.

Ryle, A. (1998) 'Transferences and countertransferences': The Cognitive Analytic Therapy perspective'. *British Journal of Psychotherapy* **14** 303-309.

Ryle, A. (2001) *CAT's dialogic perspective on the self*. ACAT News.

Ryle, A. (2004) The contribution of cognitive analytic therapy to the treatment of borderline personality disorder. *Journal of personality Disorders* **18** (1) 3-35.

Ryle, A. (2007) Keeping CAT Alive. *Reformulation*, Summer, pp.4-5.

Ryle, A., & Kerr, I. (2020) *Introducing Cognitive Analytic Therapy: Principles and practice of relational approach to mental health* (2nd Ed.). Chichester, UK: John Wiley and Sons.

Saban, A. (2006) Functions of metaphor in teaching and teacher education: A review. *Teaching Education* **17** (4) 299-315.

Schore, A. (2019) *Right-brain Psychotherapy*. New York: W. W. Norton & Company.

Schore, A., (2003) *Affect Dysregulation and Disorders of the Self*. New York.

Schore, A.N. (2012) *The Science of the Art of Psychotherapy*. WW Norton & Company.

Schore, A.N. (2021) The Interpersonal Neurobiology of Intersubjectivity. *Front Psychol.* 2021 Apr 20;12:648616. doi: 10.3389/fpsyg.2021.648616. PMID: 33959077; PMCID: PMC8093784

Schwartz, R.C. (1995) *Internal Family Systems Therapy*. New York: The Guilford Press.

Scrivener, E. (2012) *A New Name*. London, Harper Collins.

Searle, J. (1985) Metaphor. In: A.P. Martinich (Ed.), *The Philosophy of Language* (pp416-437). Oxford, England, OUP.

Seikkula, J. & Trimble, D. (2006) Healing Elements of Therapeutic Conversation: Dialogue as an Embodiment of Love. *Family Process* **44** (4) 461-475.

Serig, D. (2008) Understanding the conceptual landscape of visual metaphors. *Teaching Artist Journal* **6** (1) 41-50.

Shapiro, F. (2001) *Eye Movement Desensitisation and Reprocessing (EMDR): Basic Principles, Protocols and Procedures* (2nd ed.). New York: The Guilford Press.

Sheard, T. (2017) Embodiment as a creative resource in working with split and 'borderline' clients. *Reformulation* **48** 34-41.

Shohet, R. & Shohet, J. (2020) *In Love With Supervision: Creating transformative conversations.* PCCS Books.

Shostakovich, D. (1979) *Testimony: The memoirs of Dmitri Shostakovich.* Faber & Faber.

Siegel D. J., (2020) *The Developing Mind: How relationships and the brain interact to shape who we are*, Third edition. New York: Guilford Press.

Siegel, D. J. (2012) *Pocket Guide to Interpersonal Neurobiology: An integrative handbook of the mind.* W. W. Norton & Company.

Siegelman, E. Y. (1993) *Metaphor and Meaning in Psychotherapy.* Guilford Press.

Silent Witness (2004) Series 8, Episode 2, 42:53, Directed by Ashley Pearce, Written by Stephen Brady and Nigel McCrery, *British Broadcasting Corporation (BBC)*. [Online] Available at: www.bbc.co.uk/iplayer/episode/p02mwlj5/silent-witness-series-8-2-time-to-heal-part-2?seriesId = p02mwgqs (accessed May 2024).

Smucker, M. and Dancu, C.V. (1999) *Cognitive Behavioural Treatment for Adult Survivors of Childhood Trauma: Imagery re-scripting and reprocessing.* Hillsdale, NJ: Jason Aronson Press.

Solomon, M. (2017) Nesting dolls: A playful way to illustrate a valuable intervention in couples therapy. In: Marks-Tarlow, T., Solomon, M., Seigel D. (Eds) *Play & Creativity In Psychotherapy.* W. W. Norton & Company.

Sørensen, E. B., and Hjalager, A.-M. (2020) Conspicuous non-consumption in tourism: Non-innovation or the innovation of nothing? *Tourist Studies* **20** (2) 222–247.

Spall, B., Read, S. and Chantry, D. (2001) Metaphor: exploring its origins and therapeutic use in death, dying and bereavement. *International Journal of Palliative Nursing* **7** (7) 345-53.

Stern, D.N. (1985) *The Interpersonal World of the Infant: A view from psychoanalysis and developmental psychology.* Abington, Routledge.

Stern, D.N., (1985) *The Interpersonal World of the Infant: A view from psychoanalysis and development.* New York: Basic Books.

Stern, D. N. (2004). *The present moment: In psychotherapy and everyday life.* W.W. Norton & Co

Stern, D. N. (2010). *Forms of vitality: Exploring dynamic experience in psychology, the arts, psychotherapy, and development.* Oxford University Press

Stevens, Y.J. and Petratou, V. (2024) Creativity in CAT. In: Brummer, L., Cavieres, M. & Tan, R., (Eds) *The Oxford Handbook of Cognitive Analytic Therapy*, pp 732-753 Oxford University Press.

Stiles, W.B. (1997) Signs and voices: joining a conversation in progress. *British Journal of Medical Psychology* **70** 169-176.

Stone, S. (2022) *What's the real difference between creativity and innovation?* [online]. Available at: https://ideascale.com/blog/whats-the-real-difference-between-creativity-and-innovation/ (accessed May 2024).

Stott, R., Mansell, W., Salkovskis, P., Lavender, A and Cartwright-Hatton, S. (2010) *Oxford Guide to Metaphors in CBT: Building Cognitive Bridges.* Oxford University press.

Strong, T. (1989) Metaphors and patient change in counselling. *International Journal for the Advancement of Counselling* **12** (3) 203-213.

Such, K. (2023). *How to Heal Your Inner Child, TikTok.* 00:23. [Online] Available at: www.tiktok.com/@kristen.such/video/7195648263670877482 (accessed May 2024).

Sullivan, P. (2017) Towards a literary account of mental health from James' Principles of Psychology. *New Ideas in Psychology* **46** (2017) 31-38.

Sunderland, M. & Armstrong, N. (2018) *Draw on Your Emotions*. Chichester. John Wiley Press.

Supple, S. (2022) Seeing things differently: The creative and flexible CAT in accessibility and inclusiveness. *Reformulation* **55** pp40-45.

Swift, T. (2024) *The Tortured Poets Department*. Available at https://www.instagram.com > taylorswift@taylor swift.19.04. 2024. Accessed 20.4.24

Szasz, T. S. (1960). The myth of mental illness. *American psychologist*, **15**(2), 113.

Taylor, C., Compton Dickinson, S.J., and Maguire, A. (2022) Violence, Music Therapy and Empathy: a counterpoint of disturbance. *The International Journal of Psychotherapy, Psychoanalysis and Psychiatry: Peace and Aggression* **55** Heft1-2Nr 310-311 pp3–29.

Taylor, C.L. (1991) *Inner-child Workbook: What to do with your past when it just won't go away*. New York: Penguin Putnam.

Taylor, R. R. (2017) *Kielhofner's Model of Human Occupation: Theory and Application*. 5th edn. Philadelphia, PA: Lippincott Williams & Wilkins.

Thich Nhat Hanh. (2011) *Healing the Child Within* [online]. Available at: www.mindful.org/healing-the-child-within/ (accessed May 2024).

Törneke, N. (2017) *Metaphor in Practice: A professional's guide to using the science of language in psychotherapy*. Oakland, CA: Context Press.

Trevarthen, C. (2011) What is it like to be a person who knows nothing? Defining the active intersubjective mind of a newborn human being. *In Infant and Child Development* **20**(1):119 - 135

Trevarthen, C. (2012) "Born For Art, and the Joyful Companionship of Fiction." In Narvaez, D., Panksepp, J., Schore, A., & Gleason, T. (Eds.) (2012) *Evolution, Early Experience and Human Development: From Research to Practice and Policy*, 202-218. New York: Oxford University Press.

Trevarthen, C., Delafield-Butt, J. and Schögler, B., 2011. The psychobiology of human gesture: form, rhythm, and melody in infants' movements of narration. In: A. Gritten and E. King, eds.2011. *New perspectives on music and gesture*. Aldershot: Ashgate.Vygotsky, L.S. (1978). Mind in Society: The development of higher psychological processes. Massachusetts: Harvard University Press.

Tselikas-Portman, E. (ed) (1999) *Supervision and Dramatherapy*. London: Jessica Kingsley Publishers.

Turner JB, and Ralley R. (2019) Cognitive neuroscience, metaphor and pictures: part 1. *Mental Health Nursing* **39** (5) 16-9.

Turner, J. (2011) CAT metaphor and Pictures (part 2): An outline of the use of a pictorial metaphor in Cognitive Analytic Therapy. *Reformulation*, Winter, Issue 37, pp39-43.

Turner, J. (2014) Metaphors and therapeutic encounters in mental health nursing. *Mental Health Nursing* **34** (3).

Van der Kolk, B. (2014) *The Body Keeps the Score: Mind, brain and body in the transformation of trauma*, p283. London: Viking Penguin.

Van der Kolk, B., McFarlane, A. and Weisaeth, L. (2007) *Traumatic Stress: The effect of overwhelming experience on mind, body and society*. New York: Guilford Press.

Van der Kolk, B.A., & van der Hart, O. (1989) Pierre Janet and the breakdown of adaptation in psychological trauma. *American Journal of Psychiatry* **146** (12) 1530-1540.

van der Reyden, D., Casteleijn, D., Sherwood, W. & de Witt, P. (2019) *The Vona du Toit Model of Creative Ability: Origins, Constructs, Principles and Application in Occupational Therapy*. Pretoria, South Africa: Vona & Marie du Toit Foundation.

Van Deurzen, E. (2021) *Rising From Existential Crisis: Life beyond calamity*. PCCS Books.

Victoria, (2015). Talking myself into and out of Asperger's Syndrome: Using Cognitive Analytic Therapy (CAT) to rethink normal. *Reformulation*, Summer, pp18-22.

Vonnegut, K. (2005) *A Man Without a Country*. Seven Stories Press.

Vygotsky, L.S. (1978) *Mind in Society: The development of higher psychological processes*. Cambridge, MA. Harvard University Press.

Walker, M. (2018) *Why We Sleep: The New Science of Sleep and Dreams*. Penguin Books.

Walker, M. (2024) Incorporating eye movement desensitisation and reprocessing (EMDR) into CAT In L. Brummer, M. Cavieres, & R. Tan (Eds.), *Oxford handbook of cognitive analytic therapy* (pp. 717–731). Oxford University Press

Walters, J., LaPrairie, D. & Mason, H. (2023) *Creative Activities. In: Bryant, W., Fieldhouse, J. and Plastow, N. (eds.) Creek's Occupational Therapy and Mental Health (6th edn.)* Glasgow: Elsevier Ltd, pp278-297.

Ward, T. (2002). Good lives and the rehabilitation of offenders: Promises and problems. *Aggression and Violent Behavior*, 7, 513–528.

Warner, M. S. (1998) A client-centered approach to therapeutic work with dissociated and fragile process. In: L. S. Greenberg, J. C. Watson, & G. Lietaer (Eds.) *Handbook of Experiential Psychotherapy* (pp368–387). The Guilford Press.

Warner, M.S. (1991) Fragile process. In: L. Fusek (ed.) *New Directions in Client-Centered Therapy: Practice with difficult client populations*, pp41–58. Monograph Series I. Chicago: Chicago Counseling and Psychotherapy Center.

West, C. (2021) *We All Have Parts: An illustrated guide to healing trauma with internal family systems*. Canada: PESI Publishing.

White, M. (1997) *Narratives of Therapists' Lives*. Dulwich Centre Publications.

Wilde McCormick, E. (2012) *Change for the Better: Self-help through practical psychotherapy*, 4th Ed. Sage Publications Ltd.

Wilde McCormick, E. (2017) *Change for the Better*. 5thEd. Sage.

Wilkinson, M. (2010) *Changing Minds in Therapy: Emotion, attachment and neurobiology*. Norton.

Williams, A. (1995) *Visual and Active Supervision*. Baltimore, MD.: Norton.

Williams, C., Williams, S., and Appleton, K. (1997) Mind Maps: An aid to effective formulation. *Behavioural and Cognitive Psychotherapy* **25** 261-267.

Wilshire, B. (1982) *Role-playing and Identity: The Limits of Theatre as Metaphor*. Bloomington. Indiana University Press.

Winnicott, D. W. (1965) *The maturational processes and the facilitating environment: Studies in the theory of emotional development*. London: Routledge.

Winnicott, D. W. (1971) *Playing and Reality*. London: Routledge p54.

Winnicott, D. W. (1991) *Playing and Reality*. Psychology Press. Originally published 1971.

Winnicott, D.H. (2005) in *Playing and Reality* 2nd Ed. Routledge.

Winnicott, D.W. (1971). *Playing and Reality*. London: Routledge.

Winnicott, D.W. (1953) Transitional Objects and Transitional Phenomena. *International Journal of Psychoanalysis* **34** 89-97.

Winnicott, D.W. (1958) 'Transitional objects and transitional phenomena: A study of the first not me possession'. In: D. Winnicott (ed.) *Through Paediatrics to Psychoanalysis*, pp229-242. New York: Basic Books.

Winnicott, DW. (1953) Transitional objects and transitional phenomena; a study of the first not-me possession. *International Journal of Psychoanalysis* **34** (2) 89–97.

Witztum, E., Van der Hart, O., and Friedman, B. (1988) The use of metaphors in psychotherapy. *Journal of Contemporary Psychotherapy* **18** (4) 270-290.

Yalom, I. D., and Leszcz, M. (2005) *The Theory and Practice of Group Psychotherapy* (5th ed.). Basic Books/Hachette Book Group.

Yorke, L. (2018) The Jigsaw aka The Battle of Humpty. *Reformulation*, Winter, p43.

Yorke, L. (2021). *Reciprocal Roles – ways of relating to self and others*. Unpublished

Zatloukal, L., Žákovský, D., & Bezdíčková, E. (2019) Utilizing Metaphors in Solution-Focused Therapy. *Contemporary Family Therapy* **41** (1) 24-36. doi:10.1007/s10591-018-9468-8